Dr. Jack Newman's Guide to Breastfeeding

REVISED EDITION

Dr. Jack Newman   Teresa Pitman

pinter
&
martin

Dr. Jack Newman's Guide to Breastfeeding

Copyright © 2000, 2003, 2014 by Dr. Jack Newman and Teresa Pitman

All rights reserved

This UK/US edition published 2014 by Pinter & Martin.
Reprinted 2015, 2017

Published by arrangement with HarperCollins Publishers Ltd, Toronto, Canada

ISBN 978-1-78066-230-5

Originally published in trade paperback by HarperCollins Publishers Ltd 2000
Second revised and updated edition 2003
This third revised edition 2014

Dr Jack Newman and Terese Pitman have asserted their moral right to be identified as the authors of this work in accordance with the Copyright, Designs and Patents Act of 1988.

British Library Cataloguing-in-Publication Data
A catalogue record for this book is available from the British Library.

This book is sold subject to the condition that it shall not, by way of trade and otherwise, be lent, resold, hired out, or otherwise circulated without the publisher's prior consent in any form or binding or cover other than that in which it is published and without a similar condition being imposed on the subsequent purchaser.

Printed and bound in the UK by Ashford Colour Press Ltd, Gosport, Hampshire

This book has been printed on paper that is sourced and harvested from sustainable forests.

Pinter & Martin Ltd
6 Effra Parade
London SW2 1PS

pinterandmartin.com

Dr. Jack Newman's Guide to Breastfeeding

Dr. Jack Newman is a Toronto pediatrician who has practised medicine since 1970. In 1984 he established the first hospital-based breastfeeding clinic in Canada, at Toronto's Hospital for Sick Children. He is co-founder of the International Breastfeeding Centre located in Toronto, Ontario. He is the father of three children, all breastfed, and the grandfather of two boys, also breastfed.

Teresa Pitman was the executive director of La Leche League Canada for three years, and she has been helping mothers with breastfeeding for more than 30 years. Her articles on parenting and other topics have appeared in *Today's Parent, Pregnancy, Baby and Toddler, More, Mothering, Chatelaine* and other magazines. Teresa is the author or co-author of 12 other books on parenting topics, including, most recently, the eighth edition of *The Womanly Art of Breastfeeding.* She is the mother of four breastfed children, and the grandmother of six breastfed children.

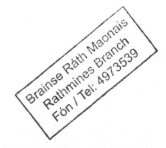

To Adele, Daniel, Elise and David Marc, without whom
I would never have understood any of this, and to Kellie,
who also helped me understand by breastfeeding
Loïc and Tevia.
J.N.

To Matthew, Lisa, Daniel and Jeremy, who taught me that
breastfeeding is about more than just giving milk.
And to Sebastian, Callista, Xavier, Keagan, Mackenzie and Dexter,
who continue our family breastfeeding traditions.
T.P.

With special thanks to Andrea Polokova, who has generously shared
her breastfeeding expertise and writing skills and
many of the photos that add so much to this book.

Contents

Quick Start:

How to Use This Book
(and Your Time!) Wisely

Picking up a book with several hundred pages about breastfeeding can feel daunting. Is there really that much to know about feeding your baby? The answer is yes—and no.

While we believe all the information in this book is valuable—and in some cases, hard to find anywhere else—not every mother or health care professional needs to know about every issue or challenge that is covered, and you certainly don't need to know about everything right away. So here's a quick reference guide that will help you find the key information for you and your situation.

Are you pregnant?

Is this your first baby? Maybe you haven't made up your mind about breastfeeding or are looking for information to help you understand the differences between breastfeeding and formula feeding. Check out Chapter 1: Why Breastfeeding Is Important. From there, you might like to go to Chapter 4: How Birth Affects Breastfeeding and Chapter 5: The First Few Days. That may give you all you need to get off to a great start with breastfeeding. We'd encourage you to keep the book handy, though, in case you do run into challenges when your baby arrives, or later in your breastfeeding experience, and need some more information.

If this is your second (or later) baby, perhaps you had difficulties or weren't able to breastfeed your first, and are hoping to be better prepared this time

around. In that case, you might want to also check out Chapter 2: Finding Good Breastfeeding Help and Chapter 3: The Sale and Promotion of Artificial Baby Milk. If you had some specific issues, you can look up those chapters or sections. These may help you in figuring out what went wrong the first time around and guide you in getting the support you need.

Do you have a brand-new baby?

Chapter 5: The First Few Days will probably be your first destination. If you are having specific challenges (perhaps your nipples are sore or your baby has jaundice), look for the chapters dealing with those issues. If you are feeling discouraged or overwhelmed, reading Chapter 1: Why Breastfeeding Is Important might give you some motivation to keep going, and Chapter 2: Finding Good Breastfeeding Help might help you get in touch with the right support person. Chapter 20: Life with a Breastfed Baby may help as well.

Are you breastfeeding but having problems?

You've come to the right place! The heart of this book is solving breastfeeding problems, and we have information about both common challenges and less-common ones, with ideas that have worked for many mothers. The more common problems (sore nipples, sore breasts) have their own chapters;

if your situation is more unusual you may need to check the index for specific information.

In discussing these common problems, we don't want to suggest that all mothers and babies will experience them; many mothers breastfeed without difficulties, especially if they've had a good start and good advice right from the beginning. Others have minor challenges they can quickly solve on their own or with a little help. And while the problem-solving sections tend to emphasize helping the baby to get more milk, breastfeeding is about more than the milk. When all is going well, it's perfectly fine—even desirable—for the baby to have some relaxed times at the breast when he's just "nibbling" and enjoying the closeness and the soothing sensation of suckling. These are the moments that encourage a long-term breastfeeding relationship.

Is breastfeeding going fine, but you've been told to wean because you are (choose one) needing to take medication, pregnant, scheduled to have some medical tests, going back to work, nursing a toddler or older child, or one of many other "reasons"?

A check through the index should help you find your situation, along with information so that you can make an educated decision about whether or not to wean (though it's almost never necessary). We also have entire chapters on breastfeeding while on medication and the normal duration of breastfeeding.

Are you a health professional, lactation consultant or La Leche League leader using this book as a reference as you work with breastfeeding mothers?

We think you'll find this book a comprehensive guide to solving breastfeeding problems. We also encourage you to look at Chapter 1: Why Breastfeeding Is Important, Chapter 2: Finding Good Breastfeeding Help and Chapter 3: The Sale and Promotion of Artificial Baby Milk. Taken together, these three chapters explain how most mothers find themselves in a situation where they want to breastfeed yet end up weaning sooner than they would like, often after weeks of struggling.

For all our readers . . .

Each of the chapters in the book (other than the first) begins with one or more of the myths or misconceptions that people often believe about breastfeeding. We highlight these because they are so common and often create barriers for women who want to breastfeed. Then we let you know the reality behind the myth, with accurate information so you can make educated decisions.

In many places, we mention research and studies that have been done on breastfeeding and related issues. Since the book is already quite thick, we haven't included them, but they are all listed at www.breastfeedinginc.ca, in case you'd like to read them. We often also refer to video clips, which are hosted on the International Breastfeeding Centre's YouTube channel (http://youtube.com/user/IBCToronto). The videos will help you see some of the techniques that can be hard to explain in writing.

Introduction

Why is this breastfeeding book unique? Surely there are enough books, articles and pamphlets on breastfeeding available that another is not necessary! Women have, of course, managed to breastfeed throughout the human race's time on earth without the benefit of "breastfeeding experts." In fact, even today there are women who do things very differently from what most lactation experts would recommend. Their babies are not latched on well, they stick to scheduled feedings, they hold the baby in awkward positions. And yet they manage to breastfeed successfully.

For too many women, though, this isn't the case. With good help, they will succeed at breastfeeding; without it, they may not. Good information is often hard to find. Mothers get conflicting advice from their doctors, the hospital nurses, their own mothers and friends, and the books they read. It can be hard to separate myth from reality.

Dr. Jack Newman's Guide to Breastfeeding will help you sort all that out.

This book is based on my understanding of breastfeeding and breastfeeding issues, which comes from the experience of my own family, learning from others interested in lactation, and more than 29 years of helping mothers with breastfeeding problems. The mothers who came to me taught me a lot as well. The knowledge I have gained over the years has helped many women breastfeed successfully, despite some difficult challenges along the way. That help is what I'm offering in this book.

I readily admit that I do not always do things as others might. I differ from many lactation specialists and doctors, for example, in my dislike of the use of the vast majority of measurements—such as absolute reliance on weighing and counting and, more recently, the baby's blood sodium level—as the approach to understanding what is going on with a particular mother and baby. I don't find it helpful to weigh babies frequently. I don't find it helps the mother overcome problems to wake her baby every three hours, either, because I believe that a baby who is breastfeeding *well* doesn't need to be woken up—he'll let you know when he is hungry, especially if he is close to you. And if the baby is *not* feeding well, his going to the breast more often won't help—drinking nothing eight times a day is no better than drinking nothing six times a day. The issue for me is whether the baby is feeding well or not.

My approach is based on observing mothers and babies, and giving them help, support and information. Even with such aid, a very few mothers will not be able to breastfeed, or will not be able to breastfeed exclusively. But for the majority of women, these factors can make the difference between breastfeeding going well, or not.

When I speak at conferences about breastfeeding, I am almost always asked how I became interested in this field. I find the question a bit strange: given the importance of breastfeeding in the health and development of a baby, surely it is a very appropriate area for a pediatrician to be interested in! In

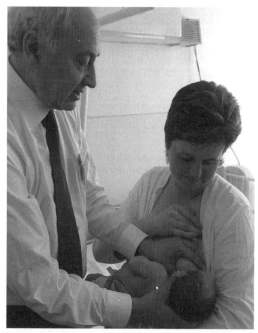

Sometimes mothers need hands-on help with breast-feeding. This mother was having significant difficulties, but with coaching on her hold and latch technique she was able to give her baby more milk from the breast.

CREDIT: **ANDREA POLOKOVA**

the past, some physicians took an interest in breast-feeding only in order to find alternatives to it; a way had to be found to feed infants whose mothers had died, for example. So infant formula was developed and through trial and error (yes, errors were common, and still are) improved so that babies usually survived and even thrived. But otherwise, physicians saw breastfeeding as women's territory. So how did I end up specializing in helping women breastfeed?

In medical school, I learned nothing about breastfeeding. We had one lecture on infant feeding. Breastfeeding was mentioned during one minute of the hour-long lecture, the pediatrician saying that breast was best because the milk was always at the right temperature and came in such cute containers (really!). During my fourth-year medical student rotation of obstetrics and gynecology, I was asked by the resident at the six-week postpartum clinic to see a new mother—ask her how she was doing, if she had any symptoms, examine her uterus and her breasts. When I examined her breasts, milk shot out

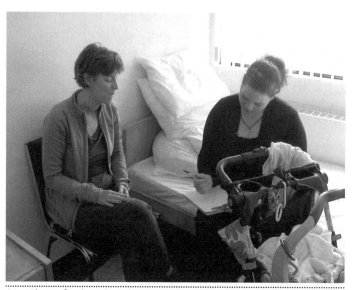

At our breastfeeding clinic, lactation consultants focus on a mother's breastfeeding history and then follow up with a feeding observation.

CREDIT: **JACK NEWMAN**

at least a metre. I was amazed. What was going on here? What was that? They hadn't prepared me for this in medical school. Surely they should have mentioned something about this secretion that occurs in the breast after birth?

I knew it was not possible for the mother to have milk, because it was routine to give the mothers an injection immediately after birth to dry up their milk.

That's all I ever got in medical school about breastfeeding. Breastfeeding was so unimportant in the curriculum that there was not a single question about it on the final exams. (Unfortunately, this hasn't changed much; even pediatric residents get little or no practical information about breastfeeding.) A few years later, I saw a woman breastfeeding in the market in San Cristóbal de las Casas, Mexico. It was such an unusual sight for me that I took a photo of her. "How Third World of her," I thought. "Good *National Geographic* photo."

Then my wife and I had our first baby in 1976. I cannot tell you why neither Adele nor I ever considered anything for our son except breastfeeding. Our experience with Daniel taught us that though breastfeeding is supposed to be natural, it is not always easy. But our baby was breastfed exclusively, except for a few bottles of sugar water here and there when he seemed to want to nurse all the time (and no, I would not recommend that today!). Since I was the only doctor in the small village where we lived at the time, and my wife was the only nurse, we didn't have anyone to ask. We muddled through. Daniel breastfed until he was almost four years old.

Because I was now the father of a breastfed baby, I became interested in the topic. I began to notice news reports about babies in Africa and other parts of the world who were dying because they were not breastfed. I realized that most of the pediatricians I was working with knew very little about breastfeeding—not even the little I had learned watching

Adele breastfeed Daniel. Breastfeeding did not come up at all as a topic of discussion; doctors never asked women if they were breastfeeding or if they wanted to, and all the babies in the special care unit were fed formula by bottle. The notion of using breastmilk for the premature babies was never even discussed.

Then I moved to the Hospital for Sick Children (HSC) in Toronto. There, breastfeeding was mentioned more often, mostly to say it was getting in the way of measuring the baby's fluid intake. One older staff pediatrician mentioned that his children had been breastfed and that he felt it was important. That impressed me. But generally, formula was used without a thought. In the intensive care unit, we wrote orders for formula without even asking if the mothers were providing milk. (The mothers were always elsewhere, since there were no births at the Hospital for Sick Children.)

After finishing my residency in pediatrics, I went to work in South Africa in 1981. The experience confirmed what I had heard about the horrors of bottle-feeding in circumstances of poverty, lack of clean water and lack of understanding about bottle feeding. Every day, babies died because they were not breastfed. Even if they were partially breastfed, they frequently got seriously ill and often died because the water used to prepare the formula was contaminated and the babies got fewer of the immune factors in breastmilk that fight infections. The mothers almost never had enough money to buy sufficient formula, so they watered it down. Starving babies and children were admitted every day to the hospital.

I realized that if we could institute three fairly simple public health measures we could reduce the flood of sick children to a more manageable level.

1. All children would be immunized. Every day children died of measles; polio was common,

tetanus not infrequent. Whooping cough was less common but devastating when it did occur.

2. All the tuberculosis contacts would be followed up and treated. Tuberculosis was epidemic.

3. All babies would be breastfed exclusively to about six months and would continue to be breastfed for two years and beyond.

I couldn't do everything, so I concentrated on helping mothers breastfeed. This seemed to me to be easier and less expensive to accomplish than tackling the other issues. Little did I know how much resistance would be put up by the formula companies and by other physicians, especially some of the physicians in the private hospital for whites.

I did get lots of support from *most* colleagues and co-workers. The nurses at the hospital were incredible. They could get babies breastfeeding who had been off the breast for weeks, and they could increase dwindling milk supplies like magic. I know now that I should have paid much more attention to what the nurses were doing, but I didn't. At the time, I thought there wasn't much to know about breastfeeding. You just put the baby to the breast, right? I'd figured out that you don't give bottles or time feedings, but that was it.

When I returned to Canada, I went to work in the Hospital for Sick Children emergency department as a staff pediatrician. Virtually every day, I saw mothers and babies suffering with breastfeeding problems. What was striking was how lousy the breastfeeding information they were getting was. Not only was the advice bad, but it often defied logic and common sense. The bad advice was widespread; I heard the same thing repeatedly from different mothers. I did what I could to help but could see that there were systemic problems.

One day, our chief of emergency suggested that we should take four hours a week to do something other than emergency—to prevent burnout. So I decided to start a breastfeeding clinic. My experiences in the emergency department had shown me that there was a definite need.

During the first full year of the clinic, 1985, only 70 mothers and their babies came. But slowly, the clinic got busier. I knew very little, really, but some of the mothers managed, and that encouraged me, and I was learning all the time. The success of the clinic created its own momentum. The word soon spread. I began to attend seminars on breastfeeding, and to learn from the mothers I worked with and other breastfeeding experts. I realized that many of the issues were caused by the lack of training of nurses and doctors in breastfeeding and how to help mothers breastfeed. I now believe that more than 90% of the difficulties women have are preventable.

Naively, I thought that hospitals, doctors and nurses would want to know how their policies and advice were causing breastfeeding difficulties for the women they worked with. I started writing letters to the hospital staff, explaining what the problems were. The response wasn't quite what I expected. I got angry letters back insisting that the mothers I had seen had not told me the truth about their experiences in the hospital. Sometimes I would simply be told to mind my own business. Sometimes people would write to the chief of pediatrics to complain about me.

But I couldn't stop being concerned about the babies who cried and suffered because they weren't getting enough milk, the mothers who struggled with agonizingly sore nipples and painful breasts, and the many other problems caused by breastfeeding mismanagement.

In 1992, the breastfeeding clinic at HSC closed and I began to see women and babies at other hospitals around the city of Toronto. Eventually, along with lactation consultant Edith Kernerman, I opened the International Breastfeeding Centre. Now we see approximately 2,500 mothers and babies every year. I speak at conferences and workshops around the world. Unfortunately, the doctors and nurses who need to be at the conferences the most are generally the ones who don't attend.

Once one takes up a cause, it becomes more and more difficult to ignore the real issues. As I learned more, I began to see how the formula companies aggressively and unethically marketed their products. I began to see how the health system collaborated, quite willingly, with the formula companies. I began to see that infant feeding was not a question of the mother making an informed choice between breastfeeding and bottle-feeding. Not at all.

I realized the whole system works against breastfeeding mothers and babies. We have stacks of research, even more than mentioned in the first edition of this book, to show that breastfeeding is important for the health and optimal development of babies and the health of the mother, and yet it is too often treated as unimportant. In my efforts to support breastfeeding, I sometimes found myself in conflict with obstetricians, pediatricians and hospital nurses—not to mention dietitians who were concerned because they couldn't measure everything, radiologists who told mothers they couldn't breastfeed after MRI (magnetic resonance imaging) scans, anaesthetists who told mothers they couldn't breastfeed after a general anaesthetic, and many other health professionals who seemed to recommend weaning in almost any situation. I found myself in opposition to child protection services that believe separation of breastfeeding mothers and babies is not a problem, and judges in family court who believe fathers deserve to have alternate weeks with their babies even if it means destroying the breastfeeding relationship.

Breastfeeding should never be expendable. Only under extraordinary circumstances should breastfeeding be interrupted. It is too important to the physical and mental health of the child and the mother for them to give it up the way one might give up ice cream.

The purpose of this book is to empower women. Their right to breastfeed, and their babies' right to be breastfed, should be paramount. It is more important than the comfort of the person sitting near them in the restaurant who is offended by seeing a baby at the breast. It is more important than the physician's desire to recommend a particular drug for the mother without bothering to find something compatible with breastfeeding, which is almost always possible. It is more important than hospital routines and paperwork that take up the time of the postpartum nurses.

My hope is that this book will help mothers and fathers understand how breastfeeding works, how it can be made a wonderful experience for both mother and baby, how problems can be overcome and how the practice is being undermined. In these pages, you will find information about getting breastfeeding off to a good start, dealing with challenging situations and handling breastfeeding in special circumstances. I also hope to counteract

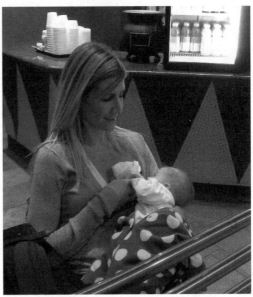

CREDIT: **JACK NEWMAN**

some widely held myths about breastfeeding—myths that can become obstacles to the new mother.

Breastfeeding is important. It is worth the effort to overcome difficulties so that it can succeed. Because it's important, we need to change our medical system and our society so that breastfeeding becomes easier and the norm.

It's been a slow process, but we're getting there. Unfortunately, after many years, there have been steps backward as well. But each mother who has a happy, successful breastfeeding experience brings us one step closer to a society where breastfeeding is, once again, the norm.

PART I:

The Normal Way
to Feed a Baby

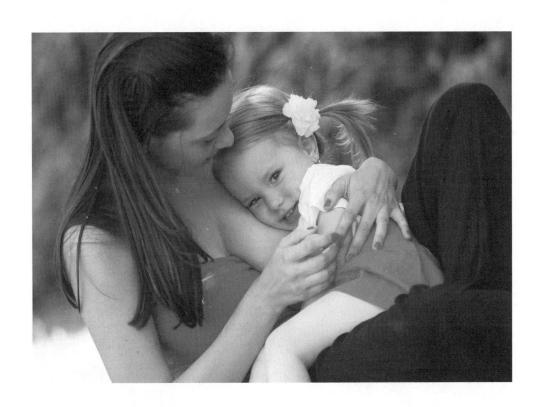

1 | Why Breastfeeding Is Important

Breastfeeding is good for the baby, good for the mother, good for the family and good for society. We have plenty of evidence to show that this is true.

The real evidence, and the real risks of artificial feeding

Health care providers, childbirth educators and others often talk about the "advantages" of breastfeeding. But to describe the differences between breastfeeding and artificial feeding this way assumes that artificial feeding is the norm. The warning messages on packages of cigarettes don't say, "Non-smokers may have lower rates of heart disease or lung cancer." They say, "Smoking increases your risk of heart disease and lung cancer." This perspective makes a difference in how statistics are presented. One study announced that women who had been breastfed as infants had a decrease of 25% in breast cancer rates when compared to women who were fed formula as infants. More accurately: women who were fed formula as infants had a 33.3% increase in breast cancer rates. Looks more significant, doesn't it?

It is breastfeeding that is the normal way to feed a baby; there are risks to artificial feeding.

We often assume that if breastfeeding is not possible—a rare situation—formula is the second-best solution. But the World Health Organization (WHO) states that second best would be the mother's own milk, pumped or expressed, and fed to her baby (perhaps with a cup or a tube). This is only second best because feeding at the breast enhances the development of neuronal connections in the baby's brain, helps with the development of the baby's jaw and facial muscles, and allows the transfer of germs back and forth between the mother and the baby, which helps protect the baby against infection and allergies. Expressed milk won't provide those important factors, or nurture the unique, close relationship between mother and baby that is also an essential part of breastfeeding. If expressing milk is impossible, the third feeding suggestion on WHO's list is screened donated milk. Only if that is also unavailable would artificial baby-milk feedings be used—the fourth-best solution.

There is also a "mutual relationship" in breastfeeding: when the baby fusses or shows he wants to feed, the mother's milk begins to let down, so that breastfeeding both fills the baby's stomach and soothes him and, at the same time, relieves the pressure of milk in the mother's breast and releases hormones that make her feel calmer and more loving. Mother an child reinforce those good feelings in each other.

Risks of not breastfeeding

The risks of feeding a baby with anything other than the milk nature designed for him are real, and they are a concern even in societies where medical care and treatment for the problems caused by not breastfeeding are readily available. In some parts of the world, the use of breastmilk substitutes means many babies will not survive. While the vast majority of bottle-fed babies in North America will live, that doesn't mean the health problems and risks are not real and potentially serious.

Let's look at some of those risks.

Contamination. The name "formula" makes artificial infant milk seem very scientific, but most formulas are just cow's milk modified with other ingredients. Some use soy milk as the basis. As with all manufactured items, mistakes are sometimes made in preparing or processing formula. Formulas have been frequently recalled because important ingredients were left out, the labels were wrong, bacteria were found in the cans, etc.

This can happen with any product, but it matters more with formula. If an important ingredient is missing, the effect on the baby can be devastating. Babies have suffered brain damage and permanent developmental delays because of chloride-deficient formulas; babies have become ill with diseases such as meningitis from contaminated formulas. A recent study of several brands of formulas found that some cans contained more than four times the amount of vitamin D listed on the label—and vitamin D in excess is toxic to infants. In 2003, three babies in Israel died and 10 were admitted to hospital because the formula they drank did not contain adequate amounts of vitamin B_1. In 2008, according to *The Guardian*, 300,000 babies in China became ill from drinking formula contaminated with melamine; 54,000 were hospitalized and died.

Parents using formula have to rely on a manufacturer's assembly line, which will inevitably produce some errors and problems. They have to hope that their baby isn't unlucky enough to get that problematic batch of formula, and that they notice when a particular lot number is recalled (and several lots of formula are recalled every year).

Uniformity of formula does not match baby's needs. One of the ways that breastfeeding is unique is that the milk constantly changes. The milk a mother produces in the morning is different from the milk in the evening. The milk also changes from day to day, and as the baby changes with time, so the milk produced for a two-week-old is not quite the same as the milk produced for a six-month-old or a one-year-old. The milk of a mother whose baby was born prematurely is different and more suitable for her tiny baby's needs than the milk of a mother whose baby was born full-term.

The milk also changes from the beginning of the feeding to the end, with generally higher levels of fat toward the end, helping to reduce the risk of obesity by making the baby feel full and satisfied. This has an impact into adulthood: research shows that being overweight at any age increases the risk of being overweight later in life.

As the baby grows into a toddler, some immune factors that kill bacteria increase in concentration in the milk, helping to keep the toddler who puts everything in his mouth healthy.

This does not mean, however, that milk donated from a mother breastfeeding a 12-month-old is less appropriate for a one-month-old than formula. The "12-month-old milk" is still closer to "one-month-old milk" than formula.

Negative effect on intelligence and cognitive development. A baby's brain is not fully developed at birth. It continues to grow and build a network of connections between brain cells for the first three or four years. Breastmilk, because it is designed for human babies, contains all the nutrients a baby's brain needs to reach its maximum potential.

Researchers have known from early on that children breastfed as infants scored higher, on average, on tests of intelligence and development, but they thought that perhaps mothers who breast-fed were more motivated to do other good things to enhance learning. Or perhaps the extra holding and skin-to-skin contact involved in breastfeeding was the reason these children were brighter.

One study that tried to reduce the effect of those factors compared mothers who gave birth in two different groups of hospitals, a group that had introduced policies to support breastfeeding and a group that had not. A higher percentage of the mothers from the breastfeeding-supportive hospitals breastfed, and the babies born in these hospitals, as a group, later scored an average of 11 points higher on tests of intelligence when compared to the babies born in the other hospitals. Incidentally, this was not a small study but one that followed many thousands of babies for several years.

A 1992 study tried to eliminate the parenting factors by looking at premature babies who were being fed through a tube in the stomach. One group was given breastmilk plus banked breastmilk if the mother was not able to express enough; the other was given breastmilk plus preterm formula if the mother was not able to express enough. When they reached school age, the children who had received only breastmilk scored an average of eight points higher on tests of intelligence. The milk itself, not extra cuddling or holding, made the difference.

Other researchers have studied babies who were breastfed for varying lengths of time, and they found that intelligence scores were higher, on average, for babies who were breastfed longer.

But it may be that the increased skin-to-skin contact and holding *is* also a factor. Mothers who are bottle-feeding usually hold their babies when they are small, but as the baby gets bigger, he may hold the bottle himself or, when he's older, even walk around with a bottle. Breastfeeding ensures the baby will be held skin to skin many times a day. This contact is undoubtedly beneficial.

Whatever the contributing factors, it's clear that babies who are not breastfed are less likely to reach their potential when it comes to intelligence.

Higher incidence of diabetes. Type 1 diabetes is the one usually seen in children, and there is clearly a genetic component that makes some children vulnerable to this illness. Some studies have shown that if a baby genetically at risk for diabetes is not given cow's milk or formula (made from cow's milk) during his first year, he's less likely to develop type 1 diabetes.

Type 2 diabetes is the kind generally seen in adults (although more and more children are affected today due to increased childhood obesity). Adults who were breastfed as children are also less likely to develop type 2 diabetes, at least in part because they are less likely to become overweight or obese. The mother who breastfeeds is also less likely to develop type 2 diabetes; the longer she breast-feeds, the lower her risk.

There is a relationship between the amount of protein a baby takes in and the risk of overweight and type 2 diabetes later in life. The amount of protein a formula-fed baby takes in during the first six months of life far exceeds that consumed by the exclusively breastfed baby. Not only does the formula-fed baby take in more, but he also absorbs more. More is not necessarily better.

Increased risk of SIDS. SIDS stands for sudden infant death syndrome, and it describes an infant death that happens for no apparent reason, usually while the baby is asleep. This used to be called crib death or cot death. No cause has been discovered, and there are probably several factors involved. (For example, doctors are now recommending that babies sleep on their backs to reduce the incidence of SIDS.)

Researchers have found that feeding a baby with formula doubles its risk of dying from SIDS.

Higher risk of later overweight and obesity. Several recent studies have found that artificially fed babies are much more likely to be overweight or obese as children and teens. Why? There are many possible reasons.

Human milk increases in fat content as the baby drains more milk from the breast. This acts as an appetite control: the baby feels satisfied and stops drinking. Breastfed babies are able to control the amount of milk they take in at each feeding, whereas bottle-fed babies are often urged to finish the bottle, leading to overeating and decreasing their sensitivity to the natural sense of being full.

A study published in the June 2010 issue of *Pediatrics* showed that the bottle itself is part of the problem, even if there is breastmilk in it: "Infants who are bottle-fed in early infancy are more likely to empty the bottle or cup in late infancy than those who are fed directly at the breast." And another quote from this article: "Bottle feeding, regardless of the type of milk, is distinct from feeding at the breast in its effect on infants' self-regulation of milk intake."

Bottle feeding may "prime" the baby to want more. A baby bottle-fed in the first few days drinks a lot more than one who is breastfeeding. One study showed that the more weight a baby gains in the first week of life, the more likely it is he will be overweight as an adult.

Exclusively breastfed babies actually take less milk than we previously thought. An exclusively breastfed, well-gaining five-month-old is taking about the same amount of milk as a one-month-old, even though the five-month-old weighs twice as much. A five-month-old formula-fed baby will usually drink twice as much as he did at one month.

Breastmilk also contains compounds such as leptin and ghrelin, which together act to control appetite. Formulas do not contain these factors.

Another factor that may help encourage healthy eating (and thus possibly prevent overweight): breastfed babies are exposed to various tastes through their mother's milk; formula-fed babies get the same bland taste at every meal. Researchers have found that breastfed babies more readily eat a variety of vegetables and fruits when they start solid foods (if their mothers have been eating these foods during the time they were breastfeeding) compared to formula-fed babies, who prefer sweet, starchy and bland foods. This early acceptance of nutritious foods gives the breastfed baby a head start on healthy eating.

Increased respiratory illnesses. Feeding a baby with formula is a risk factor for developing asthma, a condition that has increased dramatically in recent years. Babies fed formula are also at a higher risk of other respiratory illnesses, including respiratory syncytial virus (RSV) and pneumonia. As well, they take longer to recover from these illnesses than breast-fed babies.

Increased risk of meningitis. Meningitis is an inflammation of the brain that can be caused by viruses or bacteria, and the bacterial form can be fatal if not treated appropriately. Formula-fed babies are much more likely to become ill with this disease.

Increased risk of aar infections. Formula-feeding has repeatedly been shown to be a risk factor in developing otitis media (ear infection). Ear infections are often very painful and can lead to further complications, the most common of which is fluid remaining in the ear after the infection has been treated, affecting the baby's hearing and speech development. Spread of the infection to adjoining areas of the ear and even to the brain, with very serious consequences, may also occur (though, fortunately, it is not very common these days).

Higher rates of childhood cancer. At least three studies have found that formula feeding increases the risk of developing cancer during childhood. The child who is breastfed has a more mature immune system. Several cancers are caused by or facilitated by viral infections. A more mature immune system is likely to help defend the baby against these viruses. Furthermore, breastmilk contains a compound called α-lactalbumin, which is transformed in the baby's stomach to human lactalbumin and made lethal to tumour cells (HAMLET); in other words, it causes tumour cells to "commit suicide" (apoptosis).

Higher risk of gastrointestinal infections and diseases. It seems logical that the baby's gastrointestinal system would be affected by the food he consumes. Formula significantly increases the baby's risk of diarrhea caused by various germs, and babies who are fed artificially also take longer to recover, partly because they are often taken off their formula feedings and given only clear fluids while sick, so they get virtually no nutrition. A breastfed baby can and *should* continue breastfeeding and receiving high-quality nutrition plus antibodies and other immune factors to kill off the germs that are causing the illness. Diarrhea can be very serious in a young baby.

Breastfed babies are also much less likely to become constipated. It is extremely rare for an exclusively breastfed baby to have hard bowel movements. His bowel movements are usually very loose, even if infrequent. Formula is much more likely to cause constipation and painful bowel movements, a problem that can become chronic and difficult to resolve.

Constipation means hard bowel movements, not necessarily infrequent ones. Exclusively breastfed babies, after the first three to six weeks of life, *may* actually have bowel movements only every few days or even less frequently. If they are breastfeeding well, gaining weight properly and content, it is not a concern. Incidentally, I am aware of two healthy, exclusively breastfed babies who had, on one occasion, no bowel movements for 31 days and another exclusively breastfed baby who had no bowel movements for 32 days. All three were perfectly healthy, growing well and not constipated.

Decreased effectiveness of vaccines. Artificial feeding reduces the effectiveness of vaccinations by diminishing the baby's response and production of the necessary antibodies. Breastfed babies have a normal response to vaccinations, and they produce more antibodies. Some people think that breastfed babies will have a blunted response to vaccines given by mouth, such as the rotavirus. This is incorrect. A recent article suggested that breastfed babies should have a feeding delayed a few hours after vaccination because the rotavirus vaccine is less effective if feeding happens soon after the vaccine is given. This was misinterpreted in the press as a recommendation to stop breastfeeding altogether.

Inadequate development of jaw and facial muscles. Anyone who has carefully observed a baby suck on a bottle and compared it to the way a baby suckles at the breast knows that these are two very different techniques. Naturally, the development of the muscles, jaw and tongue will be different. Some people claim they can recognize a breastfed baby on sight, just by looking for the rounded, well-developed cheeks! Children who were artificially fed as babies are more likely to need orthodontic work and have related problems such as snoring and sleep apnea.

Long-term breastfeeding, in particular, promotes the development of a well-shaped jaw and straight teeth.

Higher risk of death. Babies in developing countries are much more likely to die if they are not breastfed. We tend to think that with good medical care, it's not an issue. It is. A study in the United States found that babies who are not breastfed are significantly more likely to die, from all causes, in the first year.

Increased mental health risks. Recent studies have found that children and adults who were not breastfed as infants are more likely to have depression, anxiety, alcoholism, ADHD, and schizophrenia. In their teen years, children who were not breastfed are more likely to have serious behaviour problems.

Increased risk of child abuse. The vast majority of mothers would never abuse their children. However, some parents are at higher risk of abuse, and when researchers studied some of these parents, they found that the babies fed formula were at greater risk of being abused than those who were breastfed. Why? Well, it's possible that those mothers who are less likely to be abusive are also more likely to breastfeed. Other research has shown that breastfeeding mothers, when they hear their babies cry, tend to have the nurturing and responsive areas of their brains "light up." Perhaps this is the way breastfeeding helps mothers fall in love with their babies.

Women who know they are at risk of abusing a child—perhaps because they themselves were abused as children—often find it very encouraging to know that there is something they can do to reduce that risk.

Higher risk of postpartum depression. Breastfeeding can protect mothers from postpartum depression, and it can also protect babies from the possible harmful effects of postpartum depression when it does happen. Researchers have found that when bottle-feeding mothers are depressed, their babies' brains don't develop normally. The mothers talk and interact with their babies less because of the depression. But when babies are breastfed, their brains continue to develop normally even though their mothers are depressed, and the mothers talk and interact with them in more positive ways.

Unfortunately, some researchers in postpartum depression have taken it as a given that if a mother sleeps better she is less likely to be depressed. A study is going on at present that separates mothers from their babies during the night; the babies are given formula during the night so the mothers can sleep—almost a surefire method of making breastfeeding fail.

Yes, lack of sleep can be a risk factor for postpartum depression. But there are better ways to help a mother get enough sleep while also supporting breastfeeding.

Increased risk of necrotizing enterocolitis (NEC). This is a very serious condition most often seen in premature babies; formula is a major risk factor. Hospitals in China and now some in Canada have begun giving premature babies donated human milk and have seen dramatic drops in NEC rates.

Other risks. The risks from formula feeding continue as the baby grows up. Young adults who were fed formula as babies are more likely to have high blood pressure and high cholesterol, to be overweight, and to be insulin resistant (a risk factor for type 2 diabetes). Other studies have directly linked formula feeding to heart disease in later life. Crohn's disease, ulcerative colitis and irritable bowel syndrome are more common in adults who were fed formula as babies; so are multiple sclerosis and arthritis.

Researcher David Newburg commented that he used to think of human milk as providing the best nutrition for babies, but as he continued his research he realized that its protective role against acute infections in infancy and chronic illnesses in adulthood was probably even more important. He's not the only one. Michelle G. Brenner and E. Stephen Buescher, in the abstract to a research article, write: "Human milk is not simply a food but rather a complex human infant-support system."

Risks to the mother from formula-feeding
Breastfeeding is not important only to the health of the baby, the child and the adult that child will become, but also to the mother's health. Breastfeeding helps new mothers recover after birth by encouraging the uterus to contract normally and reducing the amount of blood loss.

It also reduces the risk of developing breast cancer, cancer of the uterus and cancer of the ovaries. The more months a mother breastfeeds, the lower her risk.

Breastfeeding reduces the risk of developing osteoporosis. Although calcium transfers to the baby in the milk, resulting in loss of bone mass during breastfeeding, once the baby weans, bone mass increases and may rebound to *higher* levels than at the baby's birth.

Iron deficiency in young women is almost epidemic, despite the fact that we have iron-rich foods readily available. A mother who breastfeeds a toddler will resume her period, on average, 14 months after the birth of the baby. The mother who does not breastfeed at all will usually get her period back three months after birth. Those 11 extra menstrual periods add up to the equivalent of one unit of blood (450 ml) lost, significantly increasing the risk of anemia for the formula-feeding mother.

When a mother does not breastfeed, her risk of overweight and obesity in later life increases.

Breastfeeding helps women lose weight gained during pregnancy. The mother who does not breastfeed is at greater risk of developing type 2 diabetes and metabolic syndrome, a combination of insulin resistance, abnormal lipid profile, high blood pressure and overweight leading to a very high risk of heart attack and stroke.

Are all these risks of formula-feeding proven?
I think it is important to address some objections about studies showing that breastfeeding is superior to artificial feeding. (We will sometimes refer to formula as artificial baby milk or artificial feeding. That's a more accurate description, really. The name "formula" makes it sound scientific—but it's just an artificial substitute for the real thing, human milk.) These objections often reflect a lack of understanding about how breastfeeding actually works, as well as a bias in favour of bottle-feeding. Here are some of the comments you may have read:

The studies showing breastfeeding is superior to artificial feeding are flawed and thus prove nothing. It's true that studies comparing breastfeeding and artificial feeding do not comply with what would be considered the "gold standard": the randomized, double blind, controlled study. Good drug studies, for example, are designed this way: a group of people with high blood pressure, say, who are generally similar with regard to age, education, income, severity of their problem, etc., are divided randomly into two groups. People in one group get the drug being tested, while people in the other get a placebo (that is, a pill with no active ingredients). Neither the researchers nor the participants know who is getting the real drug (that makes it "double blind"). The study subjects' blood pressure would be measured at regular intervals and, after a given period of time, the results would be analyzed and side effects noted.

In fact, these types of studies aren't perfect either. While researchers try to make the two groups similar there may be important differences between them, especially if the numbers are small. You may know people who are very similar to you demographically but who are, essentially, very different in their ideas, politics, eating habits, etc.

Studies comparing breastfeeding and artificial feeding can't be done with randomized, double blind, controlled studies. You cannot randomly assign new mothers to breastfeed or not. It's even hard to define "breastfeeding" in a study. Often mothers who breastfeed only for a short time, or who breastfeed partially and also give formula, are included in the breastfeeding group. This tends to bias the study in favour of artificial feeding.

From multiple surveys, we know that women in industrialized countries are more likely to breastfeed if they: (a) are older, (b) have a higher level of education, (c) are more affluent, and (d) are in a stable relationship with a partner who is supportive of her breastfeeding. So the demographics of women who breastfeed and those who don't may differ in significant ways.

But those who criticize breastfeeding studies for these reasons are missing the point completely. Breastfeeding is the normal, physiologic, natural way of feeding babies and young children. Formulas are only *very* superficially similar to breastmilk. The protein, carbohydrate and fats that are in formulas are significantly different from those in human milk, not only in quantity but also biochemically. There are also dozens of components of breastmilk that are absent from formula. And there are many undesirable components, such as high concentrations of aluminum and lead, that are present in formulas that are not present in breastmilk.

Thus you don't have to prove that the normal, physiologic and natural is better than the artificial.

Demanding that breastfeeding, which is much more than breastmilk, be proved better than artificial feeding is turning the science on its head. You have to prove that the artificial is at least as good as the normal. What is interesting is that despite the challenges of accurately defining breastfeeding in these research studies, we still find in study after study that artificial feeding increases the baby's risks of a wide range of health and developmental problems.

The antibodies in milk are not absorbed into the baby's body. They stay in the gut and thus can protect the baby only against gut infections. The January 17, 2011, issue of *Maclean's* quoted Joan B. Wolf, an assistant professor of women's studies at Texas A&M University: "We do have very good evidence that breastmilk reduces gastrointestinal infections. The milk is ingested, goes into the baby's gut, and antibodies from the mother's milk fight the bacteria in the gut. What we don't have is any evidence that those antibodies have any effect anywhere else in the body." This statement makes sense *only* if you don't understand how germs get into the body and how breastfeeding works to protect against them.

First, antibodies are not the only immune factors in breastmilk. There are dozens of these factors, which interact to protect the baby from bacteria, viruses and fungi. Together, these immune components coat the linings of the gut and respiratory tract with a "shield" to prevent germs from entering the baby's body in the first place. The immune factors don't need to be in the bloodstream, because the majority of infections are transmitted through the respiratory or the intestinal tract. So breastfeeding provides a much better way of protecting the baby than having to fight off germs once they have entered its bloodstream. And the effectiveness of breastfeeding against a long list of infections and diseases has been conclusively shown in numerous studies.

Second, even if it were true that "all breastfeeding does is decrease the incidence of gut infections (gastroenteritis)," that is far from a minor accomplishment. Hundreds of babies die of gut infections in the United States every year, and hundreds of thousands die around the world. But of course, breastfeeding is important in protecting against many other conditions as well (as we discussed earlier).

"My kids were formula-fed and they're okay."
It's very true that most babies who are given formula will survive and grow and thrive. But this doesn't mean breastfeeding isn't important.

One of the reasons people don't recognize the importance of breastfeeding is that when a baby or child does get ill, it's usually not attributed to the method of feeding. For example, between 75% and 83% of children will have at least one ear infection by the time they are three years old, and 46% will have three or more. So common are ear infections that parents and doctors consider this almost normal. But it's not. Breastfed babies have far fewer ear infections than those fed with formula. Ear infections cause much suffering and may have long-term effects, but most parents would consider a child with multiple ear infections as "okay"; even if they did see it as a problem, they would not likely link it to how the baby was fed.

The formulas that people who are 30 or 60 years old were fed are very different from those of today. When I was attending medical school, commercial formulas were available, but most people made their own using homogenized whole milk (3.25% fat) or evaporated milk, water and corn syrup. Most of the adults who were fed these formulas as babies would say they are "okay" (although they may have problems with overweight, heart disease, allergies, high blood pressure and other conditions that could quite likely be related to how they were fed as infants). Yet almost everyone today would agree that those homemade formulas are not as good as the formulas of today and that they were very inadequate and should not have been used.

Every few years, formulas get "improved." A fairly recent change has been the addition of long-chained polyunsaturated fatty acids (DHA and ARA). This "improvement" has been accompanied by a huge and aggressive campaign, which employs a large A+, implying that the baby will be more intelligent and see better. Does it? We don't know. Studies not financed by the formula companies say not. Studies financed by the formula companies give different results. But if DHA and ARA do in fact make the baby more intelligent and improve his vision, does that mean that previously formula denied babies these essential nutrients?

This "formula improvement" has happened repeatedly over the years. In the 1970s, taurine (an amino acid present in breastmilk) was added so that babies' vision would be better. What about before the 1970s, when babies did not get taurine? In the 1990s, nucleotides were added, which are supposed to enhance immunity—a questionable claim. But what about the artificially fed babies before the 1990s? They didn't get this either. So, are these additions important to the baby's health or not? If not, we are being sold a bill of goods. If yes, does this mean that the health of hundreds of millions of earlier formula-fed babies has been compromised? And we know formula is still missing many components in human milk that are important to protecting and maintaining the baby's health. What new ingredients will be added in 5 years, 10 years, 20 years, that today's formulas lack?

The latest thing is the addition of prebiotics. Prebiotics, of course, have always been in breastmilk. A recent study of five-year-olds who had been given prebiotics in formula as infants showed that this did not prevent allergies, as claimed by at least one formula company.

By the time you read this book, more "amazing" ingredients will likely have been added to formula—but it still won't be breastmilk.

While no study is perfect, the accumulation of research adds up to a clear message: breastfeeding is the normal way to feed a baby and artificial feeding has risks.

The convenience and ease of breastfeeding

The topic of the first meeting in the standard La Leche League series of four meetings is Advantages of Breastfeeding. (Yes, they should probably change it to Risks of Artificial Feeding.) It is interesting that when mothers get talking at the meetings, they rarely discuss the research. Most mothers talk about the emotional side of breastfeeding and how it makes mothering a baby, toddler or young child easier and more enjoyable.

They like the convenience: the milk is always ready, always at the right temperature. It takes just a second to lift up a shirt or undo a button and offer the baby the breast. They find breastfeeding easy when travelling to places where it might be hard to store formula or find a place to heat it. They love being able to just roll over in bed and feed the baby when he fusses with hunger in the night. And they appreciate not having to spend time preparing or cleaning bottles because it means extra time with the baby.

At first, mothers are focused on the mechanics of breastfeeding. But once those techniques are mastered, some of the other important aspects of breastfeeding become apparent.

Breastfeeding is a great comfort to a baby who is hurt or upset. It soothes a baby who has to be given a vaccination and calms a baby who has been startled or stressed.

When studies came out showing that sugar water decreased the pain a newborn felt when having blood taken, sugar water was adopted with relish by the medical community. When it was shown that breastfeeding the baby worked just as well, doctors ignored it! We even see breastfed babies given sugar water instead of the breast. Some have suggested that it's not a good idea to give the baby the breast during or after a painful procedure because we don't want the baby to associate breastfeeding with pain. Does that make sense? Who would suggest that caressing the baby during a painful procedure is not a good idea because the baby would then associate caressing with pain?

Being at the breast reminds the baby of being in the womb: there's that familiar heartbeat and soothing voice, as well as the warmth and comfort. And that makes the transition to the outside world a little easier.

Mothers also talk about how breastfeeding forces them to slow down in a busy world. You can't prop up a breast and leave the baby to eat while you finish washing the dishes. Breastfeeding guarantees that mother and baby will be skin to skin or at least in close contact, relaxing together, several times a day. And those restful feeding times can help you recover from pregnancy and childbirth, and form an even closer bond with your baby.

Mothers love the smell of their breastfed baby, that clean smell that doesn't come from any soap or talcum powder. Even the baby's bowel movements don't smell unpleasant—they give off a faint yeasty odour. They talk about how breastfeeding tunes them in to their baby's signals. They tell stories about how they couldn't consciously recognize their baby's crying, but their breasts did, starting to leak milk at the sound of his voice. They talk about how often they wake up just a minute or so before the baby does. Some tell stories about how they knew their baby was ill because of a small change in the way he suckled or behaved at the breast.

In 2011, researchers did MRIs of mothers' brains while they listened to their own babies

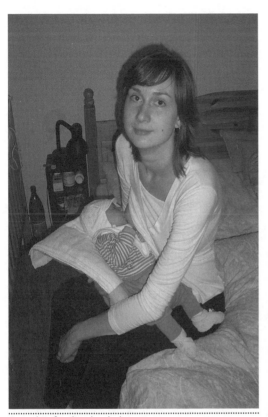

A mother feeding her baby.   CREDIT: **ANDREA POLOKOVA**

you change breasts?" The mother, surprised, said, "He was finished that side, and he wanted the other one." The nurse insisted that she hadn't seen any signals from the baby.

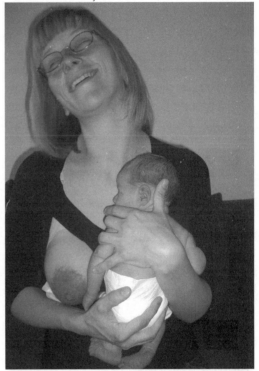

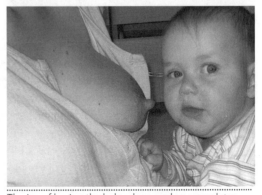

The joy of having the baby close, and one year later. This mother had considerable difficulty because her baby wasn't getting enough milk from the breast. Without any supplementation but with good help, she was able to breastfeed exclusively.

CREDIT: **ANDREA POLOKOVA**

crying. They found that the breastfeeding mothers had more response in the parts of the brain related to caregiving behaviour and empathy compared to mothers who were feeding their babies formula. These differences were apparent at one, three and four months after birth and correlated with more sensitive caregiving behaviours in the breastfeeding mothers.

Breastfeeding helps mothers learn to understand their babies' sometimes subtle cues. They learn to "read the baby," often without consciously thinking about it. One mother was nursing her baby while chatting with a public health nurse, and at one point she moved the baby to the other breast. The nurse stopped what she was saying and asked, "Why did

While in the beginning, breastfeeding usually means sitting down or lying down, experienced nursing mothers can tend to other children, prepare meals, talk with friends and still be aware of the baby's suckling so that they know when to adjust the baby's latch, when to change breasts, and when the feeding is over.

Mothers talk about the sheer pleasure of being skin to skin with their baby, and of seeing him drift off to sleep at the breast with a trickle of milk run-

---

> Taking a little one to nurse,
> watching him grow to manhood,
> that's what love is.
>
> Carol Shields, *The Stone Diaries*

---

ning down his chin. As the baby gets older, he'll begin to play at the breast, letting go to smile, patting the mother's cheek or investigating her teeth, making happy noises as he nurses. These are all part of the joy of parenting.

Mothers who work outside the home talk about how much they appreciate that bond. It's hard to leave your baby in someone else's care, but being able to put the baby to the breast at the end of the day can re-establish the connection and be relaxing for both mother and baby. These mothers like having something special between them and their babies—something the babysitter can't do.

These experiences are difficult to measure in a scientific way, but they are very real to mothers, and they are important considerations in deciding to breastfeed.

It's worth solving the problems

Twenty to 30 years ago, almost any difficulty encountered by a breastfeeding mother had one "solution": wean the baby. Sore nipples? Stop breastfeeding. Breast infection? Wean immediately. Baby isn't gaining weight well? Give him formula. Easy and straightforward for the doctor giving out the advice, but often devastating to the mother who really wanted

Mothers' Stories

Lesley

Lesley's labour was induced a week before her due date because her blood pressure was high. After a short but intense labour, her daughter was born weighing just over 3.2 kg (7 lb). The baby seemed very sleepy, and Lesley wasn't able to get her to breastfeed right away. When Lesley went home a day later, the baby had nursed a couple of times, but not well, and Lesley's nipples were getting sore. By the time the baby was three days old, Lesley's nipples were unbearably painful, and the engorgement of her breasts made it even harder to get the baby on the breast. Her doctor recommended supplementing with a bottle of formula after each feeding and suggested she take painkillers.

Quite rightly dissatisfied, Lesley called the public health department, and a nurse made a home visit. Her advice: "Put the baby on a bottle. This isn't working." Lesley wanted to breastfeed, not wean. She looked online and found information about the importance of getting a good latch, but it took several more calls before she found someone who could help her get the baby correctly latched on. Her sore nipples healed.

Lesley was well aware of the reasons breastfeeding her baby was important, but she needed more than that—she needed practical help.

to breastfeed. Many mothers have told me that they said nothing to the doctor but cried once they left the office. Doctors often believe that the mother was "asking permission to stop breastfeeding" and feel they did the right thing. I disagree. When a mother goes to the doctor with a breastfeeding problem she wishes to resolve, she is not asking for permission to quit. She is asking for help, and if the doctor did not make an attempt to help her or find help for her, the doctor has failed her. The doctor should have helped the mother with the problem and if he couldn't, he should have referred her to someone who could.

In the past, if the baby was premature or smaller than average, even if born full-term, the mother was usually advised not to even try breastfeeding, because suckling would be too hard for the baby and breastmilk wouldn't have enough calories to help him gain weight. If a baby was bigger than average, mothers were often told that their breastmilk wouldn't be enough to sustain him, and that giving formula would be better. If either baby or mother had any health issues, breastfeeding would be stopped.

Mothers today are more likely to be aware of the benefits and importance of breastfeeding, but many still have difficulty getting the help they need to make it work.

Breastfeeding and guilt

One reason that the many significant differences between breastfeeding and formula-feeding have been downplayed is that people are concerned about making mothers who do not breastfeed feel guilty.

This concern is brought up every time a positive article about breastfeeding appears in the media or when a campaign showing the risks of not breastfeeding is initiated. Formula companies succeeded in cancelling a campaign to promote breastfeeding in the United States a few years ago using just this argument, with support from the American Academy of Pediatrics (the AAP receives a lot of money from the formula companies).

We don't worry much about making mothers feel bad about their choices in other situations. If you are a smoker—or even a cat owner—and your child has asthma, you'll probably leave your doctor's

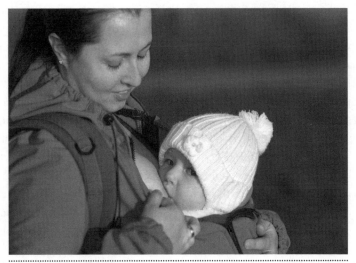

CREDIT: ING. JAROSLAV SVOBODA

office feeling that you are making your child sicker. If you are pregnant and you drink alcohol, even in small amounts, you will get stern warnings. Tell the doctor you're not going to use a car seat for your baby, and you'll get a lecture and maybe a call from the Children's Aid Society. Why isn't the doctor worried about making you feel guilty? Because he or she really believes that continuing to smoke or drink or not use the car seat is a real danger for your child.

The physician who says that we should not make the mother feel guilty for not breastfeeding obviously does not believe that breastfeeding is important for the child's or mother's health, so it's not worth making a big deal about it. There's a double standard here.

Consider this: today's formulas are better than plain whole cow's milk, in theory, but there is no clinical evidence to show that short-term and long-term differences in health result. Babies who were fed undiluted cow's milk without iron-rich solids into toddlerhood frequently became iron deficient. Babies who were fed cow's milk and developed a gut infection (gastroenteritis) often got an imbalance of electrolytes in the blood, which can be very serious. But as long as the baby got iron-rich foods, not too much whole cow's milk and didn't get sick, he was okay. Many people who were fed undiluted cow's milk from birth are now adults and they are "okay."

Breastmilk has far, far more advantages over formula than formula over straight cow's milk. Despite this, what would happen if you told your doctor that you're feeding your one-week-old baby straight cow's milk? The doctor would have a fit! You'd be told that you are putting the baby's health at risk. You'd be ordered to put the baby on formula, and you would probably feel so guilty that you would quickly comply. If you didn't, the Children's Aid Society might be called.

What if you tell your doctor you're giving your one-week-old baby formula? The doctor will probably respond, "That's fine, just make sure it's iron enriched." Most doctors will not even ask why the baby is not breastfed. Perhaps you were given incorrect information and told you could not breastfeed because you were taking medication. It may not be too late, with a one-week-old, to get breastfeeding started. But if the doctor doesn't ask for fear of making you feel guilty, then an opportunity to help you breastfeed has been lost.

The guilt question is a false and absurd argument. Many physicians ask only: "Are you planning to breastfeed or bottle-feed?" If the mother says she's planning to use formula, very few will say, "But have you considered breastfeeding? It's so much better for your baby and you." They just check off "bottle-feeding" and move on to the next question. But an important opportunity will have been missed. By not even asking the question, the doctor sends a message that breastfeeding is not important.

But this concern about guilt is, in reality, just a ploy. It allows *health professionals* not to feel guilty for their lack of knowledge about breastfeeding and their inability to help women overcome difficulties with it, many of which could be prevented in the first place. This argument also allows formula companies and health professionals to pass out formula company literature and free samples of formula to pregnant women without any guilt pangs, even though it has been clearly demonstrated that this literature and "free" samples decrease the frequency and duration of breastfeeding. (Nothing is free. The companies are repaid many times over for these "gifts.") Many mothers trust the formula-company brochures and decide to try the free samples. The formula brochures stress the "benefits" of "giving the father a chance to feed the baby," or promise their formula makes babies sleep better. Using the free samples is often the first step on the downward slope to complete weaning from the breast. The brochures make the two methods seem equivalent: for example, one brochure had a list of "pros and cons" for breastfeeding and formula. Amazingly, there were the same number of "pros" and the same number of "cons" for both types of feeding. The "pros" for breastfeeding included "baby's bowel movements smell better," a minor benefit that is easily cancelled out by one of the pros (at least in the minds of many mothers) for formula: "Father can feed the baby too." The lists are only equal because dozens of significant reasons to breastfeed are ignored.

Women should get the information they need to make an informed decision about breastfeeding. This information must not come from formula companies. (A little later, you'll read about the "information" booklet my daughter-in-law received: The business aim of these companies is to encourage formula not breastfeeding).

Women should know the truth. They can take it; they are adults, not children. If a mother opts for formula rather than breastfeeding, there is good evidence that her baby will score lower on IQ tests and will have a higher risk of many illnesses including some cancers, diabetes, respiratory illnesses, diarrhea and ear infections. She should know that her own risk of breast, ovarian and uterine cancer will be higher, as well as her daughter's risk of breast cancer. The mother increases her own risk of diabetes, high cholesterol, high blood pressure and becoming overweight by "choosing" formula feeding. There is accumulating evidence that the risk of mental illness (alcoholism, ADHD, schizophrenia) is increased by not breastfeeding. A recent study suggested that even behaviour problems in adolescents are more likely if the child was formula fed. The longer the child is breastfed, the lower the risk both for the child and the mother.

Even with this information, many will find it difficult to make an informed choice. A pregnant woman who has seen very few babies breastfeeding may find it difficult to imagine what it will be like to have a baby suckling at the breast. On the old TV show *Murphy Brown*, the star commented that having milk come out of her breast when she fed her baby was like "having bacon come out of her elbow." Honestly, I don't get the joke. Many in our society see breasts as sexual playthings only, so the idea of a baby (or, even worse, a toddler) at the breast suggests some kind of sexual abuse.

But bottle-feeding? It's everywhere—in the media, in sitcoms, in children's books. Very few pregnant women in North America have not seen babies bottle-feeding.

If a woman were ambivalent about whether to breastfeed or artificially feed, I would strongly suggest she start breastfeeding. If she finds, in spite of good help and support, that it is not for her, she can stop breastfeeding. It's easy to stop breastfeeding. But if she starts bottle-feeding and finds the baby does not tolerate formula, or for some other reason she changes her mind and decides to breastfeed, it may be difficult or impossible to go to breastfeeding. I get many emails every week from mothers who regret not starting breastfeeding, or who stopped and want to go back.

One more thing. With the vast majority of women initiating breastfeeding, who *does* feel guilty? The mother who wanted to breastfeed but for whom it didn't work out. Why are we not worried about her?

While you're pregnant

You should begin to prepare for breastfeeding while pregnant—not by "toughening up your nipples" as mothers were at one time advised to do, but by planning ahead. Some ideas:

- Attend at least one meeting of a breastfeeding

support group such as La Leche League. You will get to see babies breastfeeding and meet people who can support you once the baby arrives.

- Check out the International Breastfeeding Centre's YouTube Channel (http://youtube .com/user/IBCToronto) to see videos of babies breastfeeding so you will know how to tell if your baby is drinking well.

- If you will be giving birth in a hospital, ask about its policies and tell your doctor or midwife that you want to keep your baby with you from birth on, unless there is a medical issue that *requires* separation. (Too often, separation of mother and baby is done as a routine or for unnecessary reasons.) Arrange to have a doula with you during your labour and birth. She can help you avoid unnecessary interventions during labour and you will be more likely to breastfeed successfully.

- Plan with your caregivers how you will get breastfeeding underway if you need a Caesarean birth, if you have a premature baby or if your baby is ill. Arrange for support and practical help after the birth so you can focus on breastfeeding.

2 | Finding Good Breastfeeding Help

Myth: health professionals know more about breast-feeding than other people do.

Fact: most health professionals—nurses, midwives, physicians—say they are supportive of breastfeeding. It would be difficult for them not to be, given the evidence. All the major professional organizations, including the Canadian Paediatric Society and the American Academy of Pediatrics, have made statements about the importance of breastfeeding and the need to encourage exclusive breastfeeding for about six months and continued breastfeeding to two years and beyond. But that doesn't mean the vast majority of health professionals have the knowledge to provide practical help.

This inability to help may come from their own experiences as parents. It is difficult to provide encouragement for mothers around breastfeeding when your own breastfeeding experience (or your spouse's) involved a lot of pain, a fussy baby and early weaning to formula.

Medical training does not include much information on breastfeeding, getting things off to a good start or solving problems. Once medical school is over, it doesn't get better. The doctor is deluged with advertising from formula companies and invitations to seminars on infant nutrition—sponsored, of course, by a formula company. (While doctors claim they are not influenced by advertising, they obviously are, just like everyone else.) As soon as there are any difficulties with breastfeeding, or the baby is not fitting precisely into the growth charts,

too many health care professionals advise weaning the baby or supplementing with formula. This is almost always unnecessary if the mother gets good hands-on help.

Here is one example, shared with me by a lactation consultant, in which the doctor blamed breast-feeding for a problem and missed a serious illness. Names have been changed. (My comments appear in italics.)

When Tanya was born, her mother, Stacy, could not get her latched on. Tanya was sleepy and Stacy was told she had "bad nipples." Stacy was sent home on day four with bottle-feeding formula to reduce Tanya's high bilirubin levels. Stacy contacted me when Tanya was five days old. Tanya had never latched on and Stacy had never expressed her milk. Over the next couple of days, Stacy did everything she could to increase her milk supply. She started cup-feeding Tanya with expressed breastmilk and was able to stop formula altogether. By day 10 Tanya finally latched on and was fully breastfed from then on. When Tanya was four weeks old, Stacy called me again. Tanya's bilirubin levels were high, and her pediatrician told her this was due to Stacy's starting to breastfeed instead of continuing with formula. In addition, Tanya was not gaining well. Stacy was not ready to go back to formula after everything she had gone through. I saw Tanya and she was obviously drinking well, yet her skin was much more yellow than before. I watched Stacy change

Tanya's diaper and her bowel movement was pale and her urine dark—not good signs. I told Stacy to keep breastfeeding but to see her doctor again. She did, but her doctor refused to have the appropriate tests done, insisting that all would be well if she used formula.

"It took a month for Stacy to get an appointment with a different doctor, who quickly diagnosed Tanya with biliary atresia (a disease of the bile ducts which results in cirrhosis of the liver if not treated). Stacy and Tanya spent some time in the hospital; Stacy's milk production went down as Tanya was only allowed to breastfeed every three hours, according to that hospital's policy for sick babies (*an absurd policy*). They were then sent home to await liver transplant and were told Tanya must weigh at least 5 kg (11 lb) before surgery. Stacy started taking domperidone and Tanya began to drink very well, but she was not gaining weight. Over the next two weeks Tanya lost 40g, despite breastfeeding well. Tanya's doctor suggested supplementing with formula because, as he saw it, Tanya was not able to gain weight on breastfeeding alone since she could not process fat in breastmilk. (*This is very unlikely. Breastmilk actually contains enzymes that help digest fat.*) He also suggested giving glucose water. (*Why on earth?*) Stacy tried, but Tanya refused to drink either formula or water. Stacy was desperate.

Dr. Newman had a solution. He explained that breastmilk contains enzymes that help break down fat, protein and carbohydrate. He suggested that the baby be admitted to hospital, put on IV nutrition and continue breastfeeding. Stacy took Dr. Newman's emails to her doctor, who thought it was worth a try. Tanya was put on IV and continued to breastfeed and began to gain weight. After her surgery, she was released from the hospital and she has been gaining weight ever since on breastfeeding alone.

How can you know if your doctor or midwife is not supportive of breastfeeding? Here are some clues:

He or she gives you formula samples or literature from one or more formula companies when you are pregnant or soon after you have had your baby. What is the purpose of these formula samples and information? There is only one: to sell infant formulas. They are not gifts, they are advertising. The brochures, videos and samples of formula encourage mothers to use the formula and wean the baby early or supplement unnecessarily. Result? The mother eventually depends on a formula company for her baby's food.

The brochures and videos, subtly or not, usually undermine breastfeeding, and the handy can of formula is a powerful suggestion to the mother that she will need formula. One formula ad for a product marketed for babies older than six months says "At six months of age, your baby's nutritional needs are changing." The message mothers may take away—that after six months breastmilk is no longer doing the job—is implicit. But of course, breastmilk continues to be more than up to the job.

We know this works. The research results are clear: mothers who are given these samples of formula wean their babies earlier than mothers who are not. The formula companies are determined to get samples into mothers' hands; they offer large amounts of cash to hospitals that will use their formula exclusively. If this method of marketing didn't work, the formula companies wouldn't invest so much time, money and effort.

Mothers who are given brochures about breastfeeding written by formula companies are also more likely to wean early, compared to mothers who are given information from a source such as La Leche League.

Ask yourself why your health professional is marketing infant formula. And ask yourself why he or she is not marketing breastfeeding.

He or she tells you that breastfeeding and bottle-feeding are essentially the same. It is true that most bottle-fed babies grow up to be reasonably physically healthy and emotionally secure and that not all breastfed babies grow up to be healthy and secure. But this does not mean that it doesn't make any difference how you feed your baby.

Breastmilk is *very* different in composition from formula. Not only does it contain antibodies, living white blood cells and many other immune factors to protect babies from illness, but it changes from morning to evening, day to day and month to month. It even changes from the beginning of the feeding to the end. It is easily digested, and the nutrients are readily absorbed.

Formula is a very rough approximation of what we knew several years ago about breastmilk. It's based on the milk of an entirely different species, or based on soybeans. Many things in breastmilk can't be duplicated in formula, and formula can't be adapted to meet the baby's changing needs.

Breastfeeding also guarantees the baby a certain amount of holding and skin-to-skin contact for as long as he continues nursing.

Health professionals often describe breastfeeding and bottle-feeding as being more or less equivalent so mothers who are not able to breastfeed won't feel guilty or disappointed. If you are not able to breastfeed, you have every right to be disappointed and sad about it. To pretend that it is unimportant or insignificant is patronizing and medically inaccurate.

He or she tells you that a particular brand of formula is the best. There is no evidence that one brand of formula is better than any other for the normal, healthy baby, although individual babies do seem to tolerate some better than others. When a health professional recommends one brand, it may be because a formula salesperson gave him a brochure, or he attended a seminar, or because his own babies used that brand. Be concerned that your doctor is making recommendations based on something other than research, and not strongly supporting and encouraging breastfeeding.

He or she tells you that having your baby skin to skin immediately after birth, and giving the baby the opportunity to breastfeed, are not practical because you'll be too tired and the baby may not be interested. Skin-to-skin contact immediately after birth allows the baby the opportunity to latch on by himself, getting breastfeeding off to a good start. You may be tired, but you'll also be excited about your new baby. This is the perfect time to start breastfeeding. Your baby can breastfeed even if you have to lie flat after giving birth. Some babies are not interested immediately, but many, if kept skin to skin with their mothers, will soon begin to search for the nipple and latch on within an hour or two. If they are taken away from their mothers, many will go into a deep sleep and not show any interest in breastfeeding for many hours. Early skin-to-skin contact and breastfeeding have been shown in many research studies to be helpful in getting breastfeeding established, and the colostrum is extremely valuable for the baby.

Breastfeeding is not an exhausting activity. Even if you are tired, breastfeeding while lying down or reclining against pillows can be very relaxing. Often hospital routines such as weighing the baby, taking footprints, giving eye drops and vitamin K injections take precedence over getting breastfeeding started. There is no reason why these things can't wait for a couple of hours, while mother and baby are skin to skin and baby finds his way to the breast.

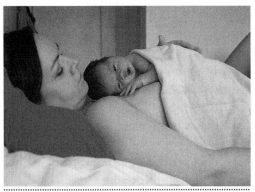

How tiring is this?

CREDIT: **ANDREA POLOKOVA**

He or she tells you there is no such thing as nipple confusion, and that you should start giving bottles to your baby early to make sure he will accept them. Why would anyone stress the importance of getting a baby used to an artificial nipple when there are so many other ways to supplement a baby's food intake (should that become necessary)? Why would it be necessary to start a bottle early if there were no such thing as nipple confusion? In fact, in Canada, where most mothers with full-time employment have 52 weeks of maternity leave, many never use a bottle. The artificial nipple has not been proven harmless to breastfeeding. Yes, some babies get bottles or pacifiers and continue to breastfeed. But others quickly develop problems, and we have no way of predicting in advance which babies will be able to cope with both, and which will not, and end up weaning early. There is an underlying assumption in this advice that your baby will eventually need to take a bottle, even though many breastfed babies never do. Health

professionals should be supporting breastfeeding without suggesting that before too long the baby will be bottle-fed.

He or she tells you that you must stop breastfeeding because you are ill, or your baby is ill, or you need medication or medical tests. There are some *rare* situations in which a mother's or baby's illness means that breastfeeding cannot continue. Too often, though, health professionals recommend weaning the baby without thinking. In the vast majority of cases, stopping breastfeeding is detrimental to the baby and the mother and completely unnecessary. A health professional who is truly supportive of breastfeeding will make every effort to find ways for the mother to continue at the same time as helping her to cope with medical conditions.

In the past, most doctors recommended that women with breast infections should immediately wean their babies, which often made the situation worse. Now most understand that continued breastfeeding on the infected breast is not only safe for the baby but helps the mother heal more quickly and reduces the risk of complications such as abscesses.

Mothers with influenza or gastrointestinal ailments are often advised to wean their babies and are warned that they risk dehydration if they continue breastfeeding. Most mothers who are sick find it easier to continue breastfeeding than to deal with engorged breasts and a miserable baby. Taking small, frequent drinks of watered-down juice or flat ginger ale will help keep the mother hydrated, and she can breastfeed her baby while lying in bed. She doesn't need to worry about passing the infection on to the baby because it was exposed to the virus before the mother had any symptoms, and the baby gets significant protection from immune factors present in the milk. See the chapter "Breastfeeding and Maternal Illness."

What about when the mother needs medication? The mother will almost always be able to continue breastfeeding because drugs get into the milk in only tiny amounts and won't affect her baby. A very few drugs are unsafe when breastfeeding, but there are almost always alternative drugs that can be used. It is extremely uncommon for there to be only one medication for a particular condition. The *Compendium of Pharmaceuticals and Specialties* (CPS) in Canada or *Physicians' Desk Reference* (PDR) in the USA are not good resources because the information comes from the drug manufacturers and suggests *all* drugs are contraindicated for breastfeeding mothers because they are afraid of liability. See the chapter "Breastfeeding While on Medication," for more information and some good resources.

If your health professional's first suggestion is a medication that requires you to stop breastfeeding, be concerned that he or she is not paying enough attention to the importance of breastfeeding. Ask for a medication that is compatible with continued breastfeeding; if the doctor is not aware of any, insist he or she get more information.

He or she is surprised to learn that your six-month-old (or one-year-old, or two-year-old) is still breastfeeding. All too typical is this story of one public health nurse who emphasized that she supported breastfeeding. In response to a call about a non-breastfeeding issue from the mother of a seven-month-old baby, she asked the mother what the baby was eating. "Oh, he's breastfeeding" was the answer. The nurse asked, "Are you giving him formula or straight cow's milk in his bottle?" The mother repeated, "No, he's breastfeeding. No bottles, no solid foods." The nurse paused briefly and said, "Well, you're brave."

The nurse's surprise that a seven-month-old would still be breastfeeding, and her expectation that he would be getting bottles even though the mother had clearly stated that he was breastfed, showed she was supportive of breastfeeding in theory but not in practice. She was suggesting that there was something abnormal or strange about a baby exclusively breastfeeding at this age. In fact, in most of the world, breastfeeding for at least two or three years or longer is common, normal and desirable. Sadly, formula company marketing is changing this. Research by anthropologist Kathy Dettwyler suggests that the natural age of weaning for humans is somewhere between two years and seven years. Breastfeeding for this length of time seems to promote optimum brain development and good development of the baby's teeth and jaw, and to reduce the incidence and severity of many illnesses and allergies; it also results in these children having strong self-esteem and feeling secure, self-confident and independent.

We often see three-year-olds with bottles or pacifiers; they may use them for naps or bedtime. Both are substitutes for the breast, so why are they seen as more acceptable than the real thing? The same professionals who think it is strange to continue breastfeeding after six months usually recommend giving babies formula until they are at least 9 or 12 months old. But formulas are only imitations of breastmilk—modifications of cow's milk (or milk made from soybeans) intended to make them "closer to breastmilk." Why should the imitation be considered acceptable while the real thing is not? In fact, the formula companies are now marketing formulas for children up to three years old!

He or she tells you that there is no value in breastmilk after the baby reaches a certain age—6 months, 12 months, or any other arbitrary age. This is simply not true. Even if breastmilk suddenly turned into white water when the baby reached a certain age, there would still be value in breastfeeding.

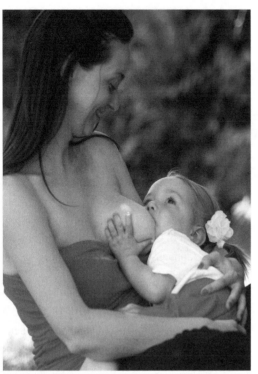

Health Canada and the WHO recommend breastfeeding for children up to two years old and beyond.

CREDIT: **ANDREA POLOKOVA**

It is an intimate relationship between a mother and a child that comforts and soothes the child and would be very important even without the milk.

However, breastmilk, at whatever age and stage the baby has reached, is still milk. It still has the calcium, fats, protein, vitamins and minerals that it always did, and these are all readily absorbed and used by the child's body. It is milk uniquely designed for humans. If there is value in a young child drinking cow's milk (or soy milk or almond milk), which are harder for the child's body to digest and absorb, in spite of the important nutrients they contain, surely there is far more value for that child in having breastmilk and *being breastfed!*

In addition, the concentration of some immune factors in breastmilk actually increases as the child

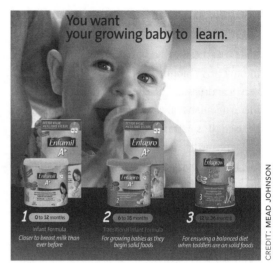

CREDIT: **MEAD JOHNSON**

Formula company advertisements push the notion that formula is necessary for up to a year and even longer—this ad suggests giving formula for up to three years. But even a baby who was never breastfed doesn't need formula for that long.

grows older, providing even more protection against illnesses such as gastroenteritis, respiratory infections, ear infections, etc. This protection is important, because older babies and toddlers are much more likely than newborns to be exposed to a wider range of germs. If your child is in daycare or around large numbers of other children, these protective antibodies and other immune factors will be very important.

He or she tells you that you must never allow your baby to fall asleep at the breast. Why not? It is sometimes convenient if a baby falls asleep without nursing, but one of the great advantages of breastfeeding is that you have a handy way of putting a tired baby to sleep. Nothing calms an overtired or overexcited baby or toddler like breastfeeding. Breastfeeding is designed to put babies to sleep when they are tired. The sweet, warm milk, the suckling, the feeling of warmth and safety in mother's arms—these all create the perfect setting for falling asleep.

What to do if the baby is tired and hungry, and likely to fall asleep at the breast? If the mother doesn't feed him, he may fall asleep on his own but wake up hungry after a short time. If she tries to keep him awake while he nurses, he may get annoyed, fuss at the breast and even bite. The mother may stop feeding before the baby is full, in order to keep him awake. Then, of course, breastfeeding will be blamed because the baby wakes up so often. Feeding becomes tense instead of being relaxed and happy. Sometimes mothers resort to using pacifiers to put the baby to sleep, which may interfere with milk production.

If you are concerned about the baby being reliant on you and on breastfeeding to get to sleep, especially as he gets older, you can certainly add other strategies for calming him and helping him to fall asleep. But never letting your baby fall asleep at the breast is a recipe for breastfeeding problems.

She or he tells you not to stay in the hospital to breastfeed your sick child because it is important that you get your rest. Babies who are ill do not need breastfeeding less than healthy babies, they need it more. Your doctor and your hospital should be making every effort to create an environment where you can rest while staying with and breastfeeding your baby. When your baby is ill, it is not the time to introduce formula to his system. This is the time when he most needs your milk, with its perfect nutrition and active disease-fighting components.

So how do you find good breastfeeding help?

When you are choosing a family doctor or a pediatrician, ask about breastfeeding. What percentage of his patients breastfeed? At three months? At six months? At a year? Two years? In what situations would he recommend weaning from the breast? (If the list is a long one, be careful.) What books or videos about breastfeeding would he recommend? (If they are from formula companies, that's a bad sign.)

If you are planning a hospital birth, look for a hospital that has earned the Baby-Friendly Hospital designation. As of the summer of 2013, there were 26 hospitals or birthing centres and seven public health units in Canada, most in Quebec, that had been designated Baby-Friendly. Unfortunately, you can't always trust the advice you get, even in a Baby-Friendly Hospital. Still, it is a step forward. To become a Baby-Friendly Hospital, the policies and routines must match the steps described in our section on getting off to a good start (plus a few more). If none of the hospitals available to you are officially Baby-Friendly, ask questions to see how close they come to meeting the requirements. Do mothers and babies stay together after birth, or is there a standard "observation period" of the baby in the nursery? If breastfeeding needs to be supplemented, how is that supplement given? What are the reasons? Are more than 10% of healthy term newborns given supplements? If you go on a hospital tour, ask questions and look around. If you see formula company posters or calendars on the wall, that's not good. If you see bottles on the night-table of many new mothers, that tells you a lot.

La Leche League (LLL) groups hold monthly meetings in most parts of North America, and they encourage mothers to begin attending while they are still pregnant. La Leche League is a volunteer organization that has provided mother-to-mother help for women interested in breastfeeding since 1956. Every La Leche League volunteer has breastfed at least one child, but she draws on more than her own personal experience in sharing information and support. She has access to a network of breastfeeding research and knowledge.

At LLL meetings you will meet other mothers, many with new babies and some with older ones. If you haven't been around babies much, here's your chance to watch them latch on, change sides, feed, fall asleep and nurse in different positions. La Leche League can be a good resource if you run into problems; if needed, the leader can put you in touch with someone with more experience. In some communities, other breastfeeding support groups have been initiated by the public health department or have sprung up informally. These can be helpful, but you may need to go elsewhere for help with serious challenges.

Lactation consultants are a relatively new group of health care professionals, having started as a professional group only in the 1980s. Right now, the name "lactation consultant" is not regulated, so anyone can call herself one. In some hospitals, any nurse who helps breastfeeding mothers is called the "LC," even if she has no additional training in breastfeeding. However, to become an International Board Certified Lactation Consultant, the person must have considerable experience working with breastfeeding mothers and babies, and must pass a written examination. So an IBCLC—and there are many in private practice, as well as many working in hospitals, clinics or doctor's offices—*should* be a good source of breastfeeding help.

Breastfeeding clinics vary considerably in their level of knowledge and helpfulness. Some are connected with hospitals or public health units, while others are run independently by physicians or lactation consultants. Clinics often have experienced, knowledgeable and interested staff, and can be a good resource.

However, a significant problem with some clinics is that policies outlining how problems are dealt with are written by committees that often include members with little or no breastfeeding expertise. So lactation consultants are forced by the clinic's policies to push a mother to supplement her baby's feeding based on birth weight, even if the baby is breastfeeding well and the consultant does not agree

with the supplementation. In some clinics lactation consultants are restricted to recommending supplements by bottle, and the use of a lactation aid (a tube that draws milk from a container of expressed breastmilk, preferably, or formula) at the breast is not allowed. Why lactation aids should be disallowed I cannot even imagine.

Good breastfeeding help is sometimes hard to find. Keep looking; keep asking. If you are told that you need to wean your baby, make sure you get other opinions. Talk to other breastfeeding mothers about the doctors, clinics or other resources they find helpful. Don't be discouraged—information about breastfeeding is spreading, and the resources available for new mothers continue to grow in number and improve in quality.

Some signs that your doctor or midwife *is* supportive of breastfeeding

- No formula company marketing materials are on display or used. For example, growth charts do not include a formula company logo.
- Schedules for meetings of support groups such as La Leche League are posted, and lists of phone numbers are readily available.
- There are no brochures or videos about breastfeeding that have been created by formula companies.
- When you ask about breastfeeding, he or she lets you know it is important. He or she refers you to La Leche League, a lactation consultant or books and other materials written by people who are not paid by formula companies.
- There are no "gift packs" with formula samples or coupons.

- Before the birth, you discuss getting breastfeeding off to a good start, starting with skin-to-skin contact as soon as possible and keeping you and the baby together so you can breastfeed according to his cues. The health care provider explains how to ensure the baby is latched on and drinking well and teaches strategies in case there are complications, such as a premature birth or a Caesarean section.
- In the waiting room, you see other mothers breastfeeding. There may be pictures or posters of breastfeeding on the walls.

It is not always easy to find a supportive doctor or midwife, but it is well worth the effort!

3 The Sale and Promotion of Artificial Baby Milk

In North America today, most mothers decide to breastfeed their babies. You are probably part of this group.

But a significant number of women do not breastfeed, and many of those who initiate breastfeeding stop sooner than they had intended to, often within a few days or weeks.

Why? The list of risks of not breastfeeding is long. Why do so many women "choose" formula or stop breastfeeding early? Research tells us that the ways in which infant formula is marketed and our culture's acceptance of bottle-feeding are major factors.

Formula company marketing not only convinces new parents and their families that formula feeding is as good or even *better* than breastfeeding; it also convinces health professionals, who often think they are too smart to be influenced by marketing.

Some people feel that companies have the right to use any methods they like to get people to buy their products, so formula marketing shouldn't be regulated. But there are many restrictions on marketing; consumers need to be protected. By law, for example, false claims about a product are not allowed. Many products cannot be advertised directly to children. Some products are available only by prescription. Many must carry warnings about side effects or risks. Some entirely legal products such as cigarettes cannot be advertised at all in Canada. Clearly, our society has determined that there are many reasons why the marketing of a particular product should be controlled or restricted.

What has this to do with breastfeeding? Why should we care about how formula is marketed? Because research shows that the marketing of formula is a major barrier to mothers' breastfeeding successfully.

Recently, an inaccurate article in a major Canadian newspaper claimed that breastfeeding advocates didn't want formula advertised because they were silly radicals who thought formula was "bad." But that's *not* the issue! Breastfeeding advocates think formula *advertising* is bad. The problem with formula is not the product itself (though there are issues, as we have already discussed), but rather the way it is presented to the public and the methods used to get people to buy it.

Baby deaths in the developing world

People first became aware of the potential for formula marketing to undermine breastfeeding in the 1970s, when photos and films of emaciated and dying babies in developing countries became public. People were shocked and demanded to know the cause.

The cause? Formula was being marketed to mothers who could not afford it, did not have access to clean, safe water, and could not read the instructions about how to prepare the formula. The mothers didn't know that giving formula would cause their milk production to dry up, or that their babies might refuse to breastfeed after getting bottles. Formula was marketed as "modern," or as "nutritional insurance" in case the mother's milk was "inadequate." Even suggesting that a mother's milk might not be "good enough" instils fear for her baby.

In both rich and developing countries, affluent women often didn't breastfeed. Everyone wanted to be like people in rich countries, with fat, happy babies. But the mothers didn't get fat happy babies; they got skinny, sick or dead babies. The cost of one day's worth of formula in many developing countries was higher than the daily income, without counting the cost of fuel to boil water. So mothers diluted the formula to make it stretch. Babies did not have the protection of the disease-fighting components of breastmilk. Formula prepared in this often unsanitary environment transmitted infection. The babies got diarrhea and respiratory illnesses. Many died. Many others were damaged for life.

I've seen it with my own eyes. In the hospital where I worked in Southern Africa there was a "drip room" where, every day, dozens of babies had to be rehydrated with intravenous fluids because of severe infections. Very few of these babies were even partially breastfed.

In 1978, a Nestlé representative told a U.S. Senate hearing that despite the company's aggressive marketing of formula in developing countries, Nestlé wasn't responsible for the illness and deaths which had resulted from this use of formula. People were shocked by the company's audacity and heartlessness.

As a result, various groups of concerned citizens and non-governmental organizations around the world organized a boycott of Nestlé products. It was suspended temporarily when it *seemed* to give in and promised to market formula only according to certain guidelines (summarized below). The boycott resumed in the 1990s when evidence accumulated that Nestlé had continued many of the marketing practices it had agreed to suspend. Ironically, as time passed and more and more

companies behaved just as badly, people became *less* shocked by the marketing tactics of formula companies and few people are still boycotting Nestlé (although both the authors continue to do so). Nestlé sells more formula than any other company in the world, but the issues of ethical marketing of formula are spread across the industry.

The WHO International Code on the Marketing of Breastmilk Substitutes (1981)

Shocked by the tragic deaths of so many babies, non-governmental organizations, the World Health Organization, UNICEF, scientific bodies *and the formula companies themselves* hammered out a code of ethical marketing of infant formula, bottles and teats (artificial nipples) and *any* food or drink that could replace breastmilk in the diet, including baby foods, gruels, teas and juices.

The WHO/UNICEF International Code on the Marketing of Breastmilk Substitutes was adopted by the World Health Assembly in 1981. It is not legally binding although some countries have legislated its provisions. Canada has not legislated them, so the code is optional. The Code bans all marketing of bottle-feeding to the lay public and sets out requirements for labelling and information on infant feeding. Any activity which undermines breastfeeding also violates the aim and spirit of the Code. The Code is intended as a minimum requirement in all countries. The final code was a compromise that included the following provisions:

Baby food companies must not:

- promote their products through hospitals or shops or directly to the general public or in the media, including the Internet. Because the Code covers *every* country in the world, getting around local laws by going "offshore" does not exempt the company from its responsibility to act ethically.

- give free or reduced-price samples of formula to pregnant women, mothers or their families.
- provide free or subsidized supplies to hospitals or maternity wards.
- give gifts to health workers or mothers.
- advertise their products to health workers. Any information must contain only scientific facts.
- promote foods or drinks for babies.
- give misleading information. In fact, they should not provide information on infant feeding at all, that being the responsibility of government.

Furthermore:

- There should be no contact between baby milk company sales personnel and mothers or their families.
- Labels must be in a language understood in the country and must include a clear health warning.
- Baby pictures may not be shown on milk labels.
- Labels must not include language that idealizes the use of the product.

All the techniques below are *contrary* to the International Code.

- In the 1970s, before the creation of the Code, formula companies in developing countries had their employees dress in white coats (like health professionals) and visit maternity hospitals. They would then lecture groups of mothers on the benefits of formula and/or visit individual mothers to convince them that their babies would be healthier if they were given formula in addition to breast milk. (In those

days breastfeeding was almost universal in many developing countries.) Today, nutritionists hired by formula companies give "information lectures" on infant feeding, often by phone, even in Canada.

- In the United States and other countries, some hospitals continue to give new mothers formula company "gift packs"—not really gifts, but advertising. The packs contain formula samples and coupons to buy more formula. Nursing staff often pass on a few bottles of formula to the mother with the whispered "I'm not supposed to do this, but I think you will need it." This suggests to the mother that she won't be able to breastfeed exclusively and gives formula the hospital's "stamp of approval." In Canada, almost all new mothers are sent a package with formula and coupons. How do the formula companies get the mother's name and address? Usually the mother herself or a well-meaning friend filled in a card for "free gifts" in a parenting magazine or at a maternity shop. But it is a violation of the International Code to give pregnant women, new mothers or their families free or low-priced samples of formula *even if* the mother intends to feed her baby formula. That's because the decision about which formula to feed the baby, *when necessary*, should be made through discussion with the baby's doctor, *not* based on samples or coupons or sales. Many physicians provide free formula to pregnant women and new mothers. Perhaps they believe they are doing them a favour. But this is also contrary to the International Code. Perhaps if they gave equal time to breastfeeding information and support it would not be so bad. But do they? Not often, because they say they don't want to make mothers feel guilty for not breastfeeding. So many obstetricians don't even talk about breastfeeding during the prenatal visits, never mind offer support.

- Sometimes ultrasound technicians give out formula packages to pregnant women. Very targeted advertising!
- Magazines rely on advertising, which pays a far higher share of the publication's bills than subscriptions. Formula companies are major advertisers in parenting magazines. No wonder the magazines hesitate to print articles that favour breastfeeding.
- Advertising of formula on television is regular and frequent in the United States, and most Canadians get these U.S. stations.
- The Internet presents new challenges. Every formula company has a website explaining how wonderful its products are. While the Code requires that cans of formula have a statement about the superiority of breastfeeding, these statements go unnoticed on websites. Formula companies use the Internet to introduce new products, such as Nestle's 2011 baby-formula machine that uses capsules to deliver warm, properly dosed servings of milk. The machine, called BabyNes, operates similarly to Nespresso and other single-serving coffee brewers. It's brilliant marketing: not only do you get people to put out big bucks for a single-function machine, but the baby, once grown up, may become nostalgic at the very sight of a Nestlé coffee brewer that reminds him of the machine that once made his formula..
- Formula companies work with search engines to ensure that their "advice sites" have high rankings. A search for "pregnancy" yields "Pregnancy information—learn about your growing baby." Sounds like a valuable resource, until you read the subtitle: "Join the Nestlé Baby Program today." It comes up even before

Wikipedia's article on pregnancy. Search for "breastfeeding and nutrition" and get the "breastfeeding nutrition" site, which turns out to be a page to sign up for the Similac baby club.

The formula companies skilfully influence media to undermine peoples' confidence in breastfeeding. While this may not be advertising as described in the Code, it is more effective because mothers imagine it is unbiased. When reporting studies showing the risks of formula feeding, journalists often feel compelled to add: "Breast is best, but for those who cannot breastfeed, infant formula is very good!" Few journalists know enough to write solid and accurate articles on infant feeding.

The Code requires that only scientific information about formulas be given to health care providers, but what they actually get are pens and writing pads with formula company logos and other items designed to sell the product. They get articles reporting studies—funded by the formula companies—"showing" how good their formulas are. They may even get free trips to exotic places where the conference speakers, paid by or connected to the formula company, praise new formulas.

Not long ago, I started to receive, every month, an information sheet from a group called Integrative Medicine (subtitled *Pediatric Nutrition*). Most of the information was about formula feeding, which is odd, given that breastfeeding is such an important part of pediatric nutrition. The April 11, 2011, issue urges the use of soy formula for bottle-fed babies allergic to cow's milk, even though both the Canadian Paediatric Society and the America Academy of Pediatrics recommend hydrolyzed formulas in this situation instead. The article (unsigned) mentions a particular brand of soy formula. In tiny type on the last page, it says: "*Distribution of this educational publication is made possible through the support of Abbott Nutrition Canada under an agreement that ensures independence."* Abbott, you will not be surprised to learn, makes the formula mentioned in the "educational publication." So how independent is this "educational publication"?

Literature on infant feeding must not be provided not by formula companies, but rather by government. Many mothers who want to breastfeed pick up free pamphlets on breastfeeding at the doctor's office or other locations, not realizing the pamphlets have been produced by formula companies, and that their goal is not to help mothers succeed in breastfeeding but just the opposite. These pamphlets take subtle and not-so-subtle swipes at breastfeeding, emphasizing that it is tiring, painful and difficult, that the father is left out, and that formula is really almost the same as breastmilk.

All donations of money or equipment by formula companies to health care facilities must be done openly, and no special benefits should be granted to the companies because of their donations. Other types of companies donate to hospitals, but they don't as a result have the right to speak to staff about their products. But formula companies usually require, as a condition of the donation, that they put up posters in the maternity ward, arrange special lunchtime seminars or informal talks, and encourage the staff to give out company gift packs and samples. They buy meals for the doctors, ensuring that when the company representative stops a busy pediatrician in the hallway to discuss a new formula, the doctor feels obliged to listen.

Remember, representatives of the formula companies were present at the table and had input into the final form of the Code. In 1981 all the countries

of the world, with the notable exception of the United States, voted to adopt the Code. But that one "nay" from the United States told the formula companies: "You don't have to take this seriously." And, from the very first, the formula companies disregarded the Code. They also undermined it with deliberate misinformation to health care professionals and media such as:

- *The Code was intended for Third World countries only.* Untrue! Both the World Health Organization and UNICEF made it clear from the beginning that the Code was meant for *every country of the world.* Actually, the Code is, in many ways, more necessary in developed countries. Many developing countries still have a breastfeeding culture; industrialized countries do not, and so mothers there are far more susceptible to misinformation. It should be mentioned, though, that breastfeeding is in decline everywhere in the world except for a few Western industrialized societies.
- *The Code is too strong for industrialized countries.* In fact, the Code was intended to define the *minimum* standard, which would be *strengthened,* not weakened, depending on the needs of each particular country.
- *The Code bans the use of formula and is too extreme.* The Code does not ban formula; there are provisions in it to protect babies who must be fed artificial baby milk. The Code requires, for example, that an expiry date be clearly visible on every tin of formula (although outdated formula is still sold in developing countries). The Code also requires that instructions on the use of formula be written in the language of the local population.

Sadly, most of the countries that signed the Code are not enforcing it. Governments have not even bothered to give the companies a little slap on the wrist for sending out formula samples to pregnant women, new mothers or their families. Every day, I get several emails from mothers who regret not breastfeeding or having stopped; often they tell me that the first step to weaning was the formula sample.

The big three formula companies in Canada (Mead Johnson, Ross and Nestlé) have done much of their marketing through the health care system. The companies vie for exclusive contracts with hospitals so that their products will be the only ones used in a particular facility. Studies show that 93% of women use or supplement with the same formula that was used in the hospital in which the baby was born, so companies are eager to pay large sums to become a hospital's exclusive provider. These exclusive contracts often last 5 to 10 years. The company gives cash (often a lot), plus money for equipment, continuing medical education and free formula for the hospital nurseries, maternity wards and pediatric departments. The hospital also receives such things as tape measures (with advertising), growth charts (with advertising) and coffee cups (with advertising), plus myriad other useful little items that show up in every office and staff room.

This system was in place for many years, but in 1989, Nestlé came onto the North American market and upset the apple cart. Nestlé couldn't work through hospitals because they were already contracted to other formula companies, so Nestlé started sending "free" formula to mothers at home. At first, the other formula companies were enraged, but soon they also started to send mothers the formula at home.

This continues today. The mothers who come to our clinic are very motivated to breastfeed exclusively. Some are resistant to giving the baby formula even if *we* say the baby needs supplementation. We ask each mother if she received free formula samples

and from whom. Almost all say yes. Some received samples when leaving the hospital; some say the doctor gave them a sample; almost all received formula in the mail, often before the baby was born.

- This booklet (**see page 34, right**), along with a coupon and a tin of infant formula, came to the home of my daughter-in-law in April 2011, only a couple of days after she gave birth. Thank you, Mead Johnson, but we don't really appreciate your "gift." Sending a package by courier with this glossy 20-page booklet and maintaining the website is clearly profitable. Included in the package are four coupons for discounts when you buy their product. How much did all this cost?

- What are the problems? Five times the booklet refers mothers to the company website and gives the phone number for the company's registered dietitian, saying: "It's like you're talking to a friend who also happens to be a Registered Dietitian." The trouble is, dietitians do not get any more training about breastfeeding than other health professionals. What advice will the dietitian give when the booklet has a whole section on "Your fuss-free guide to supplementing"?

- Breastfeeding is associated with "problems." On the contents page, the photo of the baby at the breast is captioned "Seven Feeding Problems Fixed: Can't-miss tips for relieving fussiness, gas, spit up and colic, plus tried-and-true infant soothers." Most of the "problems" could be fixed by helping the mother with breastfeeding. But the information on page seven, in spite of the photo of the baby at the breast (with the mother holding the back of his head, which is not a good idea) is all about formula-feeding problems. The only solution suggested for fussiness is "to experiment with different nipples until

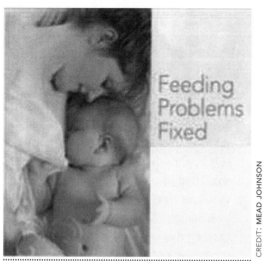

While a picture of breastfeeding is a welcome sight in a formula company brochure, as a model for breastfeeding this one isn't helpful. Any mother who attempted to feed in this position would find herself with a sore neck and limited success—creating the feeding problem this article claims to help solve.

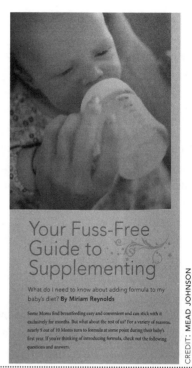

A formula company's guide to supplementing asks, "What do I need to know about adding formula to my baby's diet?" The real answer is that milk supply may decrease and the baby may stop taking the breast.

you find one that baby really latches onto." Tricky for a breastfeeding mother. A full-page ad offers only formula as an answer to gassy babies, suggesting parents "talk to the baby's doctor about ... Enfamil Gentlease A+." Since doctors have little training in breastfeeding, what will they say? (For breastfeeding-friendly solutions to colic, see the chapter "Colic (The 'C' Word).")

- The whole booklet is an ad, with ads within ads. The page opposite the contents says that Enfamil A+ supports "her normal brain and eye development." There is no evidence for this, though the ad is careful not to state that the product makes babies smarter, which is what it used to say. And the company doesn't apologize for 100 years of producing formulas without DHA and ARA and thus *not* supporting "normal brain and eye development."

- Page four emphasizes eating well in order to breastfeed. Many women contact me wondering whether they should breastfeed because their diets are not perfect: "I can't afford to follow the Canada's Food Guide, so maybe it is better to formula feed." Research is clear: even if your diet is not good, even if you eat nothing but fast-food hamburgers, your baby will get protein, carbohydrates and fat, as well as immunity, in the right proportions, just as good as the milk other mothers make. Breastmilk actually breaks the rule of "garbage in, garbage out." With breastmilk, it's "garbage in, the best for your baby out." The page goes on to tell the mother: "But when you are breastfeeding, you're

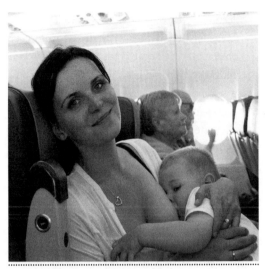

CREDIT: DURKOVICOVA ZUZANA

burning extra energy (calories) to make breast milk—this means you may need an extra two or three Food Guide Servings each day than what is normally recommended." There is no good evidence for this, and the advice may worry mothers who are looking to lose weight after the pregnancy. (I recommend that mothers should eat when hungry, according to their appetite.) The mother is also told "most nutrition experts recommend that breastfeeding women take folic acid." There is no reason for a breastfeeding woman to take folic acid. Telling mothers they need all kinds of supplements only makes breastfeeding seem complicated. But there's more. The mother is also advised to eat a diet rich in DHA and ARA; salmon and rainbow trout are listed as good sources. They apparently forget that not only does breastmilk normally have DHA and ARA, but that *no* formulas contained them until recently—and they were telling us those formulas were just fine. Mothers are told to drink two litres of water or low-fat milk each day. Wait, what about the mother who doesn't or can't drink cow's milk?

She may worry that maybe her milk won't be good enough. And two litres is a lot of water. Another reason not to breastfeed.

- There are only four photos of breastfeeding babies. When you can see the latch, it's not a good one. Usually you cannot see the breastfeeding baby's face well, but, oh, look at the formula-fed baby with his big blue eyes and cute face.
- There is information on breastmilk storage, suggesting that all mothers will need to pump and store milk, but it's inaccurate, stating that you can keep breastmilk on a countertop only six to eight hours. Breastmilk can last a longer time because of its anti-infective properties. They admit that formula is okay for only two hours at room temperature. Of course, then you have to throw it away and buy more.
- The "Fuss-Free Guide to Supplementing" page is subtitled: "What do I need to know about adding formula to my baby's diet?" as if you'll need or want to do this. It goes on: "Supplementing is giving your baby formula in addition to breastmilk, whether you replace feedings with a bottle a few times a week or several times a day." Giving a baby a bottle several times a day often leads to the end of breastfeeding. Also note that supplementing is linked to bottles, although *necessary* supplements can be given in many ways. And the answer to the question "Why do so many Moms supplement?" is "Supplementing gives you certain freedoms: you can hand off the feeding to Dad or Grandma or go back to work without the need to pump. Or if you've tried pumping but it's not working out, you can use formula a few times a day and continue to breastfeed part-time." Notice, you are part of the crowd—"so many Moms"—if you supplement. That's reassuring. But if you use a

bottle a few times a day, you are on the way to weaning the baby from the breast completely, which is, of course, exactly what the formula company wants. The real reason so many mothers supplement is that they get such poor help and advice with regard to breastfeeding. If Dad and Grandma would like to help the mother and baby, there are a million things they can do besides giving a bottle of formula.

- "Formula facts in 60 seconds flat" poses the question: "If I give my baby formula, should I worry that she's missing out on good nutrition?" The answer: "Not at all. Thanks to decades of research and scientific advancements, today's infant formulas are closer to breast milk than ever before and contain the nutrients your baby needs to grow and thrive. If adding a bottle here and there makes you a calmer, happier Mom, that will be good for your baby too." Aaaargh! The message is that giving formula makes Mom calmer and happier. But getting the mother the support, information and help she needs so that breastfeeding goes smoothly is the real solution. Breastfeeding problems are not solved by giving bottles of formula. And decades of research and scientific advancements have not made formula the equivalent of breastmilk (and certainly not the equivalent of breastfeeding, which is so much more than the milk). Yes, they are "closer than ever before"—much like Hamilton, Ontario, is closer to Vançouver than Toronto. Still pretty far!

- "Is your baby getting enough to eat?" The booklet suggests that if you feed with formula, you'll get more rest: "Generally, formula-fed babies eat every 3-4 hours during their first weeks while breastfed babies eat every 2-3 hours." Many mothers must think, "I'm so tired, it would be so nice if the baby went 3 or 4 hours between

feedings." But wait: researchers have found that breastfeeding mothers typically get *more* sleep than mothers who are bottle-feeding. They don't have to get up and prepare bottles; it takes just a second to latch baby on. Some formula-fed babies may go longer between feedings because they are overfed (the baby can't stop feeding as long as the flow of milk from the bottle is fast). This overfeeding has been linked to the current obesity epidemic. Breastfeeding works best when you don't look at the clock and when you accept that frequent feeding can be normal and even desirable. New mothers get more tired trying to stretch the time between feedings or explaining to people, "Yes, he's eating again." Having a quiet baby at the breast every hour is far less tiring than hearing a crying baby who wants to eat now, not in 20 minutes.

- The last ad in the booklet shows the different formulas you can buy. Number one is for zero to 12 months, number two for 6 to 18 months and number three from 12 to 36 months. That's right, formula for three years. There is absolutely *no* need, even for a baby who was never breastfed, to be on formula for a year, let alone three. Once the baby is eating a wide variety of foods, including iron-rich ones, in ample amounts, there is no need for formula at all: plain old homogenized cow's milk (or another kind of milk the family prefers) is fine. After the WHO Code was developed, formula companies invented the "follow-up formulas" or "grow-up formulas" to a year or longer. They said these products didn't contravene the WHO Code because the formulas for after six months did not replace breastmilk. This is rubbish, since breastfeeding is recommended by the WHO for two years and beyond. Some pediatricians have bought into this: in Europe, where they have had formulas to three years for more than 20 years, many recommend them. In Singapore, they have formula to seven years. In Indonesia, they have formula to three years, formula to seven years, formula to 12 years, formula for adolescents, formula for pregnant women, formula for pregnant women who are Muslims, formula for pregnant women with high-risk pregnancies, and formula for people over 50. I used to joke, as each new "follow-up" formula came on the scene, that we could soon be on formula from birth to death. It's no longer a joke. It's true.

In another brochure from a formula company, an ad states that after six months the baby's nutritional needs change, so they have a special formula for babies over six months. The implication is that breastmilk is no longer meeting the baby's nutritional needs because most will wrongly assume that breastmilk at seven months is no different from breastmilk at five months. But breastmilk has been changing from day one in response to the baby's changing needs. It is clear that the WHO Code is being violated.

But what does it matter? Why can't formula companies market their products just as a diaper company markets its products?

Formula is not like diapers. If a mother gets a free diaper sample and decides to use that brand, she's been influenced by the sample. If those diapers give her baby a rash or are too expensive, she can change brands or use cloth diapers. No problem. But if she starts off feeding formula, or starts breastfeeding but follows the advice in the formula ads and gives her baby a couple of bottles a day, that decision may become irreversible. Her baby may refuse to latch or latch poorly, and her milk production will drop. If her baby doesn't do well or she realizes how

expensive formula is and wants to change, it may not be easy.

Some mothers *will* be able to make the switch back to breastfeeding. Some may be able to breastfeed only partially because their milk supplies have decreased. And some won't be able to go back to breastfeeding, even with good help. The mother may find that she has no choice but to continue formula-feeding. And that's what makes marketing formula different from marketing diapers.

Formula companies argue that they are competing with other brands but they are also inevitably competing with breastfeeding. Since the vast majority of new mothers are initiating breastfeeding (95.7% in a 2009 survey in Toronto), *breastfeeding* is the *major* competitor. If the company is not competing with breastfeeding, why spend so much space in their ads and booklets stressing its inconvenience?

North American mothers considering breastfeeding are often very concerned about doing it in public, so formula companies play on this, showing images of mothers having great difficulty breastfeeding "modestly." In one ad, we see a mother who has pulled down her T-shirt to feed the baby so that the neckline is probably pushing her breast upwards and exerting pressure from underneath—not very comfortable, and leaving her very exposed.

The formula companies' solution? Giving a bottle or two a day when you go out. But milk supply can decrease even if the baby is getting only a bottle a day, even if it's breastmilk in the bottle. Here's a quote from an email that came in just as I was writing the previous sentence: "My son is 15 weeks and breastfeeds well every three to four hours. He weighs 12 lbs, is growing like a weed and has many wet diapers. Just recently, pumping breastmilk has been taking much longer than it used to and I'm getting less than I used to. I only pump when I need to take a bottle out with me, and when I do, my son is taking 7-8 ounces (and that takes me hours to pump these days). My question is: can I occasionally substitute formula when I have nothing prepared and need to go out? Also, how do I know how much formula he'll need compared to 8 ounces of breastmilk?"

So each time the mother goes out the baby gets a bottle; up until now, only breastmilk. Her supply may be decreasing since she is having trouble pumping. (See the chapter "Late-Onset Decreased Milk Supply" for information about how to reverse this situation.) And now she is asking about using formula instead. This is why the formula company booklet repeatedly suggests giving bottles.

But why is it that so many women feel they need to have a bottle to feed their babies when they are out in public? Why should they not be able to feel comfortable breastfeeding anywhere, any time? Breasts are visible on posters, billboards and all kinds of advertising.

I am an advocate of "indiscreet" breastfeeding in public, and here's why: the ads currently on billboards would have been unacceptable not long ago. But today they go unnoticed. We're used to them. If more women breastfed in public, eventually people would barely notice. And maybe more public breastfeeding would reassure women that their breasts are normal even though they no longer look as perky as they did at age 15.

Maybe one day everyone will actually see breastfeeding as beautiful. Because it is.

Things wouldn't be as bad if there was also good breastfeeding promotion. But there isn't much, and it's often not great. Years ago, Health Canada produced posters entitled "Who Says You Can't Breastfeed at the Park (or Mall)," but the photos all showed the mothers hiding their breasts. Toronto Public Health produced ads that said, "Babies were born to breastfeed" and showing cartoon babies: no mothers, no babies at the breast. (Their more recent ads, showing a baby skin to skin, are a great improvement.)

The problem is that hardly anyone makes money supporting breastfeeding. I do, but I could make more being a general pediatrician. A few lactation consultants make money, but most would make more selling hot dogs on the street with a lot less effort and aggravation. Some even lose money. Breast pump companies make money. But the potential for big profits isn't there, since pumps tend to be a one-time sale.

The Canadian government gives a risible amount to promote and maintain breastfeeding. Quebec is an exception. It has made breastfeeding a priority since 1999, and it shows what government *can* do. Quebec

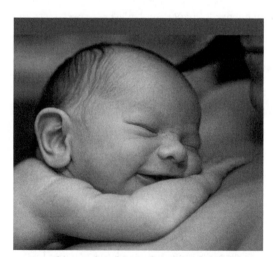

I've been looking forward to this
Skin-to-skin is the healthiest place to begin

When a mother holds her baby skin-to-skin:

Baby
- cries less and is calmer
- breastfeeds better
- stays warmer
- has better blood sugar levels

Mother
- breastfeeds more easily
- learns when baby is getting hungry
- bonds more with baby

416.338.7600   toronto.ca/health | TORONTO Public Health

Toronto Public Health got it right in 2011 with a poster advocating skin-to-skin contact.

went from a breastfeeding initiation rate of only 60% to more than 90% in fewer than 10 years. Of course, the problems have not completely disappeared. But progress has been made: the government has mandated that all maternity hospitals and health units become "Baby-Friendly." (See the section on the Baby-Friendly Hospital Initiative later in this chapter.)

Why "informed choice" is often not informed

Some of the barriers pregnant women face when making "informed choices" about how to feed their babies:

1. Bottle-feeding has become the model of infant feeding. Bottle-feeding has come to be seen as the "normal" way to feed babies and toddlers. In fact, a bottle has become a symbol that means "baby." Public restrooms with change tables in Canadian airports are indicated with a drawing of a baby bottle; congratulations cards for new parents usually show bottles. Buy your little daughter a baby doll, and it will come with a toy feeding bottle. (Yet look at the *huge* controversy that erupted when a breastfeeding doll was marketed: TV and print reports described it as "sexualizing little children.") Books for children usually show babies being fed bottles. Even books about animals show mothers bottle-feeding. In the rare book that shows breastfeeding, bottle-feeding is usually shown too. Even though most women today want to breastfeed, we live in a bottle-feeding culture that negatively influences how we understand breastfeeding.

Thus mothers often breastfeed as though they were bottle-feeding. They schedule feedings (an approach that developed when most babies were bottle-fed). Even those who say they are feeding "on demand" often assume the baby "can't be hungry already" because it's been less than three or four hours since the last feeding. Mothers imagine their breasts are like bottles and think they have to wait for them to "fill up" before feeding the baby.

2. Breastfeeding is acknowledged as "better," but formula is considered "really just as good." Today almost everyone says "breastfeeding is better," but acts as if formula is just as good. Whenever there is an article about breastfeeding on the Internet, or in a magazine, newspaper or public blog, there are always angry, resentful comments from readers saying that they hated breastfeeding, that they were "forced to breastfeed" or made to feel guilty about not breastfeeding, and that their children are just fine. I find this puzzling. Nobody has ever been *forced* to breastfeed. Women who do not want to breastfeed may resent hearing about the risks of formula, but surely it's important to be informed before making big decisions? Giving information is not the same as forcing someone to do something.

On the other hand, some women who wanted to breastfeed have actually been *forced* to formula-feed by doctors who threatened to call the Children's Aid Society if they didn't. Often the only reason for this perceived need for formula is that the doctor doesn't know how to solve breastfeeding problems.

It is a widespread belief that formula feeding and breastfeeding are so close that it doesn't matter which a mother chooses. This is untrue, and it is unfair to mothers and babies to pretend otherwise.

3. The art of breastfeeding has been lost. Today a new mother may have no close relatives or friends who have breastfed their babies. Once young girls saw breastfeeding all the time; when they had their babies, they knew intrinsically what to do. If they had problems, they had plenty of experienced friends and relatives to ask for suggestions. Today, mother-to-mother support groups such as La Leche League exist to share the knowledge handed down from generation to generation of women. Sadly, too many women struggle with false, even bizarre, notions of how breastfeeding works, and have no idea where to get help and support.

4. Health professionals share society's attitudes. Here is a recent post to a listserve by one pediatrician about another.

> *I had a conversation with a recently retired (well-respected) pediatrician today who said when he was in Zambia recently doing volunteer work, he saw for the first time the mustard-yellow "loose" stool that is normal in bf babies. He thought at first all of the kids had "diarrhea"...ha, ha. I tried to laugh along with him. But it is so sad to think a man worked with babies all of his pediatric career and not only had he never seen a normal breastfed stool, he didn't even know one when he* did *see it.*

And here is an email from a pediatric resident who finished her training in 2005 and asked me some questions about breastfeeding her own baby. They were so basic that I asked her what she'd learned in her training. Her reply: "Teaching of breastfeeding at a 'world class' 'name withheld' university for medicine and a 'world class' 'name withheld' pediatric hospital? Exactly what teaching are you referring to? I do not recall a single lecture or problem-based learning case or anything."

Doctors not only share society's misinformation about breastfeeding, they are expected to deal with mothers with breastfeeding problems despite having no training or practical knowledge.

Today the majority of medical students are women, but a female doctor is not necessarily more knowledgeable or supportive of breastfeeding. In fact, some of the most vehement anti-breastfeeding physicians are women. Perhaps some are dealing with their own baggage of past breastfeeding issues.

Most physicians, male or female, do understand the importance of breastfeeding—but without the skills to help, this is not enough.

5. Government agencies do not understand the importance of breastfeeding. Instead of protecting mothers and babies, governments protect the formula companies. They invoke rules about not interfering with free enterprise but do not apply their own rules about making false health claims (although sometimes another formula company will take its competitor to court over false health claims). Though Canada signed the WHO International Code on the Marketing of Breastmilk Substitutes, complaints of violations have been answered by form letters with platitudes about how they support breastfeeding and nothing else.

The enormous savings in money that breastfeeding would offer government health budgets is not considered important. Politicians are rarely interested in long-term planning and savings, especially if another government might get the credit down the road.

One example: a group of us met with a deputy minister of health from Ontario a few years ago to try to convince government to do more to support breastfeeding. Instead of talking about how breastfeeding protects the health of children, we tried a different approach by showing how breastfeeding decreases the risk of overweight and obesity in children and adults, the risk of type 2 diabetes, and the risk of cancers, including breast cancer. The deputy minister interrupted to say that increasing life expectancy does not save money because the longer people live, the more money they cost the system.

6. Media are usually on the side of business. Business pays for advertising, which keeps media profitable, and this inevitably influences how articles are written and slanted.

Writers sometimes gleefully describe the difficulties mothers experience with breastfeeding or a study that "proves" breastfeeding does not make babies smarter. Journalists are also looking for the controversial. Since the "breastfeeding is best" message seems to be accepted, they are eager to pounce on anything that contradicts it in order to attract attention. More information about the importance of breastfeeding? Well, that's boring; we already knew that.

7. The unethical practices of formula company advertising and marketing, which I've already discussed.

8. Everyone agrees! Everyone agrees that we should not make mothers feel guilty for not breastfeeding. I agree, too. And I believe that mothers should make an informed decision. Do they? How many women would "choose" not to breastfeed if they knew breastfeeding would decrease their risk of breast cancer? Does the woman's obstetrician share this information? Many obstetricians won't even discuss breastfeeding with pregnant women for fear of making them feel guilty if they "decide" not to or if they fail in their efforts.

The Baby-Friendly Hospital Initiative (1989)

To address the problem of lack of knowledge among health professionals and the problem of undermining policies in hospital, in 1989 UNICEF launched the Baby-Friendly Hospital Initiative. The idea was to make the immediate period after birth conducive to successful breastfeeding. To qualify, a hospital has to complete 10 steps, none of which is especially demanding, *if* the will is there to make the changes necessary.

Sadly, the routines in many hospitals that are barriers to breastfeeding are still in place, and some are worse than ever. For example, one hospital hired a new chief of pediatrics who insisted that all babies have a blood sugar test at birth. Most results were erroneously considered "too low" (see the section on hypoglycemia), so the babies were given formula. Inertia keeps other undermining routines, created at a time when most mothers bottle-fed, from being changed to support breastfeeding. And it's so easy to "fix problems," such as the baby's crying, simply by giving formula instead of helping the mother breastfeed (or preventing the problems in the first place).

Here are the 10 steps the hospital must complete, with comments.

1. It must have a breastfeeding policy that is consistent, covers the 10 points and is communicated to all staff. Sadly, many hospitals that have policies for the most trivial procedures do not consider breastfeeding important enough to warrant a policy. This often leads to the mother getting different information, much of it wrong, from each nurse, doctor or dietitian she speaks to.

2. All staff members who have dealings with pregnant women, new mothers or their families must be trained to put into practice the breastfeeding policy. No point in having a policy if the staff members don't know how to apply it! The problem is that many courses cover only theoretical issues and not practical approaches to preventing and dealing with problems. This may be the most difficult of all the steps because it costs money to train staff, and UNICEF requires 20 hours of courses, three of which must be hands on. Merely scheduling the courses can be a nightmare, given the different shifts that health professionals, particularly nurses, typically work. As a rule, physicians don't attend courses on breastfeeding because many don't think there's anything to learn: isn't it just apply Part A to Part B? They don't know what they don't know. Some staff members secretly (or not-so-secretly) wish all mothers would bottle-feed. Then there's no fuss, no bother, no worries about the baby getting enough. Others are reluctant to admit or accept that the information they have been giving out for so many years is not accurate, helpful or evidence-based. That's why, in the spring of 2011, when I gave lectures and did rounds in eight different hospitals in Slovakia, I was pleasantly surprised—taken aback, even—when a chief of obstetrics thanked me and said he was ashamed that for 30 years he had been giving out incorrect information and he would change his advice.

3. Staff must inform all pregnant women of the advantages of breastfeeding and teach them the basics of breastfeeding management. Good information allows women to make an informed choice. Obviously, no formula company literature should be given out in any hospital prenatal courses and no free samples of infant formula, bottles or nipples should be given to pregnant women or new mothers.

4. Staff must place babies in skin-to-skin contact with the mother immediately following birth for at least an hour and encourage mothers to recognize when their babies are ready to breastfeed, offering help if needed. The baby may not latch on without help and breastfeeding may not always happen, but skin-to-skin contact stabilizes the baby's body temperature, breathing, heart rate, blood pressure and metabolic processes, including blood sugar. (This is covered in more detail in the chapter "The First Few Days.") Skin-to-skin contact for at least an hour (preferably longer) will prevent many breastfeeding problems. In some hospitals, early skin-to-skin contact is initiated, but

maintained only for a few minutes instead of the hour or more that is needed. Obviously, if either the mother or the baby is too sick, their health takes precedence, but too often mothers and babies are separated "as a precaution." This is poor practice! Often mothers and babies are separated because the mother has had an episiotomy. This is wrong too! Often mothers and babies are separated because the baby has a low Apgar score. This is wrong unless the baby is not recovering quickly (fortunately, most do improve rapidly). Often, mothers and babies are separated because the baby passed meconium before the birth. If the baby is not sick, there is no reason to separate him from the mother. Dr. Nils Bergman's research shows that babies (even very premature ones) will stabilize and recover *more* quickly if kept skin to skin with their mothers.

5. Staff must help the mother initiate lactation and teach her how to maintain her milk supply if she and her baby must be separated. If separation is truly necessary, the mother should be helped to express milk, not only to establish milk production but so that the baby can have her milk, which is best except in *very rare* situations. A baby who is ill needs his mother's milk more than ever. Prematurity or illness were once considered reasons to separate mothers and babies, but research has shown that the safest, most effective approach is Kangaroo Mother Care, where mothers and their premature babies are skin to skin for much of the day. This helps to stabilize the baby, decrease breathing and cardiac problems and facilitate breastfeeding. (See the chapter "The Preterm and Near-term Baby.")

6. Staff must not give supplements of any kind to breastfed babies except when there is a legitimate medical reason. I added "legitimate" because this is an easy step to get around; many medical and nursing staff don't have the training to detect and solve problems, and the baby ends up needing supplementation.

7. Staff must allow the mother and baby to room in together. Rooming in means 24 hours a day. Taking the baby away at night so the mother can sleep will decrease milk production, creating breastfeeding problems that she may struggle to resolve for weeks to come. Keeping the mother and baby together allows the mother to learn the baby's cues, and getting breastfeeding going well decreases the risk of engorgement and developing milk supply problems. A Swedish study looked at the reasons babies were taken to the nursery in the night. The researchers found that it wasn't because the mothers wanted it; it was because they perceived that the nursing staff wanted the baby in the nursery. The mothers who did keep their babies with them were happier than those whose babies were taken to the nursery.

8. Staff must encourage breastfeeding as the baby needs it. Babies should be fed when they need to be fed, not according to a schedule. Mothers should not make babies wait for three or four hours to feed them, but it also does not make sense to say that the baby *must* feed every three hours. I disagree with the UNICEF guidelines regarding what to do if babies sleep more than three hours. UNICEF says the right answer is to wake the baby up. This misses the point. The point is to make sure the baby feeds well: get the best latch possible, observe for drinking rather than just sucking (see the videos at http://youtube.com/user/IBCToronto) and if necessary use compression to keep the baby drinking, switching sides when the baby is no longer drinking even with compression. If the baby feeds well and is in close contact with the mother, preferably skin to skin, he will let her know when he is ready to feed again. Keeping the mother and baby together is important. The baby who wakes up in the nursery may be trying to signal that he's hungry, but the busy staff may miss his cues. Some babies will cry at that point, but some will give up and go back to sleep. If the baby is feeding poorly, there is little value in waking him up to have him feed poorly eight times a day instead of five. The point is to get the baby feeding *well*.

9. The staff must give no artificial nipples to breastfeeding babies. Artificial nipples interfere with breastfeeding. If supplements (preferably the mother's own expressed milk, or, as a second choice, banked breastmilk) are needed, they are best given by lactation aid at the breast. If the baby is not taking the breast, a spoon, open cup or finger feeding can be used instead of a bottle. Finger feeding is best used to prepare a baby who is having difficulty latching on, not really as a feeding method (see the chapter "When the Baby Does Not Yet Take the Breast"). The bottle is not a good choice. Furthermore, if the baby is breastfeeding well, there is no need for pacifiers; having the baby satisfy his sucking needs at the breast helps to establish a good milk supply. If the baby is not satisfied at the breast, the mother needs help to make the breastfeeding work better; the baby does not need a pacifier. And if the baby is breastfeeding poorly, pacifiers often make the problem worse.

10. The hospital must encourage the establishment of support groups outside and ensure that new mothers are referred to them on discharge. Today's new grandmothers may have breastfed, but often not for very long or only with a lot of supplementation. La Leche League has filled this gap somewhat but does not reach all mothers. Doulas, midwives and public health can provide good support, but it's not on-going. It is sad that often the least qualified to provide this support and follow-up are physicians (though, of course, there are exceptions). It is sad that hospital staff do not always make a point of telling mothers about La Leche League (or other supports in the community). A brochure on mother-to-mother support is easily lost when it's merely inserted in a package along with dozens of other brochures, ads, coupons, doctors' appointments, and information about registering the baby's birth and name.

All this information and help should be the norm every new mother should expect from the hospital where she gives birth. Nothing radical here, except that very few hospitals manage it.

In 1999, 10 years after the Baby-Friendly Hospital Initiative began, Canada got its first Baby-Friendly Hospital. In Sweden, on the other hand, every hospital in the country with a maternity ward was designated Baby-Friendly within the first few years of the launch of the initiative. The breastfeeding initiation rate in Sweden is reported to be 99%. In North America, staff training issues present a huge stumbling block. But training is crucial to implementing the 10 steps and crucial in all areas of the hospital, not just postpartum. Even more important than staff training is attitude. If a physician doesn't believe that helping mothers breastfeed is an important part of his job, he won't bother—no matter how many hours of training he is compelled to attend. If the hospital administration cannot understand why it should reject free formula, or if the staff and pediatricians believe formula feeding is less mess and bother, nothing will change.

Why shouldn't hospitals accept free formula, especially with all the funding cuts? What's the big deal? I'd ask: How much is integrity worth? The answer will determine whether you feel breastfeeding is truly important to child and maternal health.

Research tells us that if a hospital accepts free formula, fewer babies are breastfed exclusively and fewer babies leave hospital breastfeeding. Why does this happen? When the maternity ward has lots of free formula on hand, it becomes the quick and easy solution to any problem. *The mother is tired so we'll give the baby a bottle to let her sleep. The baby isn't latching on well, so we'll supplement with a little formula.* (If the baby is not latching on well, getting a bottle won't make him latch on better.) The message the mother gets is: if you have a problem, any problem, formula is the answer. When she leaves the hospital, she gets another sample of formula, and, surprise, another sample arrives in the mail when she gets home. So on a day when she's tired or the baby is fussier than usual, it's easy to open that can of formula. That's what the hospital nurses did. And before she knows it, the baby is weaned.

Theresa recently had a call from a mother who had weaned her first baby early but was determined to breastfeed her second, now three weeks old. She said: "I'm having the same problem I had with my first. I don't seem to have enough milk in the evening—he wants to nurse on and off all evening long. Last time we ended up giving the baby formula in the evening, and that was the beginning of the end." Yes, it was the can of formula she got from the hospital that she started to supplement with last time. I reassured her that her baby's frequent nursing in the evening was common and normal and reminded her that the only way to increase her milk production is to nurse more frequently. Giving the baby formula instead will cause decreased milk production, the exact opposite of her goal. (She's still happily breast-feeding and wishes she'd understood this the first time around.)

Read any breastfeeding information or booklets you get critically. Be aware when you look around your doctor's office for subtle and not-so-subtle formula ads. Ask if your local hospital is Baby-Friendly, and if it's not, urge iy to start the process. Write to your MP and MPP about enforcing the WHO Code and making breastfeeding a priority. In the long run the only thing that will prompt change is pressure from parents.

PART II:

An Ounce of Prevention

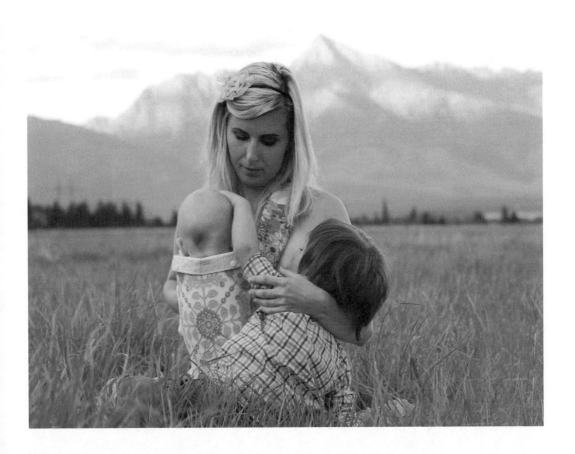

4 | How Birth Affects Breastfeeding

If you are pregnant and planning to breastfeed, you should know that what happens during labour and the birth of your baby can affect breastfeeding. You are not likely to hear this information from many other sources, but it is solidly researched.

To summarize: a natural birth without interventions helps enormously in getting breastfeeding established, and many common interventions make breastfeeding more difficult. An undisturbed birth, in which a birth attendant is present but the mother is allowed to go through her labour as her body dictates, is even better. Of course, there are times when interventions during labour and birth can prevent complications for the baby and/or the mother. Interventions can also relieve the pain of labour. But we should always keep in mind that some interventions affect breastfeeding. Pregnant women and women in labour should be able to make an informed decision about whether or not to have an epidural, for example. Interventions such as epidural or spinal anaesthesia or "elective" Caesarean section are too often presented as risk-free—relieving pain with no down side. The effects on breastfeeding, however, can be very significant.

Choosing an unmedicated birth isn't about being a martyr. Most women who choose this route find it a positive and powerful experience.

What you should know about labour, birth and breastfeeding

Interventions during birth can affect the initiation and duration of breastfeeding. If you have an abundant milk supply, as many mothers do, you can usually overcome any problems, especially if you get skilled help. Unfortunately, some mothers aren't able to get the help they need.

A quotation from Margaret Atwood's 1972 novel *Surfacing*: ". . .they want you to believe it's their power, not yours. . . They stick needles into you so you won't hear anything, you might as well be a dead pig, your legs are up in metal frames, they bend over you, technicians, mechanics, butchers, students, clumsy or sniggering practicing on your body, they take your baby out with a fork like a pickle out of a jar."

Yes, that quote is from 40 years ago, but how much has changed? Why do so many births today seem to require interventions—induction of labour, intravenous fluids, epidurals, forceps, or even a Caesarean section? The answer may be in the way we treat labouring women.

Consider this quotation from Diane Wiessinger, lactation consultant: "We have ample literature on birth in both domestic animals and zoo animals. The resounding message for helpers in all the literature is: *If possible, stay out of the way.*

"Mammalian mothers choose their own birthplace, usually somewhere secluded and quiet. They experience all the sensations of labour. They feel the delivery. They smell the birth. They smell themselves on their babies. They clean up from the birth themselves and never lose track of where their babies are. The babies follow a pre-programmed behaviour that leads them from vaginal outlet to nipple.

"When any of these links is disrupted, there is a

high likelihood that the mother will reject the baby or that the baby will be too confused to complete his role.

"The lesson that shouted out to me from all the literature I read—a lesson that took me 30 years to figure out—is that there's very little information on mammalian infant feeding. *It's all about the birth.*

"Following a normal birth, infant feeding just happens.

"Following an interventionist birth, the mother rejects the baby and there is no nursing at all.

"Our hospital births break every rule in the mammalian list of mother-baby necessities."

What does Diane mean by "Following a normal birth, infant feeding just happens"? She means that there's nothing written in the scientific literature of animal behaviour about feeding, because when the birth occurs normally and undisturbed, the baby feeds just fine.

Humans are not quite like other mammals. We have a big brain that can help us overcome many of the negative associations connected with what Wiessinger calls an "interventionist birth." The vast majority of new mothers with interventions at birth do not reject the baby. (Research by James Swain has shown that the brains of mothers who give birth by C-section are less responsive to the baby's cries than the brains of mothers who give birth vaginally. But after a few months, the brain responses of both mothers are the same.) And most babies do eventually take the breast, even if they need help.

All medical interventions, even when necessary, decrease the mother's sense of control and increase her sense of her body "not being up to the task." The message is subtle but definite. And if your body cannot birth, can you expect it to be able to nourish your baby?

After a "medicalized" birth, some mothers do not want their babies near them right away. Some mothers are at this point easily convinced that

breastfeeding is not important even if they had previously wanted to breastfeed. Some mothers say they did not at first believe that the baby was their own—there was a disconnect between having given birth and this baby who was handed to them. Are we really that different from other mammals?

And some babies, after being exposed to medications or other interventions during the birth, are not able to crawl up to the breast and latch on without help (see the chapter "The First Few Days" on breast crawl, self-attachment and skin-to-skin contact).

Sometimes a baby exposed to medication will take the nipple into his mouth but doesn't seem to know what to do. He doesn't suckle.

Many of the things done routinely in hospital births have the potential to affect breastfeeding. For example, routine electronic fetal monitoring prevents the mother from walking around (which has been shown to speed up labour and reduce the need for further interventions) or moving into more comfortable positions (which has been shown to help the baby move into a better position as well as reduce the need for pain-killing medication). We will not go into detail about episiotomies, but it can be hard for a mother to feed her baby comfortably due to pain from the incision. But we will cover in detail epidurals (which, for convenience, will also cover spinals), IV fluids and Caesarean sections, and how they affect breastfeeding.

First, epidurals. Can they really affect breastfeeding? After all, the epidural is over (or almost) by the time breastfeeding starts. Yes, epidurals can affect breastfeeding, and here's why:

1. When a labouring woman has an epidural, she also gets IV fluids, because a drop in blood pressure is a common side effect of the epidural medications. The IV fluids are intended to *prevent* the blood pressure dropping. Some women receive several litres of fluid by the time the baby is born, and this fluid also gets into the baby's body. Because of this extra fluid, the baby is born "heavier" than his true weight. The baby then starts to pee out this extra fluid and loses weight quickly. Why does this matter? Because many hospitals have a policy that if a baby loses more than 10% of his birth weight, he is given supplements, even though he may actually be doing just fine with breastfeeding.

Getting an accurate weight is trickier than most people think. In most hospitals, a baby's birth weight is measured on a scale in the delivery area. Mother and baby then move to postpartum, where another scale is used. We know that scales often vary. I have seen the same baby weighed on two different scales, minutes apart, with a 400 g difference in weight. That much of an error is unusual, but a difference of 80 g is not rare. For a baby weighing 3.2 kg (7 lb) at birth, this difference, which I have documented myself, is important if we are hung up on the percentage of weight loss, since 80 g represents 2.5% of the baby's birth weight.

Even if that weight loss were real, and a sign that the baby was not feeding well, what should we do about it? Unfortunately, often the immediate *and only* response is to give the baby formula. What *should* happen is that every possible step should be taken to improve the breastfeeding. And many babies will feed better and get more milk this way.

But helping with breastfeeding isn't usually part of the "protocol." So the baby is given formula, and what happens? The mother's confidence in breastfeeding is undermined. She gets the impression that her milk "isn't enough," that her baby was in grave danger because he was dehydrated, when, in fact, he received so much fluid he was actually *overhydrated*. If the formula is given by bottle (as it usually is) now the baby is used to getting a reward from a bottle nipple. This often means he won't latch on to the breast

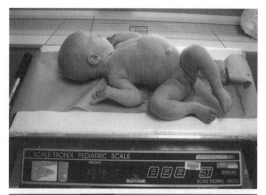
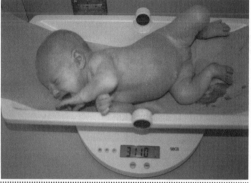

Always consider the source: two scales can produce drastically different results. On the scale in the top photo, which was shown to be accurate, the baby weighs 3.51 kg (7 lb, 12oz.). But on the scale in the bottom photo, the same baby weighs just 3.11 kg (6 lb, 13oz.), only minutes later.

well or at all. If there is a strong medical indication for giving formula, it should be given with a lactation aid at the breast, not in a bottle, a cup or a syringe or by any other method that supplements the baby off the breast. Babies learn to breastfeed by breastfeeding and when they are supplemented with a lactation aid at the breast, they are still breastfeeding.

But there's another side to epidurals. The mother also swells up from the IV fluids. Her ankles and fingers may be swollen, and her breasts may be congested with fluid as well. The accumulation of fluid is made worse if the woman has received oxytocin (Pitocin) during labour and birth. Oxytocin is very similar to the anti-diuretic hormone ADH, which causes retention of fluid by preventing the kidneys from secreting excess fluid. The swelling tends not be obvious right away, but by day two or three, with increasing milk production, breasts may be painfully swollen with fluid as well as milk, and nipples may look flat because of the swelling of the breast. It can be very hard for a new baby just learning to breastfeed to latch on to engorged and fluid-filled breasts. The mother may be told she has flat nipples and needs a nipple shield or she may just give up.

2. Epidurals often cause mothers to develop fever during labour and birth. We don't know exactly why this happens, but it is likely because the drugs in the epidural interfere with temperature regulation. So what happens when a woman in labour develops fever? A seemingly unstoppable cascade of events.

- It's difficult to figure out quickly if the fever is caused by the epidural or by a serious infection, so the mother is started on antibiotics. The mother's fever may cause the baby's heart rate to speed up, and this may suggest to the doctors/ midwives that the baby is in distress. While other steps can be taken, the goal is generally to get the baby out quickly and often the result is a Caesarean section.
- Once the baby is out, many hospital policies require that mother and baby be separated if either has a fever, since it may indicate an infection. This is so wrong! The baby is taken to the special care nursery for tests and possibly antibiotics, and he's likely to be fed formula by bottle. So breastfeeding is delayed, artificial nipples are started and the mother may not get help expressing her milk to get lactation going

and to give colostrum to the baby. Furthermore, if the mother truly has an infection, the best way to decrease the risk of the baby getting sick is by breastfeeding.
- The fact that the baby and the mother are on antibiotics results frequently in *Candida* infections (often called a thrush or a yeast infection, although thrush technically refers to the white patches in the baby's mouth). Nipple pain from *Candida* is a common reason why mothers stop breastfeeding.
- When the labouring woman gets an epidural, the baby is more likely to be born with his face toward the front of her body (called *occiput posterior* in the medical lingo), rather than toward the back (called *occiput anterior*), as is usual. When this was first noticed, some suggested that what was really happening was that mothers who had "posterior" babies experienced more painful labour and so were more likely to ask for epidurals. But further research showed the position of the babies when the mothers arrived at the hospital and again at the time of birth. No difference was found in the number of posterior babies *before* the epidurals were given. But at the time of the birth, many more of the mothers who had had epidurals had babies in posterior or other difficult positions. The problem? More than 75% of babies in posterior position are born by Caesarean section; the rest are more likely to be born using forceps or a vacuum extractor. The "posterior" baby is more likely to have a lower Apgar score, which may mean he will be separated from his mother, and the mother is at higher risk of an episiotomy or tear, making it harder to get comfortable for breastfeeding.
- Although mothers are rarely told this, there is no question that some of the medication used

in epidurals *does* get to the baby. One study measured the levels of epidural medication in newborns' umbilical cords after birth; the longer the mother had had the epidural in place, the higher the level of medication in the cord (and therefore the baby). A study looking at the effects of epidural using Fentanyl (a narcotic) on the baby showed definite negative effects on his ability to breastfeed, especially at higher doses. Those women who had the higher doses were much more likely to have stopped breastfeeding by six weeks after birth, even though all the mothers in the study had successfully breastfed a previous baby for at least six weeks. Studies that evaluated the way the baby breastfed have found that, after being exposed to the epidural medications during the labour, the baby was less able to latch on well and suckle effectively. Some studies have seen subtle effects of epidurals that lasted up to a month.

Effects of Caesarean sections

The mother who has a Caesarean section gets many of the interventions listed above: anaesthesia (usually an epidural), IV fluids and antibiotics. She has an incision that can make it difficult to get comfortable for breastfeeding. Furthermore, in far too many hospitals there is still an automatic separation of baby and mother after C-section, even though this is hardly ever necessary. Some women may be told that they can't breastfeed because of the medications they've been given. This is not true. The mother can and *should* breastfeed. (See the chapter "Breastfeeding While on Medication.")

It is said that it takes longer for a woman's milk to "come in" (increase in volume) if she has had a Caesarean section, but it may simply be that the separation and other interventions are what actually cause the delay.

How can you plan for a labour and birth experience that will make breastfeeding easier?

1. Arrange to have support people with you during labour. Studies dating back to the 1990s have shown that mothers who get good support from a birth attendant (often called a "doula") have much easier births; in fact, with *good* support, labour and birth may be enjoyable, not painful. You'll need fewer interventions and less medication, and studies show breastfeeding generally goes better. Can your partner provide this support? Perhaps, but it can be difficult if this is his or her first time at a birth. Having an experienced, knowledgeable doula at the birth may also make the experience more positive for your partner.

2. Consider home birth. Delivering the baby at home with a midwife can help you feel more relaxed and have fewer interventions. You avoid being exposed to hospital bacteria as well. For low-risk women, home birth is a safe alternative that enables a good start with breastfeeding.

3. Walk during labour as much as you can *if you feel like it*; if you decide to sit or lie down, take whatever position is most comfortable. Midwives speak frequently of mothers wanting to walk around or labour in positions that are considered bizarre by hospital staff. If a mother wants to labour for a while—or for the entire time—on her hands and knees, maybe her body knows best!

4. Eat and drink if you feel like it. This was once forbidden in case the mother needed a general anaesthetic. Nowadays, most Caesarean sections are done with spinal or epidural anaesthesia, but the restriction on eating or drinking continues in many hospitals. However, many mothers do not want to eat or drink during labour. Listen to what your body is telling you.

5. It's best to find the position that feels right to push the baby out. Many women squat. Some go on their hands and knees. I learned about the "Irish kneel" when my second grandson was born in April 2011. A woman in an "Irish kneel" position has one knee on the floor and the other knee bent with that foot on the floor. Lying on your back with your knees up in stirrups is associated with a longer pushing stage, more assisted deliveries (forceps or vacuum), more episiotomies, more second-degree tears to the perineum, more severe pain and more abnormal fetal heartbeat patterns.

6. The immediate hour or two after the birth should be considered part of the birthing process. At this time, unless there are serious health concerns, you and your baby should stay together, skin to skin. Have, at most, a diaper on the baby. Find a comfortable reclining position with pillows supporting you, and let the baby lie tummy-down on your chest, skin to skin. Your baby may crawl to the breast, pushing with his feet, latch on and start to suckle. Interestingly, many babies allowed to find the breast on their own will hold and squeeze the other nipple and areola with their hand, probably stimulating a milk ejection reflex. The fewer the interventions, the more likely this is to happen. Even if you had a completely natural birth without intervention, the baby may not do this on his own, but what a wonderful beginning to the breastfeeding relationship if he does! No need to put the baby in an incubator or under a heat lamp.

7. What begins immediately after birth continues in the hours and days after the baby is born. There is no reason, in the vast majority of

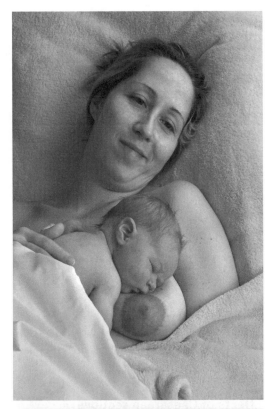

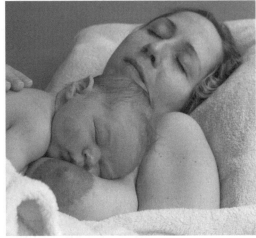

Ideally, skin-to-skin contact begins immediately after birth (top) and then continues for at least an hour or two (bottom). With the correct support and observation, a mother and her baby may rest together and the baby need not go to the nursery.

CREDIT: ANDREA POLOKOVA

cases, for mothers and babies to be separated after birth; skin-to-skin contact can and should continue. Dressing babies up in several layers does not keep them warmer than being skin to skin with the mother: research shows babies who are skin to skin have better temperature control and do not get either cold or overheated. They also breathe in a more relaxed manner and their heart rates are more regular. Furthermore, their blood sugar is more likely to be normal.

In some ways, we are not like other animals. Even the mother who feels detached from her baby won't usually abandon it. Note, however, that when babies were put skin to skin in one Russian hospital, the rate of abandonment declined very significantly.

This was also seen when Kangaroo Care was begun in Colombia. The baby who gets off to a slow start with breastfeeding will, in most cases, figure it out eventually, especially if there are some skilled breastfeeding helpers around to encourage and advise the mother. However, not all difficulties can be overcome, especially if they have been compounded by giving the baby formula supplements early on.

In Canada, more than 87% of women (it varies from region to region) decide they want to breastfeed their babies and start out doing so. Within weeks, though, that number drops dramatically. Why? Often, it is at least partly because the interventions that happened during birth prevented breastfeeding from getting off to a good start.

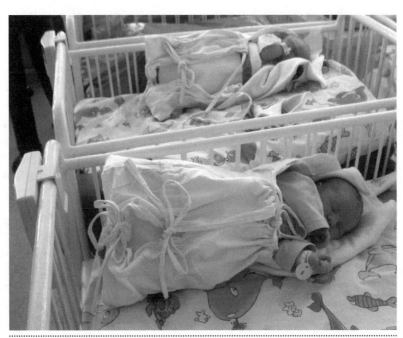

These newborns are overdressed and possibly overheated. Overheating increases the risk of SIDS, as does the side-lying position. Being skin-to-skin with their mothers would safely regulate their temperatures.

5 | The First Few Days

Myth #1: There is not enough milk to meet your baby's needs in the first few days.

Fact: There *is* enough milk. The problem is that often babies are not getting the milk that is available. Mothers are frequently told the baby is latching on well when he is not. Mothers are frequently told the baby is drinking from the breast when he is not.

The other problem is that many don't understand how breastfeeding works. During the early days, the baby is designed to feed frequently, receiving relatively small amounts of colostrum at each feeding. (Relatively small, but enough!) These frequent feedings signal the breasts to produce more milk. However, too often a mother is told that her baby is obviously "starving" and needs to be supplemented with formula, at least until her milk comes in. That supplementation means the baby will nurse less at the breast, and those important "make more milk" signals will not be received.

We live in a culture that has come to see bottle-feeding as the model of infant feeding. So if a formula-feeding one-day-old baby takes 15 ml (½ oz.) of formula, we expect the breastfed baby to take the same amount from the breast. If the breastfed baby gets less, many think he is not getting enough. But since breastfeeding is really the normal way, we are in fact, overfeeding the formula-fed baby, and there is no evidence that this overfeeding is good. Indeed, there is accumulating evidence that it can be harmful. The higher rates of overweight and obesity in artificially fed babies may be partly due to their getting used to overeating right from the start.

Myth #2: Low blood glucose is a common problem in breastfed babies and we have to watch newborn babies closely to prevent brain damage.

Fact: Glucose is a sugar found in milk that nourishes the brain, but it is only one of several nutrients in the blood that does this. Low blood glucose in healthy, full-term babies is rare; routine testing leads to unnecessary supplementation. Please see Chapter 6 for a more detailed discussion of this issue.

Myth #3: A baby who is jaundiced in the first few days needs formula and should not breastfeed.

Fact: Jaundice is a condition often seen in newborn babies (and sometimes in older children and adults, but the causes are different in these cases). A baby with jaundice looks yellow because he has high levels of a substance called bilirubin in the blood. There are several causes of jaundice in the first few days. Probably the most common reason for higher-than-average bilirubin levels in a breastfed baby is that he isn't getting enough milk. The answer is not to stop breastfeeding, but to get the baby breastfeeding better. See the chapter "Early Concerns: Low Blood Glucose and 'Breastmilk Jaundice'" for more information.

A good beginning

A mother's experience of breastfeeding can be profoundly affected by what happens during the first hours and days after her baby's birth. A good beginning can make breastfeeding easy and painless; a bad beginning can make it painful and difficult. Here are the steps that make it easier:

1. If possible, have a natural childbirth. Plan to give birth with as few interventions as possible, as discussed in more detail in the previous chapter.

2. Have your baby skin to skin with you immediately after the birth and allow time for him to start breastfeeding through self-attachment. There is no reason why the majority of newborns cannot be skin to skin with the mother within 30 minutes of birth. Babies usually experience a time of quiet alertness in the first hour or two after birth, are awake but not crying, and primed to take in new experiences such as learning to breastfeed. Yet in some hospitals there is still a "routine" separation of mothers and babies, "for observation," even if the pregnancy, labour and birth were completely normal. In many industrializing countries (in parts of Eastern Europe, India and China, for example), the separation of mothers and babies is still routine. Indeed, during a visit to Eastern Europe in 2011, I saw the complete opposite of skin-to-skin contact between mother and baby.

Observations of newborn babies going back at least 30 years have shown that babies placed skin to skin on the mother's abdomen within an hour of birth are capable of crawling to the breast and latching on without any help from anyone (watch the video at www.breastcrawl.org or on the International Breastfeeding Centre's YouTube Channel [http://youtube.com/user/IBCToronto). It shouldn't surprise us that babies can do this: newborn mammals in the wild must find the breast on their own or die. There are no tiger or moose lactation consultants around to help. Yes, the mother may help a little, but essentially the

babies do it alone. Our babies can too, if given the opportunity. Incidentally, if for some reason the baby cannot go immediately skin to skin with the mother, a few hours later or even longer may not be too late. However, immediately after birth is the ideal time.

Many of our routine birth practices, though, interfere with this: we still separate the mother and baby far too frequently. No matter how ready to self-attach the baby is, if the mother is lying on the delivery table and he is under a heat lamp or in an incubator, it's not going to happen.

Our obsession with cleanliness may also interfere. In one study, babies were allowed to crawl to the breast. One of the mother's nipples had been washed with soap and water beforehand, the other not. The baby almost always crawled to the unwashed breast. Another study showed that the Montgomery's glands (the little bumps you can see on the areola) produce a volatile (airborne) chemical that attracts the baby to the breast; washing the nipple may wipe away this chemical.

Suctioning the baby at birth can also interfere. In the past almost all babies were suctioned; if they'd passed meconium before birth they got deep suctioning into their tracheas. Research in the 1980s showed this can derail the baby's ability to find the breast and latch on. Routine suctioning has decreased considerably in the past 20 years.

Not giving the baby enough time to latch on can also prevent self-attachment. It often takes an hour or more of being skin to skin for the baby to crawl to the breast and latch on. Often he just lies on the mother for 20 minutes or more. But hospitals have other priorities: weighing the baby, putting drops or ointment in his eyes, etc. Would it really matter if the baby was weighed an hour or two later?

Ointments and drops in the baby's eyes may also affect his vision, making it harder for him to find the nipple (does he find it more easily because the areola

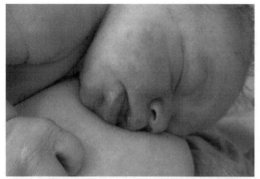

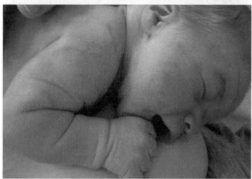

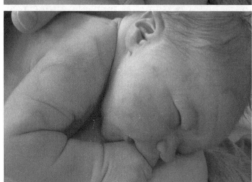

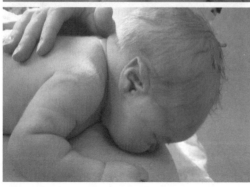

The "breast crawl" sequence: over the course of about an hour, if given the opportunity, most babies can crawl to the breast and latch on without help.

CREDIT: **ANDREA POLOKOVA**

is a different colour?). And what about the pediatrician's examination to determine the Apgar? Well, if a baby is alert and pink and breathing, and crawling to the breast, I give him a minimum of 9 out of 10. If necessary, one can put a stethoscope on the baby's chest while he's on the mother, skin to skin.

Delaying skin-to-skin contact because the baby was born by Caesarean section is common even in facilities where skin to skin is routine, but it's not necessary. If the mother and baby are well, then the baby can be put skin to skin with the mother even as the obstetrician or surgeon is sewing up the incision.

To summarize the reasons for skin-to-skin contact:

- It helps to get breastfeeding started.
- It maintains the newborn's temperature more effectively than an incubator.
- It helps the baby adapt to the new environment, especially in terms of sugar levels, acid-base balance, respiratory rate and heart rate.
- It provides comfort to the new baby after what has been said to be a stressful experience.
- It facilitates bonding.
- It causes oxytocin release in the mother, which helps her feel loving and nurturing toward the baby.
- It encourages milk ejection as well as uterine contractions (to reduce bleeding).
- It improves immediate and long-term breastfeeding success.

Not only does the baby get off to the best possible start with breastfeeding (this is true even if he does not latch on by himself), but the reaction of

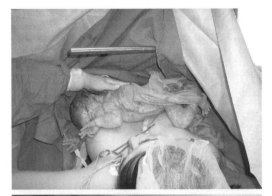

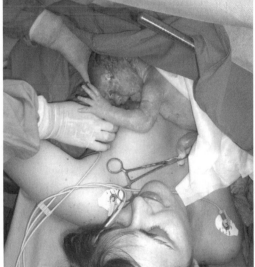

(*Top*) This mother is skin to skin with her baby immediately after a C-section. The baby lies near the breast and has almost latched on, while the obstetrician is still sewing up the incision. (*Bottom*) Moments later, the baby has fully latched on to the breast.

CREDIT: **ANDREA POLOKOVA**

the mother to the baby's presence can be dramatic. Mothers often say that it was at that moment that they fell in love with their babies. This physical connection between mother and baby is incredibly powerful.

The mother is usually emotionally ready to make this breastfeeding connection with her baby. Even if the labour has been hard and exhausting, she may find that holding the baby is the perfect reward. She may need some help getting into a comfortable position, but even if she must lie flat, the baby can still be held skin to skin and allowed to find the breast.

At first, the baby may just lick or nuzzle the nipple. That's okay; it's one step in the natural process. Forcing babies to the breast or continually pushing it to the breast probably causes many babies to refuse it. When the mother can relax and enjoy this time with her baby, he'll let her know when he's ready to eat. It might be 10 minutes, 30 minutes, an hour or more. If the mother and baby are in a chilly delivery room, they should be moved *together* to a warmer room, though being skin to skin keeps the baby warm most of the time. This initial time of quiet alertness is a special window of opportunity for establishing breastfeeding. Some babies, if separated from their mothers before this first feeding, seem to "shut down." They become sleepy and may show no interest in feeding. The longer they go without feeding, the harder it may be to get them interested in taking the breast.

Even worse is the situation in which the baby does not get a chance to breastfeed—perhaps because medical staff are concerned that the mother is too tired—and is instead given a bottle of formula

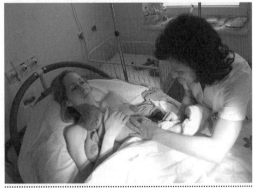

A health care provider takes a baby's temperature while it remains skin to skin with the mother.

CREDIT: **ANDREA POLOKOVA**

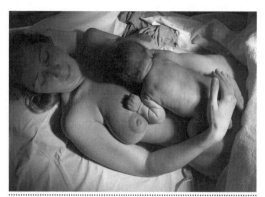

Mother and newborn skin to skin.

CREDIT: **ANDREA POLOKOVA**

> The benefits to the mother of immediate breastfeeding are innumerable, not the least of which after the weariness of labour and birth is the emotional gratification, the feeling of strength, composure, and the sense of fulfillment that comes with the handling and suckling of the baby.
>
> —Ashley Montagu, *Touching*

or sugar water. This often has a negative effect on the baby's suckling. Here he is, primed to learn to breastfeed, and he is given a rigid bottle nipple and expected to form his lips and tongue to manage its rapid flow. Because the baby is so sensitive at this stage, even one feeding from a bottle can create long-lasting problems. True, one bottle does not *always* cause problems, and most problems can be fixed with good help. But why create problems in the first place? It does neither the mother nor the baby any favour to separate them. If the baby needs to be fed, he should be breastfed. How tiring is it, really, for a mother to lie in bed with her baby lying across her body, sucking at her breast? In fact, the hormones produced when the baby nurses create a sense of relaxation and blissful contentment—just the reward a tired new mother needs.

Especially for a baby born in a hospital, feeding right away is important because he benefits from the protection against infection provided by the colostrum. Also, sharing the mother's bacteria prevents him from becoming colonized by hospital bacteria.

Some babies will take a few hours to decide they are ready to breastfeed. It is harmful to force a baby to the breast when he is not ready, since forcing will only make him angry or upset or he will simply "shut down." As long as the mother and baby are together, there is no rush. The mother can cuddle him, skin to skin, and feed him when he shows interest.

3. You and your baby should "room-in" together.
And rooming-in means 24 hours a day, not just daylight hours. Sometimes mothers are encouraged to send the baby to the nursery at night because nurses think mothers will get more rest. But this isn't so. Mothers and babies who are together will get "in synch" as they sleep and wake at the same time.

Mothers often find that they wake up just before their babies. When the baby starts to wake, his breathing changes, becoming more rapid. The mother who is attuned to her baby from birth, even when she's asleep, will respond to these subtle changes. Her milk will begin to let down; she'll start to wake up. By the time the baby has progressed from the change in breathing to moving around or perhaps turning his head to the side or making quiet noises, his mother will be awake and ready to feed him. Because he isn't ravenously hungry yet, he can be patient if getting latched on well takes a couple of tries or if the mother needs to arrange some pillows or her clothes to prepare for feeding. He will take the milk he needs and fall asleep again and his mother can sleep as well.

It's very different when the baby is in a separate room at home or in the hospital. When his breathing changes, the nursery staff won't notice. His mother is far away, in a deep sleep. He turns his head from side to side and tries to suck. Again, probably nobody notices. When the baby finally starts to cry loudly, the nurse may have another baby to tend to before she can take the first one to his mother. Finally, she brings him to the room and wakes the mother from a sound sleep. The baby continues to cry, and his mother, groggy from being woken up and struggling to deal with a frantic baby, will try to feed him. But her milk hasn't let down yet, and even when the very hungry baby latches on, he doesn't at first get anything to drink. He gets more upset, and in his frustration may even refuse to take the breast.

Today's hospital stays are short, but they can still be a good time for mother and baby to get to know each other while other people are providing food and care. But it's important for mother and baby to stay together to make it work.

4. Don't give the baby artificial nipples. You only need to watch babies suck on a bottle nipple and suckle at the breast to see that these are two very different processes. The baby at the breast must use his mouth and tongue quite differently from the baby sucking on a plastic bottle nipple, a nipple shield, or even a pacifier.

Here's what Japanese researchers Mizuno and Ueda stated in an article in *Pediatric Research* in 2006: "It is evident from the results of this study that bottle-feeding is a completely different feeding method regardless of attempts to make bottle-feeding more closely resemble breastfeeding."

During the first few days after giving birth, mothers produce only small amounts of milk, called colostrum. Colostrum has a very high concentration of antibodies and other immune factors and is also a laxative, preparing the baby's intestines to handle the more mature milk that the breasts will soon be producing. The breasts of a new mother are fairly soft, making it easier for the new baby to learn to latch on. Sometimes, though, a new baby only "allows" the breast into his mouth and is actually not latched on. A baby who "latches on just fine for the first few days" and then cannot latch on when the mother's milk comes in and she becomes engorged probably didn't latch on in the first few days: he pretended to. If a baby breastfeeds well in the first few days, the mother may feel full when her milk "comes in," but she should not be so engorged that the baby cannot latch on.

At first, the baby doesn't get a lot of milk. That's good; it's what nature intended. If the baby gets a bottle, though, he gets a lot more milk, and the rigid bottle nipple must be forced into his mouth, so he has to suckle very differently. Some people will say that giving a baby a bottle isn't a problem because they know babies who take both the bottle and the breast. True, some do seem able to do both. But for many others, bottles cause problems, and nobody can know in advance which baby will have problems. However, if the baby is already having problems latching on, a bottle or a pacifier will probably make it worse. And even babies who are doing fine at the breast can have problems if they are given bottles. Even one bottle can create problems if it is given early on. This is sometimes called "nipple confusion," although the babies are not really confused. They just want milk. If they go to the breast and don't get much milk (because they aren't supposed to get much in the first few days or because they are not latched on well) and are then given a bottle and get a fast flow of milk, they will develop a preference for the bottle. Babies don't have to be Einsteins to figure it out.

For this reason, many will describe this situation as "nipple preference" rather than "nipple confusion." This term can be pretty upsetting to the mother who may already be feeling emotional about the problems she is having breastfeeding and now is told that the baby "prefers" the bottle. She may feel as if the baby is rejecting her. "Nipple confusion" suggests that the baby really does want to breastfeed (and he does! Really!) but is temporarily not sure what to do.

The solution? Help the baby latch well so he gets as much milk as possible. However, the flow of milk at the breast, unlike that in the bottle, will always be variable. So if the baby does need supplementation, it should be given with a lactation aid at the breast. Then there's no room for confusion. Even when babies seem to be able to feed both at the breast and at the bottle, bottle-feeding is often the first step to early weaning. Breastfeeding may go "well enough" in the early weeks when the mother's milk supply is very plentiful, but may become more difficult with time and the mother's diminishing milk supply. The milk diminishes because the more bottles of formula the baby gets, the less stimulation the breasts receive to keep up her milk production. As it gets harder for the baby to get milk from his mother's breasts, he begins to prefer the bottle. Recognizing that her milk supply is down, his mother gives him additional bottles, and her milk supply decreases further. Before long, the baby may refuse the breast altogether. I remember a mother who came to LLL meetings for several months, mentioning each time that she was giving bottles as well as breastfeeding and having no problems. When her baby was seven months old, she showed up at the meeting in tears. He was now refusing to breastfeed.

Many mothers say that the baby is not "nipple confused" because he will take both the breast and the bottle. But complete breast refusal is only the most extreme manifestation of nipple confusion—along with poor weight gain, high bilirubin levels, sore nipples, colic, pulling and crying at the breast (often misdiagnosed as "reflux") and breast infections.

I'm surprised when people say nipple confusion doesn't exist. They'd certainly agree that a baby may prefer one kind of bottle nipple or pacifier over another, or one breast over the other. Why is it surprising that babies might learn to prefer the bottle nipple to the breast, or at least prefer to latch on less well and thus drink less well?

A mother recently emailed me to ask for help with her situation. She'd been advised to "top-up" her baby's feedings at the breast by giving expressed breastmilk in a bottle after each feeding. A couple of weeks later, the baby was refusing the breast completely. When the mother contacted me, the baby was four weeks old and she'd been expressing her milk and feeding it in a bottle for two weeks. She wanted to get her baby feeding at the breast again but didn't know how. Another contradiction: many of the people who say there is no such thing as nipple confusion are the same ones who urge parents to give their babies a bottle early on so that he will be willing to take one. They warn parents that if they delay introducing a bottle, the baby may always resist it. In other words, their concern is that the baby will have a persistent preference for the breast. But a bottle is not the only way to supplement a breastfed baby, should that become necessary (see the chapter "Increasing the Baby's Breastmilk Intake").

5. Don't restrict the frequency or length of feedings. One book from 30 years ago said that the most important piece of equipment needed for successful breastfeeding was a reliable clock. That's a sad legacy from the days when babies' lives were tightly scheduled, and those schedules frequently led to breastfeeding failure. For millenia mothers have breastfed their babies without clocks, watches or schedules. In many parts of the world this is still true, and these mothers almost universally succeed at breastfeeding.

So how will you know when to feed your baby? You'll learn his cues. If you're not watching the clock, you'll be able to watch your baby and see his individual ways of showing hunger. Maybe he'll move around in a restless way, or make sucking motions with his lips, or try to put his hands in his mouth, or start searching for the nipple. Soon you'll recognize his signals without even thinking.

In traditional societies, it is common for babies to nurse frequently for short periods of time. Anthropologist Kathy Dettwyler describes babies in Mali nursing for a few minutes at a time, several times an hour, with some longer stretches between feedings when the baby is in a deeper sleep. The shorter, more frequent feeding pattern lets the baby get milk with a higher fat content; when there is a longer time between feedings, the milk has a higher water content. These babies are undoubtedly "snacking" at the breast, drinking only small amounts at each feeding, so they want to return to the breast frequently. *There is nothing wrong with this.* North Americans do not consider this "efficient," and many breastfeeding problems result from trying to "fix" this.

However, it is important to remember that a baby who is *not* feeding well and not really getting milk will also want to come to the breast frequently. You want to be sure that the baby is well latched on and drinking at each feeding. See the video clips at the International Breastfeeding Centre's YouTube Channel (http://youtube/glCYw1uTiG4).

Limiting and scheduling feedings can also increase the risk of sore nipples. If the baby is ravenously hungry when he comes to the breast, he may grab the nipple and not be patient enough to wait until his mother gets him well positioned. His frustration when the milk doesn't flow quickly enough may make him pull at the breast, often coming off and relatching poorly, causing more pain. If the mother gives him bottles or a pacifier to help him wait until the next scheduled feeding time, his latch and the way he sucks may get even worse, and the mother will be even more likely to have nipple pain.

What about the baby who is at the breast for hours? Most often, this means he is not properly latched on and is not really getting milk. He is at the breast, but he is not actually drinking a lot of the time. These babies normally use a rapid, fluttering kind of suck that may stimulate some milk to let down so they are able to drink a little bit; however, they don't do the slow suckling with distinct pauses that indicates a good flow of milk. Once the baby is latched on well, his sucking usually changes dramatically, his stomach gets filled up and he no longer spends hours at the breast.

There are babies who seem to want to spend more time at the breast than others, even if they are getting plenty of milk. Some seem to need the extra comfort that breastfeeding gives them. Some are just "high-need." It's important to watch the baby at the breast to figure out what is really going on.

> Never again, never in the future
> that dawned later on, were we so sated.
> We were suckled and suckled. Always
> superabundance was flowing into us.
> Never any question of enough is enough
> or let's not overdo it. Never were we
> given a pacifier and told to be
> reasonable. It was always
> suckling time.
>
> —Günter Grass, *The Flounder*

6. Don't give the baby water, sugar water or formula unless necessary—and that should be rare. Many hospitals used to routinely supplement all breastfed babies' feedings with water or sugar water for the first few days. That's supposed to have changed, but a 2009 Toronto study found that one-third of breastfed babies in the hospital received a supplement, even though the average stay was less than two days! A national Canadian study found the rate was 48%. Babies born in hospitals with high supplementation rates are likely to be weaned much earlier.

There are very few medical reasons for giving supplements to babies, and if one is needed, it should be given by a lactation aid with the baby on the breast so that he gets milk from the breast and the supplement at the same time. If the mother and baby really need to be separated, the baby can receive his supplement from a cup.

In most cases, though, the best way to provide extra milk for the baby is to get it well latched on. Breast compression (see video clips at http://youtube/glCYwluTiG4) is another option.

7. Do not accept free or reduced price samples of formula. The World Health Organization has specifically advised against this, for good reason. These "gifts" are simply a marketing technique. They undermine breastfeeding and many studies show they decrease its exclusivity and duration. They also undermine the mother's confidence and become a too-easy "solution" to breastfeeding problems.

8. Focus on proper positioning and latching on; they are crucial to success. "Latching on" refers to the way the baby takes the breast into his mouth. A good latch means pain-free breastfeeding; it also means that the baby will usually get the milk he needs. That's the foundation of successful breastfeeding. But sometimes it's hard to do. Most women have seen many more bottle-fed babies than breastfed babies, and the images imprinted on their brains of "how babies are fed" include babies lying on their backs, turned away from their mothers, with a rubber nipple pushed into their mouths.

The hospital staff who are trying to help the mother breastfeed may not be experienced or have the skills to recognize a good latch or help correct a bad one. While some nurses have taken courses in breastfeeding or developed the ability to deal with stumbling blocks, many have not. It can be hard for some nurses to accept that they may have been teaching new mothers incorrect breastfeeding techniques for many years. Many insist that it is inevitably painful and don't recognize that they are contributing to that painful experience by not helping the mother and baby to get breastfeeding well established. A Toronto lactation consultant told me that when she pointed out to a nurse that her nipples were not sore during breastfeeding, the nurse responded, "You are just lucky." What would this nurse say to the mother who does have sore nipples? Perhaps "Well, you wanted to breastfeed; suck it up." If this sounds unlikely, I can only say that mothers have reported to me that this is just what they were told.

The exact technique of getting the baby on the breast is not always as simple as "Apply Part A to Part B." Babies are individuals, and every breast is different—even the breasts on the same mother! Sometimes a baby takes one breast easily, but not the other. Sometimes mothers use a cradle hold for one breast and switch to the football hold for the other. Some women find it easier to get breastfeeding going if they are lying down instead of sitting up.

Blanket rules—such as, "The baby should take the whole areola into his mouth as well as the nipple"—don't apply to everyone. Some women have small areolas, and if the baby takes even the whole areola into his mouth, he may *still* not have enough of the breast in his mouth. Other women have very large areolas that cover much of their breasts, and it simply isn't possible for the baby to take the entire areola into his mouth. Some women also have very large nipples that fill the baby's mouth and limit the amount of additional breast tissue that he can take in.

Babies are different, too. Some are eager breast-feeders from the very first day; some are calm but efficient; and others take a day or two before they really figure out what's what. Some are sleepy because of medications their mothers received in labour. Some have a tight frenulum (the thin piece of flesh that attaches the tongue to the bottom of the mouth) that limits the movement of the tongue.

People who help mothers with breastfeeding need to be aware of these differences and know how to manage them, even if that just means reassuring the mother that her baby is normal. If a mother is feeling more than minimal breast tenderness when the baby is breastfeeding, he is probably not latched on well—no matter what anyone may say. If, once the milk becomes abundant, the baby is still making only small sucking motions and not doing the "open mouth wide–pause–close mouth" type of suckling that shows he is getting mouthfuls of milk (http://youtu.be/CrysrsFzBWY), he is probably not latched on well and the mother needs good, hands-on help. And if the baby is spending long hours at the breast and still seems dissatisfied, the mother and baby need good help. Good help means helping the mother latch the baby on well.

A good latch means the baby will get more milk. A baby may be able to get enough milk even with a bad latch if the mother has an abundant supply, but often the mother will have sore nipples, or the baby will nurse very frequently, or the mother's milk supply will decrease over time. To give a bottle-feeding comparison: when the baby latches on poorly, it's as though he's being bottle-fed with a bottle nipple with tiny holes. The bottle may be full of milk, but the baby will struggle to get that milk. The smaller the nipple hole, the less milk he will get, and the

longer it will take for him to get it, even though there is plenty available.

Why do we say the latch is important, when clearly mothers all over the world and throughout history have breastfed their babies without paying much attention to how the baby was latched on? Part of the reason is that mothers in breastfeeding cultures didn't need to analyze the latch: they'd seen babies breastfeed all their lives and knew how to hold and position the baby without even thinking about it. It's very different in our society, where mothers are much more likely to see babies being bottle-fed. As well, in traditional cultures nobody worried much about the baby who was on the breast many hours a day. If the latch wasn't perfect and the baby needed to breastfeed more often, nobody accused the mother of spoiling the baby or having inadequate milk. With free access to the breast, most babies gained weight just fine and as they got bigger usually figured out how to improve their latch. Thanks to an obsession with numbers and the clock, and with "scientific" medicine's increasing involvement in infant feeding, this more relaxed and usually successful approach has been largely discarded in our society.

By the twentieth century, pediatricians were advising mothers to feed by the clock—so many minutes on each side, every so many hours. "Scientific" infant feeding (from which the special-ity of modern pediatrics grew, incidentally) often did not work, so that, more and more, supplemental milk was "required."

It may be more surprising that sometimes breast-feeding *did* work, despite these obstacles. When the mother's supply is abundant, sometimes even the most bizarre rules will not derail the process. And of course there have always been some mothers who simply ignored their doctor's advice. This is lucky; otherwise, the art of breastfeeding might have been lost completely in the industrialized world.

We now know that there are more efficient and less efficient ways of having a baby take the breast. When the amount of time the baby spends at the breast or the frequency with which he takes it are not considerations, how well he does it may not be that important. But the less milk a mother has, even if the amount is sufficient to nourish her baby adequately, the better the latch must be in order for her baby to get that milk.

One reason women worry so much about not having enough milk is recent media coverage of cases in which "breastfed" babies became dehydrated. But in my experience, most of the mothers whose babies became dehydrated had plenty of milk; once they were helped to improve their technique they could continue breastfeeding exclusively. But even if the mothers did not have enough milk, the problem was that they were *not* breastfeeding and that's why they became dehydrated.

If you are a nursing mother, you can try this test yourself. Pretend your thumb and index finger are your baby's gums. Put your thumb over the top of one of your nipples, and your index finger under the nipple. Now squeeze. You may feel pain, and notice how little milk comes out—at best, probably drops.

Now move your fingers back two or three centimetres (an inch or so) and squeeze. You probably feel no pain, and quite possibly your milk will spray. Notice what a big difference such a short distance can make. See the video at the International Breastfeeding Centre's YouTube Channel (http://youtube.com/user/IBCToronto).

What is a good latch?

The answer to this question has changed over the years as more and more observations of babies breastfeeding have been made by knowledgeable people. Mothers and babies will have an easier time if the baby comes to the breast and latches on *asymmetrically*, covering more of the areola with his lower lip than with his upper lip. In this position, he can extract milk from the breast in a more efficient manner. He will usually get the milk he needs and breastfeeding will usually be painless for the mother. (However, while pain usually indicates a problem, a pain-free latch doesn't necessarily mean a good one.)

How do you achieve this asymmetrical latch? I usually suggest mothers start by using the cross-cradle hold. Most mothers find this the easiest way, especially with a newborn. But it is not

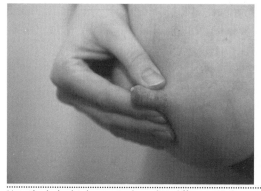 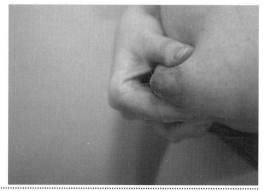

How the baby latches on makes a big difference in how well he gets milk. With a shallow latch on only the nipple (*left*), the baby may get very little. But when he takes more of the areola in his mouth, milk flows more easily. (http://youtu.be/V2qKjEOaK5A)

CREDIT: **ANDREA POLOKOVA**

the only way. The best latch can also be achieved using the cradle hold or the football hold or while lying down.

The cross-cradle hold

If you are putting the baby to your left breast using the cross-cradle hold, here's our approach:

- Hold the baby with your right arm and push the baby's bottom into your chest or upper abdomen with the *side* of your right forearm. This pushing in of your baby's bottom is very important and will ensure that he gets an asymmetrical latch. The baby's weight will be supported by your forearm, not your hand or wrist. Your right hand will be palm-up toward the ceiling, underneath the baby's face like a pillow, not on his shoulder or neck.
- When you move the baby toward the breast your nipple will automatically point to the baby's upper lip or even his nose.
- Lightly brush the baby's upper lip *from one corner to the other* with your nipple until he opens wide, and then bring the baby onto the breast, keeping the nipple pointed at the roof of his mouth. The baby should be brought onto the breast with a fairly brisk movement using your whole arm, but be careful not to push the baby's head forward so that the nipple ends up in the middle of his mouth. In other words, don't scoop the baby's head around.

If the baby has latched on well:

- he will cover more of the areola with his lower lip than his upper lip
- his lips will be turned outward
- his chin, but *not* his nose, will be touching the breast

- his whole body, not just his head, will be slightly rotated upwards so that he can look at your face

If the baby hasn't latched on well, check for these problems:

- You used your hand or wrist to push the baby's head to the breast, rather than using your whole arm to push his whole body, and the baby ended up with his nose buried in your breast. His chin may be pulled away from the

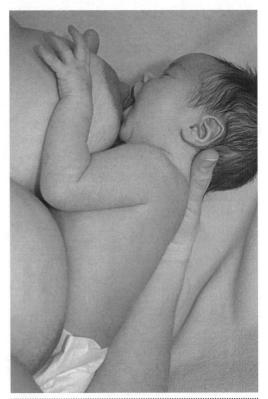

Getting the ideal latch: The baby is held in a cross-cradle position while the mother pushes his bottom into her body with the side of her forearm. The four fingers of her hand are under the baby's face, not on his neck or shoulder. He approaches the breast, and the nipple points toward the roof of his mouth.

CREDIT: **ANDREA POLOKOVA**

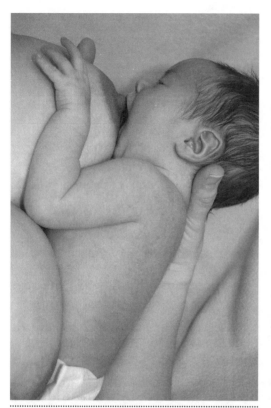

As the baby comes to the breast, the nipple stays pointed toward the roof of his mouth. His chin touches the breast first.

CREDIT: **ANDREA POLOKOVA**

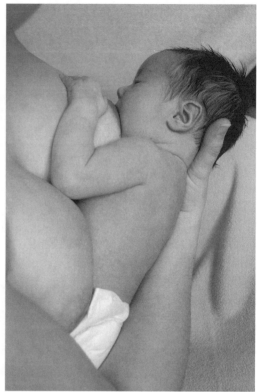

The baby is latched on. His chin is in the breast and his nose is not, and he covers more of the areola with his lower lip than with his upper lip. This asymmetrical latch is often easiest for mother and baby.

CREDIT: **ANDREA POLOKOVA**

breast.

- The baby was positioned too far over to your left side. The baby should be positioned with his mouth just at the nipple or even to the right of it.
- The baby was lying too much on his back or not turned slightly upward at all.
- You didn't wait for the baby to open his mouth wide enough. It can be hard to be patient, especially if the baby is hungry, and babies who have had bottles and pacifiers may not be used to opening wide. Take your time, stroke the baby's upper lip and wait. It will happen. You may have tried to put the breast in the baby's mouth (as you would a bottle) rather than bringing the

baby onto the breast.

The football hold

Some mothers find the football hold, where the baby is tucked under the arm, easier to manage than the cross-cradle.

- To latch on the left breast, push the baby's bottom into your left *side* at waist level or higher with the *side* of your *left* forearm. The baby's weight will be supported by your forearm, not your hand or wrist.
- The baby's feet will now be behind you, perhaps against the back of the chair.

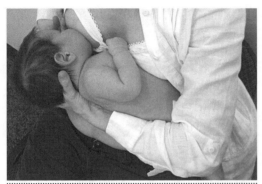

This woman demonstrates a good cross-cradle position. She holds the baby's bottom against her chest with her forearm, and her hand supports his face like a pillow. The baby's chin is in the breast, but his nose does not touch it.

CREDIT: **JACK NEWMAN**

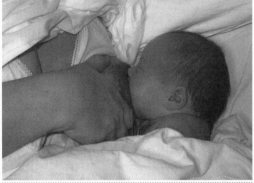

This mother could improve the latch by moving her baby closer to the centre of her body so that his nose is not buried in her breast. Compare this photo to the one above.

CREDIT: **ANDREA POLOKOVA**

- Support your left breast with your right hand, fingers underneath, thumb on top, as far as possible from the nipple and areola.
- Again, your left thumb is on the side of the baby's face, the web between the thumb and fingers is in the nape of his neck and the other four fingers are on his face.
- You want the baby to come to the breast with the nipple pointed to the roof of his mouth, upper lip or nose. Tickle the baby's upper lip, lightly, *from one corner of his mouth to the other*

and when he opens up, bring him onto the breast with a brisk arm movement.

- Two challenges with the football hold: one, it is hard with a bigger or older baby; two, it is easy to unintentionally push the baby's head forward and get a symmetrical latch (not the asymmetrical latch you want), or one where the baby is nose-first into the breast.

The "cradle hold"

The cradle hold is the position seen in thousands of classical paintings and the method used by most mothers once they have the hang of breastfeeding.

To feed the baby on the left breast in this position, hold the baby in your left arm, with his head just below the crook of your elbow and your left hand supporting his bum. Use your right hand to support your breast; the baby should be at the level

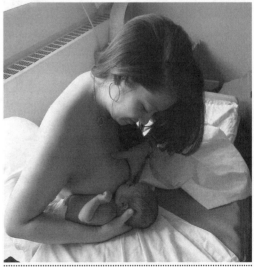

In football hold the mother holds the baby in much the same way that a football player carries the ball. The baby is beside the mother rather than across hers. But she still holds the baby's body against hers with her forearm, while her hand is underneath his face like a pillow. Notice that the baby has an asymmetrical latch. The latch would be even better if he were slightly farther back.

CREDIT: **JACK NEWMAN**

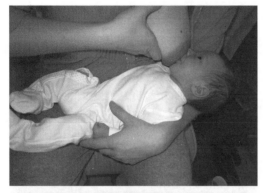

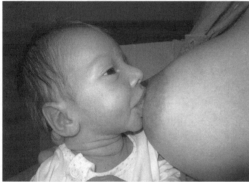

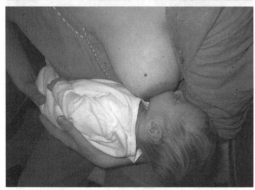

of your nipple. Stroke the baby's upper lip lightly from corner to corner with your nipple. When the baby opens wide, use your left arm to bring him in close as he latches on. You can also latch him on in the cross-cradle position and then switch arms to hold him in the cradle hold.

I believe the cross-cradle hold is the easiest way for mothers to learn latching on, but I expect that once they've got that, they will switch to a cradle hold. In the long run it's easier and more practical. It's also very practical to be able to breastfeed lying down. In the evenings, when many babies are fussy, feeding while lying down can help the baby be calmer and feed better.

Latching on the baby while lying down

To breastfeed on the left breast lying down, lie on your left side and position your baby on his right, facing you. Have the baby's mouth at the level of your nipple. You may want a pillow or rolled up towel under your breast or a pillow under the baby, or both. You can also use a pillow behind your back or your head so you're comfortable.

Support your breast with your right hand. Your left arm goes behind the baby's back, your hand on his bum. Lightly stroke his upper lip with your

The right hold can make a big difference. (*Top*) The baby is lying on his back with his mother hunched over him. His nose is in the breast, and you can see that his latch is very shallow because his mouth and jaw are not open wide and he has very little areola in his mouth. (*Middle*) Although he appears to be feeding, his shallow latch and the milk dripping out of his mouth suggest he may just be pretending. (*Bottom*) By adjusting the cradle hold, both mother and baby are more comfortable and breastfeeding is successful, although the baby could be a little closer to the centre of the woman's body.

CREDIT: **ANDREA POLOKOYA**

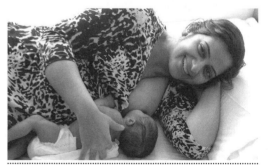

Lying down to breastfeed. This position is especially helpful during those evenings when babies want to feed frequently and mothers are tired. The baby has an asymmetrical latch even in this position.

CREDIT: **JACK NEWMAN**

nipple and move him in to latch when he opens his mouth wide. If you tuck his feet and legs toward your abdomen, he should be in a good position to latch on asymmetrically. This is a good time for the father or grandmother to help out by holding the baby while you get into position and then putting him in place next to you.

Another position often recommended when the baby is having difficulty taking the breast is the "laid-back" position, called the "biological nurturing" position by Suzanne Colson (www.biologicalnurturing.com). This extends the "self-attachment" process we have described with newborns: you find a comfortable semi-reclining position (using pillows as needed) and place the baby tummy-down on your body. Usually the baby is at an angle across your body, but he can be vertical. (If you had a Caesarean section, you may want a pillow over your incision to protect it.) You can be skin to skin with the baby, or one or both of you can be dressed lightly with your breasts accessible. Because gravity is holding the baby against you, your hands are free to stroke him or provide a little help as needed. The baby typically begins by bobbing his head as he searches for the breast but will usually latch on well with only minimal assistance.

Feeding the baby this way can be especially helpful if he has come to resist breastfeeding, perhaps because the hospital staff tended to push his head into the breast at feeding time or because he received artificial nipples. The laid-back position allows the baby to do the latching on himself.

The baby is latched on: How do you know he is actually getting milk?

Once you know how to tell if a baby is drinking from the breast, it is easy to recognize. The baby who is getting milk in substantial quantities will demonstrate a very definite pause in the movement of his chin as he opens his mouth to the maximum while sucking. The baby opens his mouth wide, keeping it wide open for a second or two, then closes it again before opening it wide once more, pausing while his mouth is open, then closing it again.

As he pauses, his mouth is filling up with milk. The longer the pause, the more milk he is getting. The baby who is *not* getting much milk will have a fast sucking pattern without many of these wide-open-mouth pauses. He will mostly just open-close, open-close, open-close (with very few or no pauses). We have some very good video clips on the International Breastfeeding Centre YouTube Channel to demonstrate this (http://youtube.com/user/IBCToronto).

In the first two or three days, you may not notice the pauses because they are often very short. That's because colostrum is produced in fairly small (but adequate) quantities. However, as early as minutes after birth you can see the pauses if you know how to look for them. You may find, if you have lots of colostrum and your latch is very good, that there are lots of pauses and swallowing even in the first few days. You should definitely see these pauses once your milk "comes in."

How else to know if the baby is getting enough milk

1. The baby is losing weight. Babies normally lose weight in the first few days after birth. But in many hospitals or doctors' offices, there are concerns if the baby has lost a certain percentage of his birth weight (most commonly 10% but in some places the magic number is 7% or even 5%). I believe this to be a completely meaningless way of evaluating breastfeeding. On top of being useless, it is *harmful*. We've already mentioned that in hospitals with high intervention rates, babies are born with extra weight because of the intravenous infusions that the mother gets during labour and birth. We've

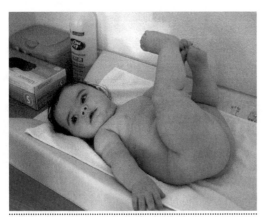

This healthy six-month-old baby breastfed exclusively, except for a formula supplement that was given two days after birth because of a 10% weight loss. It is unlikely that a mother who produces enough milk to make a baby grow like this doesn't have enough colostrum. Breastfeeding help, not formula feeding, should always be the first solution to weight loss.

CREDIT: **JACK NEWMAN**

also already mentioned that even the best electronic scales do not always give the same reading. In addition, humans make mistakes. Numbers have been read incorrectly; numbers have been written into the charts incorrectly or typed incorrectly into electronic records. And each time the baby is weighed, error is possible.

In one case I know of personally, a baby's birth weight was recorded as 2.58 kg (5 lbs, 11 oz.). Five hours later, the baby was re-weighed and the result was 3.1 kg (6 lbs, 13 oz.). What happened? We don't usually weigh babies every five hours. But someone looked at the baby and thought: "There is no way this baby weighs only 2.58 kg. He's too big. Let's weigh him again." But what if it had been the other way around? What if the baby's birth weight was first recorded at 3.1 kg and the next day the weight was 2.58 kg? That's a decrease in weight of 17%. You can imagine the panic that might have ensued!

(In fact, I recently helped a mother when this happened: her baby's weight at 24 hours after birth showed a drop of 15%. Panic ensued, and the mother was urged to give formula. Then concerns grew because other babies at this small hospital were also showing dramatic weight loss. Several women had started giving formula before someone figured out that the scale was broken.)

On the other hand, we have seen babies getting very little milk who lost less than 5% of their birth weight. The real question is: is the baby breastfeeding well or not? If he is drinking well, he'll make up the weight loss even if it's more than 10% of the birth weight. If he's not drinking well, he won't, even if he's lost only 4%.

2. There is red urine in the baby's diaper. This is often considered a sign that he is not getting enough milk. Early in the 20th century, red urine in the diaper was considered normal. At the time, mothers were told to feed babies just two or three minutes per breast, every four hours, for the first day. In some places, the babies were not fed at all for the first 24 hours. Not a good way to get breastfeeding established! But what does that red urine mean today? I think it is best to forget the colour of the urine and make sure the baby is drinking well. If he is, then this is not a problem. If he is not, then we should fix the breastfeeding. In the photo that follows, a three-day-old baby had this red stain in his diaper. We made sure he was breastfeeding well, and by day 10, he weighed significantly more than at birth and continued gaining weight well.

3. Tests show that the baby's serum sodium is "elevated," a sign of dehydration. But the level of the sodium has no more value than the red urine or the percentage of weight lost. If the baby is feeding well, then the problem will be resolved; if the baby isn't feeding well, we need to fix that. If the baby is dehydrated, it may be prudent to admit him to

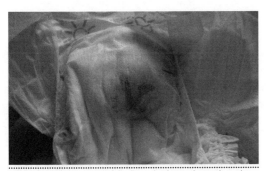

It's not easy to see in a black-and-white photo, but this diaper of a three-day-old baby has a reddish stain. Adjusting the baby's latch and making sure the baby was drinking milk resulted in both the mother and the baby doing well. No supplements were ever given. The baby was breastfed exclusively for more than five months and is still breastfeeding at over a year old.

CREDIT: JACK NEWMAN

hospital, but the focus should be on helping him to breastfeed more effectively. The fact that so many health professionals dealing with new mothers and babies don't know how to evaluate breastfeeding is scandalous and has led to tragic results. With regard to serum sodium, the question that has not been asked is: what is the normal sodium in a three-day-old baby (for instance) who is breastfeeding exclusively and doing well? Nobody knows; a study has never been done. It does not follow that the normal range of sodium should be the same as that of a 10-day-old baby doing well or a five-year-old child or an adult. (In those cases, 130-150 meq/litre is the normal range, depending on the normal values, which can vary from laboratory to laboratory). The normal range for the three-day-old, exclusively breastfed baby who is getting small but adequate amounts of milk could be, say, 145 to 155 meq/litre. Nobody knows.

4. The baby is weighed before and after the feeding to see how much milk he's getting. But what does this really tell us? Consider this: a baby who is exclusively breastfeeding and gaining weight well at

five months is not getting any more milk than a one-month-old who is exclusively breastfed and gaining weight well, even though the older baby weighs at least twice as much as the younger. This is quite different from formula-fed babies, who increase their intake over time.

But in the first few days of life, babies are getting only small amounts of colostrum. What amount is ideal? We cannot say he should get as much as he will take if fed formula by bottle. That's not physiological. But that is exactly how most hospitals determine what the baby should get; they are using the formula-fed, bottle-fed baby as the standard. What standard should we use to determine how much a baby should get at a single feeding, especially when the amount he normally takes will vary throughout the day, whether he is two days or two months old?

5. The baby wants to be on the breast *all* the time. A baby can be on the breast a lot for reasons other than hunger. Babies get pleasure and security from being at the breast. Being skin to skin with the mother reassures the baby, and the smell of his mother's milk will encourage him to take the breast and suckle.

But what if the baby is hungry? There is not a lot of milk available to the baby in the first few days but there is enough, *if the baby gets it*. When there is not a lot of milk, the baby needs to latch on very well to get that milk. As well, if the latch is not good, the mother's nipples may get sore. So it is very important the baby latch on well. Compression of the breast to help the baby get more milk can help. See the video clip at the International Breastfeeding Centre YouTube Channel (http://youtube/g1CYw1uTiG4) showing a 40-hour-old baby drinking well at the breast after the mother started using compression.

6. The baby sleeps a lot and hardly goes to the breast. It is a problem if they go to the breast "too often" and also a problem if they don't go often enough. What is often enough? Some people say 8 to 12 times a day in the first few weeks. But where did this number come from? It seems to me it was invented, probably based on the idea that the baby should eat every two to three hours. When I ask midwives about the behaviour of babies in the first 24 hours after birth, they say that babies feed and sleep in completely unpredictable patterns. Most will breastfeed in the first hour or two after birth; some will continue to feed very frequently (*more* than 12 times in 24 hours), while others may sleep six or more hours without wanting to breastfeed again, and still others will be somewhere in between. They are all different.

The problem is that in the first few days, babies who want to go to the breast and suck but do not get milk can become very sleepy. Their going to the breast, falling asleep while suckling and then staying asleep may lull inexperienced helpers and mothers into believing all is well. A baby who feeds well and is in close contact with the mother, preferably skin to skin, will let her know when he is ready to feed again. If this is four hours after the previous feed, well, so be it. If the baby is not feeding well, waking him up to feed again won't help—fixing the breastfeeding is necessary.

So how do we fix the breastfeeding?

1. Mothers need help to get the best latch possible. The better the latch, the less likely the mother is to have pain and the more milk the baby will get. If the baby is getting milk well (see video clips at the International Breastfeeding Centre YouTube Channel) and the mother has no pain, it's working. We've described how we teach latching on in the previous section (see pages 64–70).

2. It is essential that mothers know how to recognize when the baby is getting milk. Once mothers know this, they realize that feeding the baby for 10, 15, 20 minutes (or any length of time) makes no sense. If the baby is still drinking—actually getting milk— 10 minutes after the feeding began, why take him off? If the baby is sleeping at the breast, keeping him there not drinking will not increase the "high-fat" milk everyone seems to be concerned about (see the chapter "Increasing Breastmilk Intake by the Baby"). The baby won't get the high fat-milk because he isn't getting any milk at all if he's only "nibbling."

3. When the baby is not drinking, only nibbling, or drinking very little, breast compression usually works to keep him *drinking*. Babies tend to fall asleep at the breast when the flow of milk is slow, and this is particularly true in the first few days and weeks after birth. If things are going well, and it is obvious the baby is drinking well, breast compression need not be done. However, it is a useful technique to get more milk into the baby. See the video clips at the International Breastfeeding Centre YouTube Channel. It is best to start while the baby is not yet sleepy and mostly nibbling but still drinking a little. If the baby is not sucking at all, it is best to wait until he starts again. That way, the rhythm of suckling is maintained, with active sucking alternating with periods of rest. If the mother compresses while the baby is sucking but not drinking, she and the baby are working together.

4. When the baby is not drinking even with compression, switch sides and repeat the process.

5. If the baby truly needs supplementation, it should be done with a lactation aid at the breast. Because the baby is still *breastfeeding* when getting the supplement, he will not refuse the breast; he continues to get milk from the breast, and both mother and baby learn to breastfeed by breastfeeding.

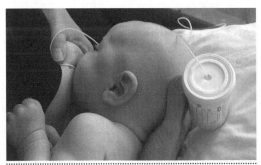

There is more to breastfeeding than milk. In this case, a mother uses a lactation aid to supplement her baby's diet with formula. The baby is still breastfeeding, and the risk of breast rejection is much lower.

CREDIT: JACK NEWMAN

What is the best supplement? Not formula. The *first* choice is always the mother's own milk. Hand expression during the first few days, when there is not a lot of colostrum, is often more effective than the best pumps. Colostrum is fairly thick, and if there is not a lot it can be diluted with water or 5% glucose water so it will flow more easily in the tube of the lactation aid. Or it can be expressed directly onto a small spoon and given with the spoon.

The *second* choice is banked breastmilk. Every hospital dealing with new mothers and babies, or older babies and toddlers, should have banked breastmilk on hand.

The *third* choice is 5% glucose water alone. Given in small amounts, this can help when the mother's nipples are very sore or if the baby is becoming dehydrated. With a lactation aid at the breast, the baby gets some colostrum too.

Some have expressed concerns that the 5% glucose might cause a rapid rise in the baby's blood sugar, stimulating insulin release and then causing a rapid drop, but a 5% glucose solution is not enough to raise the healthy newborn's blood sugar that high that quickly.

Some also worry that the baby's level of bilirubin could rise with the use of 5% glucose, causing higher levels of jaundice. However, if the 5% glucose is given at the breast with a lactation aid, the baby also gets colostrum, helping to prevent these problems.

Formula is the fourth choice—and is hardly ever necessary.

Other reasons babies are unnecessarily supplemented or taken off the breast

1. The baby won't "settle." This excuse may be one of the most common reasons babies are given supplements in the hospital. But babies *do* settle if they are just allowed to nurse as long as they want. The idea is still out there that 20 minutes on each side is enough, or that there's no more milk in the breasts after that, so the baby is taken off before he's finished. If the baby feeds well, he will be relaxed and content. If the baby is unhappy but doesn't want to breastfeed, being skin to skin with the mother is a very good way to soothe him.

2. The mother has sore nipples. The way to prevent sore nipples is to get the best latch from the very first feeding. Preventing engorgement is important, too, because it's harder for the baby to latch when the nipple and areola are swollen. (see page 190). The solution is not to give the baby supplements and/or take him

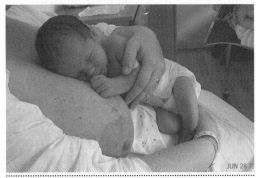

At several hours old, this baby was fussing and didn't want to take the breast again, but he settled with skin-to-skin contact.

CREDIT: JACK NEWMAN

off the breast to "rest the nipples," or give the mother a nipple shield. The solution is to fix the way the baby takes the breast. The baby should also be checked for a tongue tie, a frequent cause of nipple pain.

Some mothers with sore nipples are told that if they latch the baby on and it hurts, they should un-latch the baby and try again; if it hurts again, un-latch the baby and try again, and again, and again. Unfortunately, each time the baby is relatched poorly, more damage is done to the nipples. The mother is in pain and frustrated, and the baby may get so frustrated that he refuses to latch on at all. It is often possible to improve the latch without taking the baby off the breast. The mother pushes the baby's bottom into her body, which makes the latch more asymmetrical. And she can gently pull down the baby's chin to get more of the breast into his mouth. Even if these "tricks" don't help, the pain usually improves as the feeding goes on (if it doesn't, the baby may have a tongue tie). So if she can get through this feeding, she can try again to fix the latch when the baby takes the other side.

3. The mother needs to take medication or have certain tests done. Almost no medication requires the mother to interrupt breastfeeding. The amount of drug that gets into the milk is tiny, and the risks of giving the baby formula are almost always greater than the risk of this tiny amount of medication.

This issue is discussed more completely in the chapter "Breastfeeding While on Medication." There are some special considerations for the first few days, however. It is said that the junctions between the cells of the breast are "leakier" in the first few days and thus more drug can get into the milk. This is possibly true, but the amount of drug in the milk still depends on the concentration of drug in the mother's blood, which is usually very low. Since the amount of milk the baby gets is small in the first few days, he's still getting only a tiny dose of the drug.

The mother should not interrupt breastfeeding for a CT scan, or an MRI scan. Radioactive scans are a bit of a problem, but instead of doing a radioactive scan the mother may be able to get an MRI or a CT scan. For example, a CT scan is often better for the diagnosis of a pulmonary embolus (a blood clot in the lung) than the usual scan with radiation.

Avoiding the barriers

Understanding some of the potential problems of breastfeeding can help you be prepared to get off to a good start. Remember that even if you experience some of the potential challenges we've discussed in this chapter, with good help you can still succeed in meeting your breastfeeding goals. It's what both you and your baby are designed to do, and with a little assistance you'll navigate your way through the difficulties.

6 Early Concerns: Low Blood Glucose and "Breastmilk Jaundice"

The problem of hypoglycemia (low blood glucose)

Concerns that a baby might develop low blood glucose have become a major stumbling block for some mothers trying to establish breastfeeding. Yes, severe hypoglycemia can cause brain damage, but the worry has gone beyond the limits of the rational to the point where we can qualify the attitude of many pediatricians and neonatologists as "hysteroglycemia." In some hospitals in North America, especially in the United States, every single baby is screened for hypoglycemia at birth, even though studies have shown that the risk in the vast majority of healthy full-term babies is vanishingly low. For example, in one study, the authors concluded that "the occurrence of low blood glucose concentrations in healthy, breastfed, term infants of appropriate size for gestational age is very rare, and screening in these infants is not indicated." In other words, by testing every baby:

- We are wasting nurses' and technicians' time.
- We are adding unnecessary costs.
- We are causing the babies pain.
- We are causing the parents anxiety.
- We are giving babies formula and bottles unnecessarily.
- We are increasing admissions to special care units (NICUs) at considerable cost to the health system, separating mothers and babies and causing yet more anxiety for parents.

- We are increasing the rates of breastfeeding failure.

In fact, nobody has identified the lower limit of normal blood sugars. Every pediatrician or neonatologist has his or her own definition of what is too low and the tendency is to raise that limit higher and higher, "just to be safe." Not that long ago, in the 1990s, we considered a blood glucose concentration of 2.2 mmol/litre (40 mg%) the lower limit of normal. Then it got raised to 2.6 or 2.7 mmol/litre (47 mg%). Now, in some places, including at least two hospitals in the Toronto area, the lower limit is 3.4 mmol/litre (61 mg%). As a result, more and more babies are receiving formula, usually by bottle, and/or being admitted to the special care unit for intravenous infusions of glucose.

Glucose nourishes the brain, and without nourishment the brain can suffer damage. But glucose is not the only nutrient that can nourish the brain. If blood glucose decreases, other nutrients such as ketone bodies, almost certainly, and free fatty acids and lactic acid, probably, will increase in a healthy baby. Things to know about hypoglycemia:

1. It has no universally accepted definition. There is no quick, useful test to tell if the baby's blood glucose is too low. The test is usually done by pricking a baby's heel and putting the blood on a paper strip. But the glucose level in the plasma (the part of the blood without red blood cells)

would be more accurate because the glucose in the plasma that nourishes the brain. A test for glucose in blood, especially in a newborn, gives a lower number than glucose in the plasma. Many hospitals now understand this and send blood to the laboratory for verification, but often, in the meantime, the baby is given a bottle of formula *just in case.*

2.   There is no evidence that "asymptomatic" hypoglycemia causes damage to the baby's brain. Neonatologists will argue that seizures in newborn babies are subtle and hard to spot, and thus they cannot take chances. The reality is that a healthy full-term baby is at very, very low risk. Breastfeeding (or breastmilk) is the best approach to prevent and treat hypoglycemia.

3.   We know that glucose levels *normally* fall immediately after birth. In some hospitals, the routine is to measure the blood glucose at birth, then again in an hour. If the plasma glucose has dropped, the baby is given formula. Almost every baby shows a drop, because the drop in blood glucose is *normal.* As experts in neonatology and hypoglycemia reported in the May 2000 issue of *Pediatrics,* "In the majority of healthy neonates, the frequently observed low blood glucose concentrations are *not* related to any significant problem and *merely reflect normal processes of metabolic adaptation to extrauterine life*" [my emphasis]. In the same article: "During the first two hours of postnatal life, there is a decline in plasma glucose levels followed by a rise, reaching a steady state glucose concentration by two to three hours after birth." They continue, "Breastfed term infants have lower concentrations of blood glucose but higher concentrations of ketone bodies than formula-fed infants."

Here is yet another example of taking the formula-fed/bottle-fed baby as our model of normal and applying it to breastfed babies, to the detriment of breastfeeding. Because the formula-fed baby tends to have higher levels of glucose, we assume this is normal.

However, breastfeeding protects babies' brains by increasing the ketone bodies in the blood (and probably also lactic acid and free fatty acids, all derived from fat). The graph on page 79, which was published in *Pediatrics* in March 2002, shows the various concentrations of ketone bodies in babies born small for gestational age (a term baby who weighs less than 2.5 kg [5 lb, 8 oz.] is considered small for gestational age, but if he is born prematurely he can also be small for gestational age and there are growth curves to spot this). The open circles represent babies who are exclusively breastfed, the open squares breastfed babies supplemented with formula and the black triangles exclusively formula-fed babies. Note that the scale along the left side of the graph is a *logarithmic* scale and thus each level is 10 times the concentration of the level below it. All the exclusively breastfed babies (except one) with a blood glucose of 2.7 mmol/litre (46 mg%) or less have concentrations of ketone bodies 10 or more times those of the exclusively formula-fed babies with the same blood glucose.

As the authors emphasize, giving formula does not necessarily prevent low blood glucose, yet, at the same time, it inhibits the formation of ketone bodies. Thus the exclusively formula-fed baby who is also small for his gestational age is doubly at risk, having a low concentration of both glucose and ketone bodies. This is also *the* problem for infants of diabetic mothers; they are at risk of having low concentrations of *both* glucose and ketone bodies. This is what insulin does; it lowers glucose *and* ketone bodies, free fatty acid and lactic acid levels, thus risking brain damage because the concentrations of all the molecules that protect the brain are lowered.

One way to increase the baby's blood glucose is for the mother and baby to be skin to skin. This is true even if the baby is born premature or small for his gestational age and even if he isn't fed.

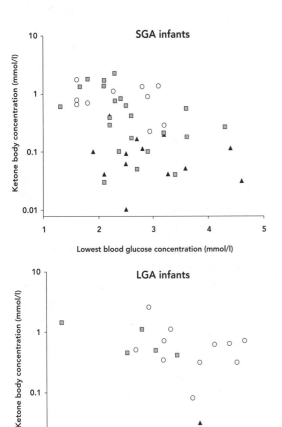

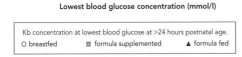

This chart shows normal blood sugar levels in newborn babies. The glucose level is high at birth and then drops in the first hour or two, sometimes to a level that could be considered hypoglycemic. However, this is normal. After about an hour the blood sugar will rise, even if the baby has not been fed!

SOURCE: **PEDIATRICS.ORG**

Note that a baby who is *large* for gestational age but whose mother is *not* diabetic is *not* at risk for low blood glucose. Even in Baby-Friendly hospitals it is sometimes assumed that a baby of 4 or 4.5 kg at birth is at risk for low blood sugar, but this is false.

Why is the infant of the diabetic mother particularly at risk?

When a pregnant woman has diabetes that is not well controlled, she risks having elevated blood glucose, which also raises her baby's blood glucose. The baby responds by producing insulin. Insulin is a growth hormone, so the fetus tends to grow bigger than average. When the baby is born, he no longer gets glucose from the mother, but his insulin stays high for 24 hours or more. The insulin removes glucose from his bloodstream, so now his glucose levels will drop and he may become hypoglycemic. On top of that, insulin inhibits the breakdown of fat to make ketone bodies. So, not only may the baby's concentration of plasma glucose be low, but also he cannot compensate, *as normal babies would*, by increasing the production of ketone bodies, putting this baby at risk.

Controlling the pregnant woman's glucose levels helps prevent this problem. It also helps to avoid giving the mother intravenous glucose during labour. Having the baby skin to skin and starting feeding immediately after birth, the mother can help prevent and treat hypoglycemia in her baby. A little colostrum is much better to prevent low blood glucose than a lot of formula, because, unlike formula, colostrum does not stimulate the baby's production of insulin.

If the baby needs to be treated, I would prefer an intravenous infusion of glucose rather than formula. There is some research indicating that supplementation with cow's milk formula increases the baby's risk of later developing diabetes. The mother can still breastfeed while the baby has an intravenous. On the other hand, a baby stuffed with formula may

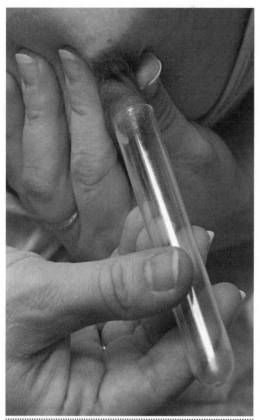

Prenatal expression of colostrum.

CREDIT: **ANDREA POLOKOVA**

"I had a woman last week with insulin depen-dent diabetes mellitus (gestational, but probably pre-existing too) who had unstable blood sugars in pregnancy and labour. She expressed colostrum into microcollect tubes (for blood), which store about 1.5 ml each. She birthed a baby weighing 3.8 kg and the baby was given 3 ml of colostrum immediately. He was kept warm and had a very good breastfeeding soon after birth. Blood sugars never went below 3.4 mmol/litre (61 mg%) and he never had formula, only the stored colostrum and breastfeeding. Each 'top-up' was very small—no more than 3 ml at the most."

Some health professionals are concerned that expressing colostrum before the baby is born may lead to premature labour. At the hospital in New Zealand mentioned above, in response to this ques-tion, the chief of obstetrics wrote that they have not had an increase in premature births since starting prenatal expression of colostrum in 2005. Since breastfeeding a toddler several times a day during pregnancy (as many women do) doesn't increase the risk of premature birth, why would a few minutes of hand expression do so?

Does the baby of a diabetic mother need to be in the special care unit?

Not necessarily. A recent study stated: "Neonatal care with rooming-in mothers with type 1 diabetes and their newborn infants seems safe and is associated with reduced neonatal morbidity when compared with routine separation of infants from their moth-ers." To assure adequate feeding and prevent hypo-glycemia, it is best for the mother and baby to be skin to skin rather than separated.

What about the mother who has gestational diabetes?

Gestational diabetes is different from type 1 dia-betes, but if the mother's blood glucose levels are

not take the breast, and a baby used to a bottle nip-ple may have trouble latching.

Prenatal expression of colostrum

I encourage mothers whose babies are at risk of low blood glucose after the birth to start expressing milk *before* the baby is born. They can start at about 35 or 36 weeks gestation, and even if they get only 1 ml per day, that's 14 ml (1/2 oz.) in two weeks. (Can't get any? That does *not* mean there won't be enough milk later.) Here is an email I received from a lactation consultant in New Zealand, where this approach is now routine for pregnant women with high-risk pregnancies:

high, the baby is at risk of hypoglycemia. However, once again, this does not mean that he should be separated from the mother and given formula. The mother with gestational diabetes could also consider prenatal expression of colostrum.

A study published in the *Journal of Human Nutrition and Dietetics* in 2009 showed that infants of mothers with gestational diabetes who were breastfed in the delivery room had *higher* levels of glucose than babies who were given formula. This is completely contrary to what most pediatricians believe—that breastmilk is inadequate to maintain the baby's glucose and that babies at risk must be given formula. But breastfeeding itself and close skin-to-skin contact maintain the baby's glucose better than formula and separation from the mother. Here are a couple of quotes from this study:

- ". . . Infants breastfed in the delivery room had significantly higher mean blood glucose levels compared to infants who were not breastfed in the delivery room."
- ". . . Breastfed infants had a significantly higher mean blood glucose level compared to those who were formula fed for their first feed."

The "problem" of jaundice

Jaundice is another condition that often leads to babies being separated from their mothers in hospital and/or getting formula, often by bottle.

Here's what happens when a baby is jaundiced. Bilirubin (the pigment that causes the yellow colour of the skin) comes mostly from the breakdown of red blood cells. The bilirubin, which is fat soluble (or unconjugated), is not easily disposed of, so it is carried to the liver and changed to a water-soluble (or conjugated) form, then excreted with the bowel movements. However, there is always a small percentage of bilirubin that

Bilirubin Metabolism

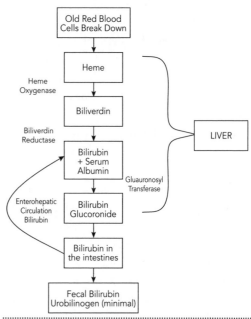

A simplified chart showing how bilirubin is metabolized and how poor breastmilk intake in the first few days can lead to higher bilirubin levels. Stopping breastfeeding is not the solution to higher-than-average bilirubin levels—in fact, providing breastfeeding help should be the first indicated option.

becomes fat soluble again and is reabsorbed into the body from the intestines.

Newborn babies get what is called physiological jaundice ("physiological" means normal) because their red blood cells break down more rapidly than an adult's—a newborn has more red blood cells per millilitre of blood than an adult—and his liver has less of the enzyme that converts the bilirubin that can be eliminated from the body. This is normal, and no treatment is needed.

If jaundice is normal, why do people worry so much about it?

Because *sometimes* it's a sign of a more serious problem. In the past, for example, when rhesus negative (Rh-) mothers had rhesus positive (Rh+) babies, the mother's antibodies might destroy the baby's red blood cells, causing severe jaundice. This happens because sometimes during pregnancy some of the baby's blood gets into the mother's system, and the mother's body creates antibodies against the Rh+ factor on the baby's red blood cells. These antibodies enter the baby's blood and attack his red blood cells, which break down and cause severe jaundice at birth, often leading to brain damage. This severe condition has almost been eliminated thanks to the injection of Rhogam given during pregnancy to Rh- mothers, but fear lingers. Furthermore, there are other serious conditions where jaundice is a symptom.

Today, there is increasing evidence that bilirubin, in small amounts, is an anti-oxidant and *beneficial*. A recent study showed that premature babies whose bilirubin levels were high, but not too high, had less damage to the retina (a problem for very premature babies) than if the bilirubin levels were lower.

What is the link between jaundice and breastfeeding?

Many pediatricians and other physicians believe that breastmilk causes higher levels of bilirubin in the first few days of life. Not true. But the reason that some breastfed babies are more jaundiced is that they are *not* breastfeeding well and are not getting enough breastmilk. That means the baby will also not have substantial enough bowel movements to remove the bilirubin in his intestine and prevent it from being absorbed back into the body. The answer is not to give formula, but to help the mother with the latching on of the baby and making sure he is breastfeeding well (see how this is done earlier in the chapter). Then he will poop more (because colostrum is a laxative) and the bilirubin will decrease. In

most cases no supplementation is needed; if it does become necessary it should be given by a lactation aid at the breast, in this order of preference:

1. The mother's own expressed breastmilk.
2. Banked breastmilk.
3. The mother's own expressed breastmilk with added 5% glucose so that there is enough volume.
4. Formula. This should be used only if we cannot get the baby breastfeeding well and the first choices do not work.

There are other causes of higher-than-average bilirubin levels in the first few days, but none require the mother to stop breastfeeding.

Phototherapy ("light therapy") for newborn babies with jaundice

Phototherapy involves exposing the baby to light (using special lights) that will change the bilirubin into the water-soluble type we described earlier. The baby is usually naked, or wearing just a diaper, and his eyes are covered to protect them from the bright light. Most often phototherapy is done with the baby in an incubator but blankets with lights in them are available in some hospitals.

Over the past 10 to 15 years, it has been recognized that phototherapy has been overused as a treatment for jaundice. Sometimes it is very useful, but if the problem is that breastfeeding is not going well, phototherapy is not the solution.

Too often the baby is admitted to the hospital, phototherapy for a day or two brings down the bilirubin, and the baby is discharged—but the real problem is not fixed. Hospitalization *may be* necessary for babies with significant jaundice in the first week of life. Since infection can sometimes be the cause of increased bilirubin and weight loss at the same time, the prudent pediatrician will want to bring the newborn into the hospital for tests and treatment. Jaundice and dehydration often go together. What is surprising is that many pediatricians still think the jaundice is due to something in the breastmilk and that the dehydration is due to the fact that the baby is not getting breastmilk, *at the same time*. How does that work?

Phototherapy can interfere with breastfeeding if the baby is kept in an incubator and separated from his mother. What can be done?

- There is no need for the baby to be constantly under the lights, so he can be removed from the incubator and fed as often as he shows interest. However, the lack of stimulation (the baby's eyes are covered to protect them) and the heat in the incubator may make the baby sleepier and less likely to signal hunger. He may also sleep more because he is not feeding well. Many health professionals believe that jaundice itself makes the baby sleepy, but unless the bilirubin level is extremely high, this is probably not true. If the baby feeds well, he'll wake up.
- Phototherapy should be done in the mother's room, rather than in the nursery, so she'll be able to watch the baby for cues that he wants to eat. There are "bili-blankets" that wrap around the baby and deliver phototherapy without him being in the incubator. With these, the mother can hold her baby, although not skin to skin because of the blanket. The baby in the blanket also doesn't need a blindfold to protect his eyes, as he would under overhead lights, so he may be more alert. The blankets may be somewhat less effective, but since the main problem in most cases is that the baby is not feeding well, improving breastfeeding should be the priority.
- Phototherapy is said to increase the baby's requirements for fluids by about 15%. For this reason, mothers are told they must give the baby a supplement, usually formula. However, many of the babies admitted for jaundice and dehydration are already on intravenous fluids, and IV is a better way to rehydrate the baby than formula. If an IV is not in place, supplementing with 5% glucose water (using a lactation aid at the breast) would be more appropriate to replace fluid loss than formula. But still, the first choice would be the mother's own milk, and the second choice would be banked breastmilk.

"Breastmilk jaundice"

Breastmilk jaundice, by definition, does not occur in the first days of life, but it seems best to continue the discussion of jaundice here.

Many mothers are told to discontinue breastfeeding at 3 to 10 weeks because their babies continue to be jaundiced (they have "elevated" bilirubin levels, also called hyberbilirubinemia).

The baby who is fed formula is rarely jaundiced after the first week or two of life and when he is, something is likely medically wrong. So doctors assume that if the exclusively breastfed, well-gaining baby is still jaundiced after the first week or two, there must be something wrong. But this, again, is turning the world upside down.

So-called breastmilk jaundice is actually the *norm* for exclusively breastfed, well-gaining babies for as long as three months or more after the birth. Most of the time the jaundice is not very obvious, but if you look carefully, you can often see a subtle yellow tinge to the baby's skin. In some cases, especially if at least one parent is Asian or Native Canadian, the jaundice is more obvious, and then doctors worry.

Here is the most important statement in this whole section: if the baby is exclusively breastfed (or breastmilk fed), gaining weight well and abnormalities causing jaundice are ruled out, jaundice is normal.

What are some abnormalities that can cause higher levels of bilirubin after the first week or two?

There are, essentially, two types of jaundice that occur in babies after the first week or so of life. One is due to increased levels of indirect reacting bilirubin (also called fat-soluble or unconjugated bilirubin). This is the most common type of jaundice, both during the first few days after birth as well as in the weeks after. When it occurs after the first week or so, and if the baby is breastfeeding well and gaining well, it is normal.

The other type of jaundice is due to a build-up of direct reacting bilirubin (also called water-soluble or conjugated bilirubin). The most common cause of this type of jaundice is a problem with the baby's liver.

The two types of jaundice can be distinguished clinically. The direct reacting bilirubin appears in the urine and turns it brownish or even brown if there is enough. The colour is not due to the urine being highly concentrated. A baby with only elevated indirect reacting bilirubin will have clear or slightly yellowish urine if he is well hydrated. If the baby has a liver problem, the liver and often the spleen will be enlarged, a finding that any physician should be able to note on physical examination.

Jaundice caused by elevated direct bilirubin

This type of jaundice is *always abnormal* and frequently very serious and needs immediate investigation to find out the cause and get treatment underway. If the baby's urine is brownish or brown, especially if he is drinking well, the doctor should see him as soon as possible. Here are *some* causes of this type of jaundice:

1. **Biliary atresia.** Blockage of the duct from the liver to the intestine is called biliary atresia. Conjugated bilirubin cannot get to the gut and so it regurgitates into the bloodstream and comes out in the urine. There are variations on the classical complete blockage of the duct (partial blockage, for example). Treatment as early as possible to prevent cirrhosis of the liver is necessary.

2. **Galactosemia.** Galactosemia is a rare problem due to a hereditary inability to metabolize and use galactose, one of the two sugars that make up lactose (the other is glucose). Liver disease due to galactosemia should be rare now because most jurisdictions screen for galactosemia in the days after birth, before liver damage can occur. With galactosemia in which the baby has little or no enzyme to metabolize galactose, breastfeeding is contraindicated. There are milder forms which may allow for continued breastfeeding. Some other inherited metabolic problems, even rarer than galactosemia, can also cause liver disease and an elevated level of direct bilirubin. Tyrosinemia, still very rare but apparently more common in French Canadians, is one of these.

3. **Hepatitis.** Hepatitis, a viral infection of the liver, causes jaundice of this type. It is rare in newborn babies but it can occur.

4. **Drugs, toxins.** Drugs and toxins can cause injury to the liver. This would be unusual in the newborn baby, but it can sometimes be caused by drug use by the mother during pregnancy.

Except for galactosemia, *none* of the above causes of direct hyperbilirubinemia requires the mother to stop breastfeeding. On the contrary, a baby who is sick needs breastmilk and breastfeeding even more than one who is in good health.

Why is it not a bad thing to be jaundiced even six weeks or longer after birth?

Although "breastmilk jaundice" is not a bad thing—and is, in fact, normal—many pediatricians worry about it. However, there is now ample evidence that being jaundiced for six weeks or more is not dangerous for the breastfed baby as long as he is gaining well. Since the breastfed baby is the norm, what is abnormal is *not to be jaundiced*. I call this abnormality "absence of jaundice in the artificially fed baby."

There is evidence that breastfeeding protects the baby's cells from damage from oxygen free radicals. This is a good thing.

What else besides breastmilk jaundice might cause a two- or three-week-old baby to be jaundiced, aside from liver problems?

1. **The baby is not getting enough breastmilk.** Just as a baby can have jaundice because he is not getting enough milk at two or three days of age, a baby who is not getting enough milk at three weeks can be jaundiced. The jaundice is a marker for the real problem.

   Actually, babies who are exclusively breastfeeding but *not* gaining well often are *not* jaundiced. This is yet more evidence that it is a good thing, not a bad thing, to be jaundiced. The solution is not to stop breastfeeding, but to fix the breastfeeding so that the baby gets more breastmilk. If supplementation is necessary, it should be done with a lactation aid at the breast. See the chapter "Increasing Breastmilk Intake by the Baby."

2. **The baby could be breaking down red blood cells even weeks after birth.** This would be unusual, but it can occur. For example, a baby who has a condition called G6PD deficiency will break down his red blood cells if given or exposed to certain medications. There would be no reason at all to interrupt breastfeeding for this reason (but there is a reason to stop, or switch, the medication).

3. **There are some inherited enzyme deficiencies that can result in prolonged jaundice.** Gilbert's syndrome is probably the most common cause of slightly elevated bilirubin and prolonged elevated levels of bilirubin aside from normal breastmilk jaundice. People with Gilbert's syndrome have a lifelong elevation of bilirubin that often increases due to stress or infection. People with Gilbert's syndrome have a significantly decreased risk of atherosclerosis (hardening of the arteries, now thought to be an inflammatory disease), again suggesting that bilirubin, at least when elevated only slightly, actually protects the body's cells from injury. There is no reason to interrupt breastfeeding for Gilbert's syndrome for the much more severe problem called Crigler-Najjar syndrome.

Should breastfeeding be interrupted to prove the diagnosis of breastmilk jaundice?

The baby with "breastmilk jaundice" is usually thriving, content, drinks well at the breast and happens to have a yellow colour to his skin and eyes. Because there is no evidence that the jaundice causes the baby any short-term or long-term harm, and may actually be good for him, why interrupt breastfeeding even for 24 or 48 hours? Twenty-four to 48 hours on the bottle may result in problems with breastfeeding after. Even if the baby does not refuse the breast, he may fuss when the flow of milk slows, whereas before he would wait patiently for the milk to flow again. The mother may develop sore nipples because the baby does not latch on as well as he did before, because he has adopted the bottle-type sucking after 24 to 48 hours of artificial nipples. If there were a reason to bring down the bilirubin, that would be one thing, but there isn't. The baby in the next photo is six weeks old and still jaundiced. But he is also exclusively breastfed,

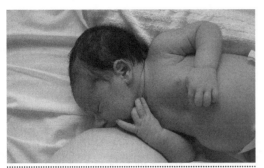

This six-week-old baby has jaundice. He has been exclusively breastfed, he is gaining well and there is no suggestion he might have liver disease. Jaundice is normal and not of concern!

CREDIT: JACK NEWMAN

gaining weight at a terrific rate and alert, content and developing normally. His urine is clear as water, his liver and spleen are not enlarged, he breastfeeds beautifully. Does he have breastmilk jaundice? Well, he has *normal* jaundice. Should we interrupt breastfeeding for 24 to 48 hours? Absolutely not!

A few tests, perhaps to rule out an infection in the urine, to make sure the problem is not in the liver, might be helpful to reassure everyone, but exclusive breastfeeding should continue. Stopping breastfeeding is not a treatment for urinary infection. In fact, withholding the immune factors found in breastmilk from the baby may actually make the situation worse.

So, let's not panic about breastmilk jaundice. It is normal and it may even be good for the baby to have an elevated bilirubin.

Should we put the baby under bilirubin lights (phototherapy) if he has breastmilk jaundice?

The guidelines for treating jaundice issued by all pediatric professional societies that I know of say the need for phototherapy depends very much on how old the baby is and how quickly the bilirubin

rises. The older the baby, the less we need to be concerned about the high level of the bilirubin. So, for example, a rate of 350 µmol/litre (20 mg%) at three days of age is much more worrisome than the same level at three weeks of age, *if* the baby is gaining well and otherwise healthy. With typical breastmilk jaundice, the bilirubin does not rise quickly, if at all. After the first few weeks of relatively slow rise, it tends to decrease slowly until it is gone by three months of age, often sooner. Only if the bilirubin is extraordinarily high would phototherapy be indicated (plus appropriate tests to determine the cause), and breastfeeding should continue.

The following email clarifies the odd situation in which mothers of babies with breastmilk jaundice find themselves. This woman was told to stop breastfeeding for *three* days (longer than I'd ever heard). "I think it is a bit odd that the doctors were really adamant about feeding him every three hours (*by the clock!*) in the hospital and making sure he was nursing really well before we went home, and now they think that is what is making him *sick*. I guess what I am emailing you for is to see if I can get a more clear explanation for this and for my child's *affliction*."

The word "affliction" makes the baby's jaundice sound like a problem of biblical proportions. Imagine how stressful this is for the parents! The mother believes her baby is sick, when in fact he is fine. This whole question of breastmilk jaundice has caused so much pain and heartache for parents. And all for nothing.

While it's worrying to be told your baby has hypoglycemia or jaundice, in the vast majority of cases he can continue to breastfeed exclusively and the situation is far from dire. In fact, most of the time, these babies are just normal.

7 | The Preterm Baby

Myth #1: Premature babies cannot breastfeed exclusively.

Fact: Of course they can. A very premature baby may not be able to actually feed at the breast at first, but he can have his mother's milk until he is ready to breastfeed—and he is ready long before most neonatologists think. With good help and encouragement, the mother can produce enough milk and soon have the baby breastfeeding. Unfortunately, most neonatal intensive care units (NICUs) do not provide this help.

Myth #2: Premature babies need to be cared for in incubators.

Fact: The data are clear. Premature babies are *usually* better off when cared for in Kangaroo Mother Care (KMC), where they are skin to skin with the mother. The baby is usually more stable with regard to his breathing, heart function, blood pressure, blood sugar and temperature when skin to skin than in an incubator. The mother produces more milk and the baby is more likely to get breastfeeding earlier and better.

Myth #3: All premature babies need to have their mother's milk "fortified."

Fact: Rubbish. Perhaps the most premature of prematures, those who in the past would never have survived and for whom breastmilk was not designed, require "fortification" of their mother's milk. However, in some places, virtually any baby born before 37 weeks gestation receives "fortified"

breastmilk (if he is lucky). The less lucky ones get only formula. Some babies are even receiving "fortified" breastmilk after they leave the hospital. Surely if the baby is big and healthy enough to go home, he should do fine on breastmilk alone. Many mothers don't realize that breastmilk "fortifier" is made from cow's milk. There's no reason, really, why it can't be made from human milk.

Myth #4: Premature babies cannot start breastfeeding until they are 34 weeks gestation.

Fact: Outside North America (where this myth is taken as gospel), particularly in Scandinavia, babies start at the breast by 28 weeks gestation. In Sweden, for example, babies are often breastfeeding exclusively by 34 weeks gestation, before we even "allow" them to start in North America.

Myth #5: Breastfeeding is tiring, particularly for the premature baby, much more tiring than bottle-feeding.

Fact: This is not true. This notion arises from the fact that too often too many do not understand how breastfeeding works. Research has shown that breastfeeding is less stressful and less tiring than bottle-feeding for the premature baby.

If we're not good at helping mothers of full-term babies breastfeed, it's not surprising that we're even worse with mothers of the premature babies. Often, especially with a very premature or sick baby, the attitude is "We are dealing with life and death issues here. Be glad your baby is alive. Breastfeeding is of minor importance in the scheme of things." But doctors can do everything necessary to save the baby's life and still not sabotage the breastfeeding. *If the will is there.*

There is often great emphasis on making sure the baby gains weight at the rate he would if still in his mother's womb. But there is no proof that this rate of gain is necessary or even desirable. In fact, there are studies in the medical literature that suggest that too rapid a weight gain is harmful. Nobody really knows how babies would gain if they were born at, say, 32 weeks gestation instead of 40 weeks. Doctors tend to assume that breastmilk alone is not good enough because premature babies don't gain weight as quickly when fed only breastmilk and we can make them gain more if we add "fortifiers." Thus, adding "fortifiers" is deemed a good thing. But we could make a full-term baby gain weight faster by giving only high-calorie formula. Is that a good thing? Given the increasing rates of overweight and obesity in wealthy countries, it is definitely not good by any means.

The importance and the value of Kangaroo Mother Care

Kangaroo Mother Care should be the standard of care for premature babies (and full-term babies as well). Since KMC was spearheaded in the 1980s by Dr. Nathalie Charpak in Bogotá, Colombia, this approach to keeping babies warm, metabolically stable and breastfeeding has been consistently shown to be superior to incubator care, and it results in earlier latching on and better breastfeeding. Because the initial work was done in Colombia, it was often ignored by North American neonatologists, but more and more work in "developed" countries has shown that KMC stabilizes the baby's temperature, blood sugars, heart function, breathing and blood pressure better than an incubator. And the babies cared for with KMC are more likely to breastfeed earlier, better and continue longer and more exclusively.

Premature babies are not in incubators because they are unstable. Premature babies are unstable because they are in incubators. Research shows that unstable babies stabilize more quickly in KMC than in an incubator.

Many of the staff in the special care unit are not comfortable with the whole notion of KMC. It's a big change from the days when babies were in incubators and the staff did all the care. Of course, the smaller and/or the sicker the baby was, the more easily parents were convinced they knew nothing. Often they were and still are intimidated into not advocating for themselves and their babies.

When Teresa's first grandson, Sebastian, was born at 32 weeks, the NICU nurse's first comment to his mother was, "You may be getting pressure to breastfeed, but you should know that breastfeeding isn't always the best thing for a premature baby." Many women would have been intimidated by that comment and, still shell-shocked from the unexpected early arrival of their babies, would have gone along with the "expert's" recommendation to give formula. Fortunately, Sebastian's mother simply introduced the nurse to Teresa (who politely shared some information with her) and continued with her plans to breastfeed (Sebastian never had a drop of formula).

South African doctor Nils Bergman has stated that a baby lying in an incubator, a tiny premature one perhaps even more so, needs the comfort skin-to-skin contact provides. If he doesn't get it, he goes into *despair* and demands nothing; he just lies there not responding—not because he is premature, but because he is not getting the comfort, regulation and stimulation of skin-to-skin contact. All sorts of technological "advances" have been put in place over the years to simulate skin-to-skin contact (though probably not with skin-to-skin contact in mind).

For example, to prevent babies from developing apneas (interruption of breathing for too long) and bradycardias (too slow beating of the heart), rocking beds have replaced non-moving ones. These rocking beds apparently work, but skin-to-skin contact also does this and so much more! A baby skin to skin with mother (or father) moves up and down with every breath the mother takes. If the baby is no longer attached to intravenous lines or monitors, the mother can walk around, further stimulating the baby's breathing and heartbeat.

KMC should be done throughout the day. The baby is naked, except for a diaper, against the mother's bare chest. The baby is kept in place with a special wrap that holds him with his head fixed and face free. In order to keep the baby's trachea open, his head is slightly tilted back in what some call "sniffing position."

As Bergman says: "Skin-to-skin contact and breastfeeding is the means whereby the premature infant continues its gestation."

So what are the benefits of KMC?

1. The baby is likely to have fewer bradycardias and apneas.
2. The baby is less likely to have significant decreases in his oxygenation and thus may need less oxygen. Very premature babies can have serious injury to their retinas, called retinopathy of prematurity, if given too high a concentration of oxygen.
3. The baby's body temperature is better maintained in the normal range.
4. The baby is less likely to have low blood glucose.
5. The baby is less stressed.
6. The baby's immunity is increased and he is more likely to develop the same bacteria as the mother. This is better than being colonized with the "super" bacteria that exist in NICUs.

7. The baby is less lethargic and more aware of his surroundings. His sleep cycles are regulated better and thus after a good sleep he is able to be awake to breastfeed.
8. It helps the baby's brain development.
9. The baby is less likely to cry and be distressed (although of course if his hunger cues are not responded to, he will become distressed).
10. It provides comfort and probably pain relief during painful procedures.
11. The baby benefits from smelling the mother, hearing her voice, feeling her skin, feeling her chest moving and having the opportunity to make attempts at latching on to the breast, all of which eventually lead to breastfeeding.
12. The baby is likely to be discharged earlier from hospital.
13. A better parent–child relationship develops. It is known that babies born prematurely are more likely to be neglected and/or abused. It is very likely that the separation of the parents and the baby (who passes his time in the incubator) and the lack of responsibility given to the parents in the care of the baby have a lot to do with this.
14. The baby is more likely to achieve exclusive breastfeeding in hospital and continue after discharge. KMC increases the desire of the mother to breastfeed and the volume of milk she makes.

Why do premature babies need breastmilk (and breastfeeding, which is not the same thing)?

There is no question that breastmilk is best not only for babies born at term, but also for babies born prematurely. This was not always understood: when I was a resident in pediatrics from 1978 to 1981, we never asked mothers of premature babies if they wanted to breastfeed. The babies were automatically

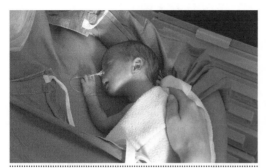

A one-week-old baby born at 28 weeks gestation in skin-to-skin contact with the mother.

CREDIT: **ANDREA POLOKOVA**

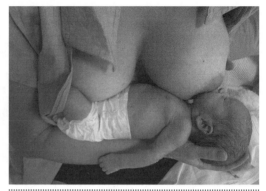

A baby born at 28 weeks gestation, about two weeks old now and actually drinking from the breast. Babies fall asleep at the breast when the flow of milk is slow, but this one is awake—notice the open eyes. The mother's hold would be better if her hand were not on the back of the baby's head, but if it works, it works!

CREDIT: **ANDREA POLOKOVA**

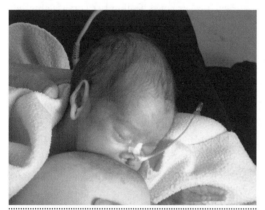

A two-week-old baby born at 28 weeks gestation, latched on!

CREDIT: **ANDREA POLOKOVA**

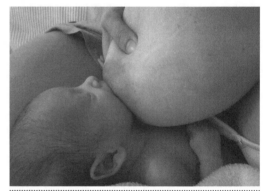

Using compression to get more milk to a 28-week-gestation two-week-old baby.

CREDIT: **ANDREA POLOKOVA**

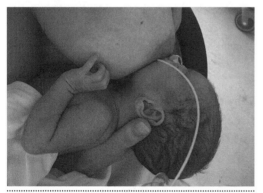

Supplementing the two-week-old premature baby at the breast with a lactation aid. A mother's expressed milk is the preferred supplement. Banked breastmilk is the second choice.

CREDIT: **ANDREA POLOKOVA**

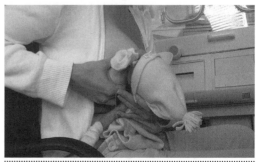

At 30 weeks gestation, this baby is latched on and drinking. No need for test weighing!

CREDIT: **ANDREA POLOKOVA**

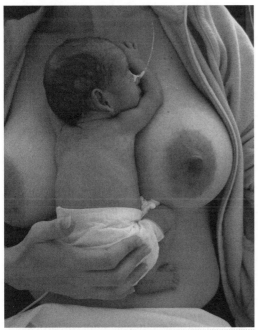

Kangaroo mother care of a 30-week-gestation baby whose body temperature is normal.

CREDIT: **ANDREA POLOKOVA**

given regular formula. Special premature formulas or fortifiers didn't exist. In the six months I spent in the neonatal intensive care unit of Toronto's Hospital for Sick Children, I didn't see one mother putting the baby to the breast. Yes, many of these babies survived and probably developed normally. So why bother with breastmilk anyway?

1. Breastmilk protects against infections. This is crucial for a tiny baby in an NICU, where infections can spread quickly. Infection is thought to be a factor, if not necessarily *the* cause of necrotizing enterocolitis (NEC), a very serious intestinal problem in which parts of the gut actually die. The evidence that breastmilk protects against this is strong. A study from Norway showed that the earlier a baby gets breastmilk, and the sooner he gets it exclusively, the less likely he is to die of sepsis (a blood infection which can affect all parts of the body). This was a study remarkable in its completeness. It looked at the entire population of premature babies born under 1,000 g (a little more than 2 lb) for a whole year in the entire country.

2. Breastmilk contains growth factors that help the baby's body to mature and develop, including epidermal growth factor, which helps the gut develop. That means the nutrients in the milk are absorbed better. Epidermal growth factor may be one of the reasons breastfed babies are less likely to develop NEC. Other factors in the milk include insulin-like growth factor, nerve growth factor and granulocyte colony–stimulating factor, to name just a few.

3. Breastmilk varies according to the gestational age of the baby. It contains what the baby needs at the time he needs it. It is possible that at the extreme of viable prematurity (presently 24 to 25 weeks gestation) this is not the case, but certainly for larger premature babies it is. The baby gets appropriate amounts of docosahexaenoic acid (DHA, an omega-3 fatty acid) and arachidonic acid (ARA, an omega-6 fatty acid). These polyunsaturated long-chained fatty acids seem to be important for the development of the baby's brain and retina and may partially account for why breastfed babies, including premature ones, do better on cognitive tests. Belatedly, these fatty acids have been added to formula, but particularly in premature babies, DHA and ARA are not absorbed well from formula. This is important, as they need to be absorbed in a particular ratio or they may be toxic.

4. In addition to KMC, providing breastmilk is another way the mother participates in the care of her baby. Nothing is as good for the baby as the mother's expressed milk, and she should

know what an important and valuable thing she is doing for her baby. Her milk is the best medicine, her body the ideal habitat.

But aren't preterm formulas and fortifiers designed for premature babies?

These are intended to fix the "deficiencies" of breast-milk, but these "deficiencies" are, in large part, a function of how we feed premature babies. For example, the amounts we give them are very restricted much of the time. Prematures are often fed by the clock, typically every two or three hours. This is not normal for the baby born at term and I don't see why it would be appropriate for the baby born prematurely. When I worked in southern Africa for 18 months, a large part of my work involved overseeing the special care nursery. About 10% of babies born there were premature or small for gestational age, so we had many patients. No formula or bottles could be used in the hospital; both were forbidden, no exceptions. So I couldn't use high-calorie formulas to help the babies grow. What could I do?

I could increase the amount of breastmilk the baby received. In most NICUs, babies are allowed only up to 180 ml of fluid/kg/day. In some NICUs, it's even less than that. For babies on respirators, it makes sense to limit their intake of fluids because with their respiratory problems large amounts of fluid could cause heart failure or aggravate it, making it difficult to get them off the respirator. But given the lack of high-tech facilities in Africa, our small babies were generally quite healthy and vigorous (if they weren't, they usually died). Believing at that time that the baby should grow at intrauterine rates, I started increasing the amount of breastmilk. At first, very nervously, I went up to 200 ml/kg/day. When that worked for some, I went up to 225 ml/kg/day or even 250, and then 300 for those who still didn't grow as I had wanted. We fed babies through a tube in the stomach, but 24 hours a day, drop by drop, so they never had too much in their stomachs at one time. And most grew quickly.

The "need" for fortifiers and preterm formulas disappears for some babies if we simply give them more breastmilk. It worked in Africa and there is no reason it won't work in North America or Europe.

Fortifiers are also used to provide more calcium and phosphorus to prevent the baby from developing osteopenia (bones with little calcium). This problem often leads to fractures, particularly in the ribs of very premature babies. But the extra calcium and phosphorus can be added to the breastmilk. Vitamin D, if necessary, can also be given to prevent osteopenia.

Some babies do need fortifiers. However, they can be made from human milk rather than cow's milk. There is one company in the United States that makes fortifiers from human milk. Unfortunately, although the mothers who donate their milk are not paid, the formula is very expensive. If we had support for breastmilk banks, perhaps we could use some of that milk to make affordable human milk fortifiers for those cases where it is needed.

How soon can premature babies go to the breast?

It has been "traditional" in North America to wait until the baby is 34 weeks gestation before attempting to put him to the breast, because it is wrongly believed that only then can he coordinate sucking, swallowing and breathing. Kerstin Nyqvist, a Swedish midwife, wrote the following in a study published in *Early Human Development* in 1999: "Restrictions in breastfeeding policies for preterm infants are commonly *based on studies of bottle-feeding* (emphasis added), where it has been established that infants with immature cardio-respiratory control show a less coordinated suck-swallow-breathe pattern, resulting in apnea, hypoxia and bradycardia."

In Nyqvist's study, many babies were latching on by 28 weeks gestation. By 31 weeks, many were drinking milk from the breast. In the article describing the study, it is noted that "Sixty-seven (out of 71) infants were breastfed at discharge. Fifty-seven of them established full breastfeeding at 36.0 weeks (33.4-40.0)." Look at that! At least one baby was fully breastfed (not fed breastmilk in a bottle or by tube, but actually *at the breast*) by 33.4 weeks, a few days before we even start them at the breast in North America.

Is breastfeeding really more tiring for the baby than bottle-feeding?

Many mothers are told this but it simply shows lack of understanding of how breastfeeding works.

Babies respond to milk flow. If flow is fast, the baby will drink and usually remain awake. In other words, it's not the baby who "works" at getting the milk. Of course, the baby does his part by stimulating the breast by sucking, but once the milk flows, the baby drinks, doing less work than if he were drinking milk from a bottle.

At the breast, the baby's sucks stimulate the milk to let down and flow into his mouth. Not much work to that. So why do so many think breastfeeding is harder for the baby? In an NICU, here's how they feed a premie: The amount the baby should get is determined by his weight (perhaps 30 ml per feeding). The baby is weighed. The mother is told to breastfeed no more than 15 or 20 minutes. The baby at some point falls asleep at the breast and is weighed again; he got only 20 ml. The baby is then given the rest by bottle; he wakes up and sucks vigorously. The staff conclude incorrectly that breastfeeding is too tiring because the baby fell asleep before getting "enough."

To start with, is that calculation of 30 ml per feeding correct? The amounts are based on what formula-fed babies get, and formula is not breastmilk. The real story is that babies respond to milk flow, not to what is in the breast. To observe this phenomenon, see the video "Inserting a Lactation Aid" at the International Breastfeeding Centre YouTube Channel (http://youtu.be/g1CYw1uTiG4).

So how do we help the premature baby get more milk? The same way we do with any full-term baby:

1. Get the best latch possible. See the chapter "The First Few Days."
2. Know how to recognize when the baby is getting milk rather than just sucking. See the video clips of babies drinking well at the breast, and not, at the International Breastfeeding Centre YouTube Channel (http://youtube.com/user/IBCToronto).
3. Use compression to keep up the flow. See the video clips that show mothers using compression and the description in the chapter "Increasing Breastmilk Intake by the Baby."
4. If the baby needs more, supplements can be given with a lactation aid at the breast (not finger feeding). See the chapter "Increasing Breastmilk Intake by the Baby."

Latching the premature baby on to the breast

Latching a premature baby on to the breast is really no different from latching on a full-term baby. If the baby is skin to skin with the mother, the mother will notice that he is showing interest in feeding and she won't have to wait until two or three hours have passed to feed him. She can let him find the breast on his own, with a little guidance. If this doesn't work, the description of how to latch on a full-term baby can be found in the chapter "The First Few Days"; the process can work just as well with a premature baby as with a full-term one.

What about using a nipple shield to help the baby latch on?

A baby on a nipple shield is not latched on. He can't get a good amount of breast into his mouth so at best he's sucking on the nipple with a plastic covering. At worst, he is just sucking on the shield and there is virtually no breast tissue inside the nipple part of the shield. I believe that a nipple shield for a premature baby is just as bad as for a full-term one. The ultimate result, in many cases, is a decrease in milk production so that it becomes very difficult to get the baby on the breast. As the milk supply decreases, the mother starts giving formula and the situation just continues to deteriorate.

If we were not in such a rush, if we did more Kangaroo Mother Care, if we really helped the mother with latching on, we wouldn't "need" nipple shields.

Weighing the baby before and after a feeding to see how much he got

This is not helpful. We don't know how much a breastfeeding baby is supposed to get at a feeding anyway. Instead, watch for the open-pause-close type of sucking to know if the baby is feeding well.

Does "nipple confusion" exist in the premature baby?

Mothers are frequently told that "nipple confusion," where the baby prefers the bottle nipple to the breast, just does not exist in premature babies. Clearly this is not true; we see it all the time. In too many NICUs, mothers are told that the baby has to show he can feed from a bottle before he can go home. Why not make sure the baby can feed well at the breast? There is no reason bottles need to be used. Premature babies are often fed at first with a tube in the stomach. By 28 or more weeks, some can start drinking from an open cup and, at the same time, can start going to the breast. The bottle will not be necessary. And if the baby needs to be supplemented, it should be done with a lactation aid at the breast.

The near-term baby (born at 35 to 37 weeks gestation)

I've heard these babies called the "great pretenders," presumably because they "pretend" to breastfeed. Since they are not really getting milk, they run into problems of dehydration and/or jaundice.

Mothers of near-term babies also often don't get good help with breastfeeding. Teach the mother how to know what a good latch is and how to get the best one possible. Show the mother how to know if her baby is drinking at the breast. Use breast compression to increase the flow of milk to the baby. If the baby needs supplementation, it should be done with a lactation aid at the breast.

This approach works for more premature and more mature babies. Why should the situation be special if the baby happens to be born at 36 weeks gestation?

PART III:

Common Problems and Solutions

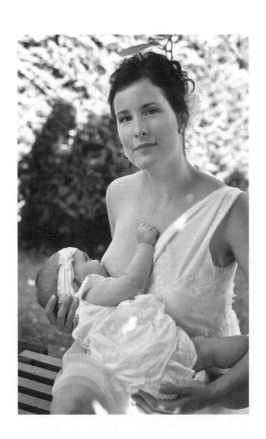

8 | Increasing Breastmilk Intake by the Baby

Myth #1: Many women cannot produce enough milk.
Fact: Many women *seem* not to produce enough milk, but could produce enough if they were given the help and support they need.

Myth #2: If the mother cannot produce enough milk, it is better to just formula feed.
Fact: Unfortunately, too many people, including health professionals, feel this way. But why is *some* breastmilk worse than none at all? Must it be said? Some breastmilk *is* better than none. True, there are undoubtedly some women who really cannot produce enough milk, but they should be encouraged to breastfeed, supplementing (ideally with donated breastmilk) at the breast with a lactation aid. Breastfeeding is much more than breastmilk!

Is it really a problem of milk supply?

We mention this first because often mothers believe that they are not producing enough milk when in fact they have plenty.

When a mother brings a baby in for a well-baby check, the baby is weighed and measured, and these two numbers are plotted on a graph. For many years, the graphs came from the U.S. Centre for Disease Control and were based on records of babies who were primarily *fed formula* (and who grew into a population of children and adults with very high levels of overweight and obesity). More recently, the World Health Organization (WHO) has developed growth standards based on *exclusively breastfed babies*.

Growth charts are marked with curved lines that indicate percentiles. A baby boy whose weight is at the 25th percentile for his age, for example, weighs less than 75% of other boy babies, and more than 24% of them.

The percentile is not a score on a test: it is not better to be at the 99th percentile, or worse to be at the 3rd percentile. All the babies whose weights are recorded are healthy and normal, so if one is on the 3rd percentile and following that curve, his weight gain is normal. Somebody (a healthy, normal somebody) *must* be on the 3rd percentile!

Generally, over time, the baby's weight follows one of the curved lines. But he won't necessarily follow it exactly, because the lines are averages of hundreds of babies. Dr. Adriano Cattano, an Italian epidemiologist who has been involved with creating the WHO growth charts, points out that about 18% of these normal, healthy babies will drop down one or two z-scores (essentially, one or two standard deviations) at some point during their first six months.

So sometimes a mother brings her baby for a weight check and is told that he has dropped down to a lower curve on the growth chart. This may be because the doctor is still using the older charts, not the WHO charts. Or it may be that the baby is one of the 18% who drop a few percentiles normally. But the mother may be told she needs to supplement with formula or even wean. In reality, there may not be a problem at all.

A mother might worry that she doesn't have enough milk because the baby nurses "frequently." Yet many babies feed more often than every three or even every two hours.

Peter Hartmann and other researchers in Perth, Australia, have suggested, based on their research, that some mothers have a greater milk storage capacity than others. A mother who has a greater milk storage capacity can offer her baby more milk at each feeding, so he nurses less often. A mother who has a smaller milk storage capacity will need to feed more often because the baby will get less at each feeding. The babies of both these mothers will get more or less the same amount of milk over 24 hours but the mother whose storage capacity is smaller will need to feed more often.

Mothers also worry when their babies seem to cry a lot. Sometimes this is because they've been told to feed the baby for 10 or 15 or 20 minutes on each breast, every three or four hours. This leads to a lot of crying for many babies. If the mother has a lot of milk, the baby may still grow well, so the crying is interpreted as colic. Sometimes mothers are told to feed the baby on one breast at each feeding so the baby gets more "hind milk" (higher-fat milk), or to feed on one breast for two or more feedings in a row. Or worse, something called "block feeding" is recommended, which means that the mother is told to feed the baby on the same breast for several feedings (sometimes for as long as 12 hours). Feeding the baby on just one side can decrease milk production to the point where he is not getting enough. Or a mother may be told that her baby cries because he's allergic to her milk and she should switch to formula. The sad thing is that often when the mother gives formula, the hungry baby now becomes happier, and the mother is convinced that something was wrong with her milk. All this comes from poor teaching of breastfeeding, silly rules about how to breastfeed, and undermining the mother's confidence in breastfeeding.

Are there women who truly cannot produce enough milk?

Yes, there are, but we don't know how many. Until every mother gets a good start with breastfeeding and receives the help and support she needs, we won't know how common true insufficient milk supply is. It *seems* that in tribal societies insufficient milk supply is a rarity, but we really don't have research to back this up. Maybe there are women in such societies who do not produce enough milk, but their babies are fed some of the time by other mothers in the community, so that the babies gain weight just fine.

It was a woman about to adopt a new baby who helped me understand that not having enough milk is a disappointment for many women, but that *breastfeeding is about much more than the milk*. She was the first woman I encountered who wanted to breastfeed an adopted baby. When I said that I didn't think she could produce a lot of milk, her answer was (and I remember her words as if it were yesterday), "I don't care. I want to breastfeed my baby and if the baby also gets breastmilk that will be a bonus."

Some causes of insufficient milk
Breast surgery

Breast reduction surgery, as it is often done, can be a problem. I believe it is the incision around the areola, cutting through some of the ducts leading to the nipple, that is the reason for milk production problems. It is also possible that cutting the nerves to and from the nipple and areola plays a part. Removal of breast tissue likely also has some effect, but I think the incision is significant because women who have had breast augmentation with a similar incision have milk production problems despite not losing breast tissue. Also, women who

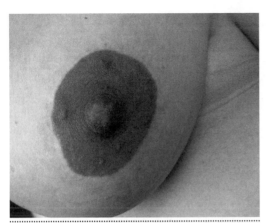

The appearance of the breast after surgery for breast reduction. The incision around the areola seriously compromises milk production. This type of incision, for any reason, should be avoided. Even an incision around part of the areola may decrease milk supply.

CREDIT: **JACK NEWMAN**

have a biopsy of a breast often notice a difference in milk supply from the affected breast even though no breast tissue was removed and the incision around the areola is only partial.

There does seem to be a relationship between how complete the incision is and how much milk production declines. An incision around the whole areola is associated with a significant decrease; an incision only a centimetre or two is associated with a lesser effect on milk supply.

The photo below, left, shows exactly how *not* to make an incision to drain a breast abscess. The mother's milk supply on that side may be compromised for this baby and also for future ones. Furthermore, she will probably not be able to feed on that side for several days because it would be quite painful. See the chapter "Sore Breasts" on the best treatment for a breast abscess.

The photo below, right, shows an incision done for a biopsy of a breast lump. If this incision had been done perpendicular to the actual incision, and farther away from the areola, it would have helped to protect breastfeeding. Surely surgeons should try to maintain the function of the body part they are operating on. What is the function of the breast? Making milk! It is certainly worth at least an attempt not to sabotage future milk supply.

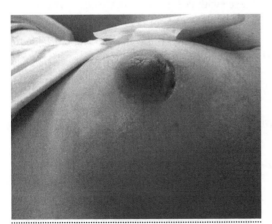

A periareolar incision for a breast abscess. The mother had asked the surgeon not to make this sort of incision, but he did it anyway! See the chapter on sore breasts for a much *better* way of treating a breast abscess.

CREDIT: **ALISON BARRETT**

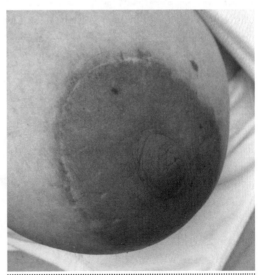

This incision was made for a biopsy of a lump. The woman's milk supply is very decreased on this side. Making the incision further back would have allowed for more normal breastfeeding function.

CREDIT: **JACK NEWMAN**

On the other hand, even if a mother has had breast reduction surgery, she may produce enough milk. In 2007 we had a mother of twins breastfeed exclusively for six months, even after breast reduction surgery.

Too often hospital staff assume the mother who has had a breast reduction won't make enough milk, and encourage supplementation. But these mothers *seem* to produce enough colostrum, even though they might not get a full milk supply. Supplementation should never be automatic and is *not usually* indicated in the first few days. Good help during this period will increase the mother's chances of making enough milk.

I try to help mothers with breast reduction have realistic expectations, without ruling out the possibility that they will produce enough milk. If supplementation is necessary, it should be given with a lactation aid at the breast, because then the mother and baby are breastfeeding. If the mother wishes, we suggest she start fenugreek and blessed thistle from the day of the baby's birth, as well as domperidone, three tablets (30 mg) three times a day. Though domperidone does not usually work well in the first few weeks, it does *sometimes*, and I think it is worth a try.

Retained placental fragments

If a piece of placenta remains attached to the uterus after the baby is born, it may continue to produce pregnancy hormones and the milk won't "come in."

One sign of a retained placental fragment is recurrence of vaginal bleeding and/or cramping, sometimes days or weeks after the baby was born.

A problem with milk production associated with a return of bleeding and cramps suggests the doctor should check (with ultrasound) to see if any fragments are left. A blood test (showing elevated HCG) can also suggest a piece of retained placenta.

Endocrine Syndromes

Sheehan's syndrome. Sheehan's syndrome occurs when blood loss during the labour and birth is so great that the mother's blood pressure falls dangerously low. When this happens, the pituitary gland, which secretes prolactin, oxytocin and other hormones, is damaged or even dies, so there are no hormones to make the milk or cause letdown (milk ejection reflex). I have not always been enamoured with modern obstetric practice, but certainly one huge improvement has been the virtual elimination of Sheehan's syndrome. Rapid intervention when blood loss is significant can prevent it.

Some lactation consultants feel that significant blood loss, even if it is not so great as to cause a drop in blood pressure, can also cause a decrease in milk supply. But if the pituitary is not damaged, there should be no problem with milk supply simply because of blood loss.

Polycystic ovarian syndrome (PCOS). This syndrome, which is quite variable in its manifestations, is associated with multiple hormonal abnormalities. Women with PCOS may be overweight, have hirsutism (excessive body or facial hair), acne, infertility, glucose intolerance (difficulty metabolizing glucose without necessarily having diabetes), an elevation in male hormones in the blood and cysts in the ovaries. The primary abnormality, apparently, is a problem with the ratio of two hormones from the pituitary gland, luteinizing hormone (LH) and follicle stimulating hormone (FSH). These hormones regulate the development of the ova (eggs) in the ovary and the release of the eggs during the cycle. PCOS is now being diagnosed in more and more women, and I have heard of an incidence as high as 15%.

Women with fertility problems due to PCOS are often treated with a drug called metformin. Because metformin decreases male hormones in the mother's blood, it could, at least in theory, increase the mother's milk supply. We have tried using metformin in women with PCOS. The dose we use is one 500-mg tablet per day for a week, then two tablets a day for a week and so on to a maximum of four tablets per day. Metformin causes considerable stomach upset in many women, which is why we increase the dose gradually and suggest it be taken with food. Because it takes several weeks for metformin to have an effect, we suggest the mother start it toward the end of her pregnancy, around 36 weeks gestation. We are not sure how much metformin helps; however, we never treat "not enough milk" only with metformin, so it's never easy to say what, if anything, is the solution.

Hypothyroidism (low-functioning thyroid gland). Hypothyroidism is frequently cited as a cause of insufficient milk production, but I have never seen any evidence to back this up. Profound hypothyroidism could, presumably, cause problems with milk supply because, essentially, all the body functions slow down in this situation.

Insufficient glandular tissue

Some women's breasts appear not to have developed fully and often these mothers do not produce a full milk supply. However, we have seen many mothers with apparent insufficient glandular tissue who did produce enough milk and whose babies gained well without supplementation. The photo above show a mother with breasts that truly can be classified as having insufficient glandular tissue. This mother did not produce enough milk, but was able, by using a lactation aid, to continue to breastfeed her baby.

Drugs

There is no question that some drugs can decrease milk production. Birth control pills with estrogen

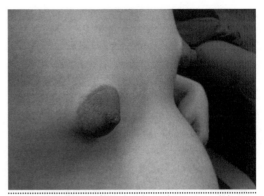

Breasts that did not fully develop. The woman did not produce enough milk but was able to breastfeed using supplementation given by lactation aid at the breast.

CREDIT: **JACK NEWMAN**

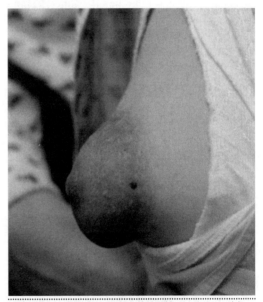

This mother, also with undeveloped breasts, was able to breastfeed exclusively once she received help. The baby gained well, breastfeeding exclusively until four months of age, when solids were added.

CREDIT: **JACK NEWMAN**

and progesterone, or even just progesterone, and IUDs containing hormones, have this effect. Women should at least be warned that this is a possibility, despite what the manufacturer may state.

Two drugs that decrease prolactin and therefore

"turn off" milk production, usually completely, are bromocriptine (Parlodil) and cabergoline (Dostinex).

Drugs used as fertility treatments. Clomiphene (Clomid) does indeed decrease, and even turn off, milk production by increasing maternal estrogen levels. But very little will get into the milk, therefore any worry about exposing the baby is not a reason to interrupt breastfeeding. Other drugs for fertility treatments are usually hormones, given by injection because they are not absorbed when given by mouth. They can also decrease milk production, but the baby won't get any hormone because the hormones are too big to get into the milk. The milk supply will decrease, but if the mother becomes pregnant her milk supply will decrease anyway, so there is no reason to stop breastfeeding. Usually, toddlers who breastfeed mostly for the milk rather than the comfort will stop breastfeeding when the mother becomes pregnant and the milk supply decreases, but many will continue breastfeeding even if little milk is present.

Antihistamines. Antihistamines do, I am fairly certain, decrease the milk supply. Whether they do so in every mother or whether all antihistamines can decrease the milk supply is not possible to say, but many mothers have given a very clear story of antihistamine use followed within only a few days by a decrease in milk supply. If it happened only once, I wouldn't include this information here, but every spring and autumn the emails come in. There are alternatives to oral antihistamines. See the chapter "Late-Onset Decreased Milk Supply."

Other drugs. Other drugs that may decrease milk production are mentioned in the chapter "Late-Onset Decreased Milk Supply."

Poor Breastfeeding

This is the most common cause of a reduced milk intake. In our clinic, since most of our mothers and babies are seen weeks after birth, we cannot always tell which came first: poor breastfeeding resulting in a decreased milk production, or a decreased milk production resulting in poor breastfeeding. In fact, the two can both contribute and reinforce a difficult situation. If the mother's milk is not abundant and the baby is not latched on well, he will mostly nibble at the breast and fall asleep, meaning the breast is not stimulated to make more milk. Mothers (or nurses) sometimes call these babies "lazy." But babies are *not* lazy; they respond to milk flow. See the video clip called "Inserting Lactation Aid" at www.breastfeeding-inc.ca (also on YouTube), which shows how the baby's behaviour changes when he gets more milk.

So how do you increase the milk the baby gets?

How to increase breastmilk intake by the baby
Step 1: Achieve the best latch possible
Our approach to latching on a baby is outlined in the chapter "The First Few Days." What are the features of the ideal latch? I call it an asymmetrical latch. Looking at the baby latched on you see:

- The baby's chin touches the breast but the nose does not. The fact that babies can breathe even if the nose is buried in the breast does not mean it is desirable. An asymmetrical latch seems to work better.
- The baby covers more of the areola with his lower lip than with his upper lip.
- The baby's whole body is tilted slightly upwards so he can look up at his mother.

You can get this ideal latch in any position you choose, but we find the cross-cradle is easiest for

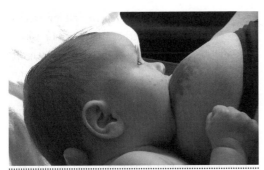

Not a bad latch at all: it's asymmetrical, and the baby is covering more of the areola with his lower lip than his upper lip. The areola is large, and much of it is showing, but the baby has a fair amount of breast in his mouth. His lower lip may be tucked in a little, which can be fixed by pressing gently on the chin for a few seconds while the baby is sucking.

CREDIT: JACK NEWMAN

most new mothers and babies. Many newborns will find the breast and latch on by themselves. Usually, if you start with the cross-cradle hold, you'll want to switch to a cradle hold within two or three weeks naturally if the breastfeeding is going well. If the baby gets a good latch, you are unlikely to have nipple pain, and he will get more milk even if the supply is low. Indeed, the lower the milk supply, the more important it is for the baby to get a good latch.

Sometimes mothers and health professionals will say, "I didn't latch my baby this way—I just latched on any old way and my baby did fine." If you have an abundant milk supply, the baby can latch on "any old way" and still get milk, although you may have sore nipples. However, a poor latch initially, even if the baby gets milk, may cause your milk production to slow down later.

A Swedish study published in *Birth* in 1992 looked at the importance of sucking technique in breastfeeding success. Only exclusively breastfed babies (97% of them in hospital) were included in the study. Babies were classified by a skilled lactation specialist into two groups: those babies who had a good latch and those who didn't. This second

group was then divided randomly into two smaller groups: one whose latch was corrected and another whose latch was not. All groups received the same general information about breastfeeding.

The combined group of babies who had a good latch *plus* those whose poor latch was corrected was compared to the group whose latch was not corrected. The authors stated: "A change-over from breast to bottle within the first month was *10 times more common* in the nipple-sucking group (36%, 9/25) than in those with a correct technique" (my emphasis). Furthermore, "The respective proportions of mothers still breastfeeding, exclusively or partly, were 64% vs 96.5% at one month, 48% vs 84% at 2 months, 44% vs 79% at 3 months, 40% vs 74% at 4 months." Those with a good or corrected latch were far more likely to continue breastfeeding. The researchers commented, "A striking finding in this study was that it was possible to identify and correct a faulty sucking technique (latch) in the maternity ward, and thereby improve the women's chances of achieving successful breastfeeding."

If the mother has problems, the latch usually can be improved. The video clips that show good latching can help mothers learn how. Many lactation consultants teach latching on differently from the way we teach it. I don't have an emotional attachment to the asymmetric latch. I didn't invent it. But when I saw that it worked better, I changed what I was doing.

Step 2: Learn how to recognize when the baby is drinking from the breast and not just sucking

See the video clips that show babies drinking well at the breast, or not (http://youtube.com/user/IBCToronto). Once a mother recognizes that the "pause in the chin" means the baby just got a mouthful of milk, and that the longer the pause the more milk he got, she understands that instructions about how long to breastfeed make no sense. Why stop feeding on the first side after 10 or 20 minutes if the baby is still drinking? Why keep the baby on the breast to get "hind milk" if he is not drinking and is therefore getting very little milk of any kind?

Step 3: Use breast compression

Breast compression can be a very useful tool to help the baby get more milk. While working in South Africa, I would see women walking along the street with the baby at the breast and pressing that breast with their hands. I didn't think much about it until a woman from Chile came to the clinic with her baby, gently squeezing or compressing her breast while the baby was breastfeeding. I asked why. Her first response was that her mother had suggested it. That is a good reason, since the passing on of breastfeeding knowledge to the new generation used to be the domain of more experienced mothers. When I asked why her mother had suggested it, she looked at me as if I were from a different planet and said, "Because the baby gets more milk." And the penny dropped for me. Of course the baby gets more milk!

It is necessary to know when the baby is drinking (step 2) and when he is not. Compression shouldn't be used when the baby is drinking very well or even not too badly. But as the feeding goes on, babies will nibble more and drink less—this is a normal response to the slowdown in milk flow. Of course, mothers can have more milk ejection reflexes later in a feeding so that just as it appears the baby is hardly drinking anymore, he may suddenly start to drink very well again for a period of time.

It is important to understand that, particularly during the first few weeks, babies tend to react to a slow flow of milk by falling asleep, even if they have not yet had enough. After the first few weeks, they tend to pull away rather than just fall asleep. But many babies may vary in their response at different times and even at the same feeding. Some babies pull away when the flow slows, even in the first week or two, whereas some always tend to fall asleep at the breast even at four months or older. For this reason we recommend the mother initiate compressions when the baby is mostly nibbling but still drinking so that he doesn't get too sleepy or pull off the breast when the flow slows down. Here's the technique:

- Be sure you know the difference between when the baby is drinking and just nibbling (step 2). When the baby starts to nibble much of the time but is still having some pauses as he sucks, start compression. Don't compress when the baby isn't sucking at all, or when he's drinking well.
- Put your thumb on one side of the breast and your four fingers flat against the other, as far away from the areola as you can comfortably manage. *As the baby sucks, squeeze your thumb and fingers together, compressing your breast. Pressure should be firm but not painful.* If compression works, the baby will start drinking again. Keep up the steady pressure as long as the baby is drinking, then release once he is not drinking even with the compression.
- After you release the pressure, your baby will probably stop sucking. Wait for him to start again—there is no need to encourage him, he'll start on his own. If he starts to suck and actually drinks (pause!), there's no need to use compression. When the drinking starts to slow down, you can start compressing again.
- You can continue using compressions this way until the baby is falling asleep and stops drinking, or lets go of the breast.

Step 4: Once the baby no longer drinks even with compression, offer the other breast

Repeat the same process, using compression when the baby is sucking but not drinking.

When the baby is not drinking on the second side even with compressions, offer the first breast again if he seems interested. If your nipples aren't sore, you can go back and forth between breasts several times if the baby is willing. The breasts make milk continuously, so the baby *may start drinking again.*

Step 5: Use drugs that increase milk supply (galactogogues)

We recommend both herbs and pharmaceuticals, depending on the situation. Herbs are not necessarily safer than medication made in a factory. If herbs can change something in the body for the better, they can change something for the worse (an undesirable side effect). It is better not to need medication, but I believe strongly that if the baby can get more milk from his mother and/or avoid formula or use less, it's worth using it.

I used to see galactogogues as a last resort. But sometimes an immediate boost in milk supply provided by a galactogogue can turn things around quickly. However, galactogogues should not be suggested without also using the first four steps above; they are important.

Fenugreek (*Trigonella foenum-graecum*). Fenugreek is an herb classified as a food by Health Canada. It is a traditional medicine for making more milk in much of the Middle East, but we do not have good research to show that it works.

In the clinic, we usually start with a dose of three capsules of fenugreek three times a day. Fenugreek comes in several different capsule sizes and, like most herbal remedies, it's not standardized, so the ingredients can vary. A mother who is getting

enough fenugreek will smell of it. If not, she should increase the number of capsules.

Our experience suggests that fenugreek works best in the first days after birth, so that starting it at six weeks does not seem to help much. On the other hand, *some* mothers who have had late-onset decrease in their milk supply say fenugreek helped even months after the birth.

Studies of rats getting very large doses of fenugreek (up to 1 g/kg) injected into the abdominal space developed low blood sugar. A mother weighing 60 kg, taking nine 500 mg capsules a day of fenugreek, would be taking 0.075 g/kg/day, much less than the rats got, so what does this study mean, since we don't inject it into mothers' abdomens? As for human studies, there are a few, but only in diabetics, that showed a possible mild lowering of blood sugars. If a breastfeeding diabetic is taking medications to lower her blood sugar, she should make sure to test it regularly.

Another issue that has come up is that fenugreek may interfere with thyroid function. I have tried to find the sources for this concern and have not found a study that proves such a connection. If the mother is worried, she should have her thyroid function tested.

Finally, it has been suggested that because fenugreek is in the same family as peanuts, those allergic to peanuts should not take it. However, just because two foods are in the same family does not mean a mother who is allergic to one food will be allergic to all.

Side effects that mothers have reported while taking fenugreek include abdominal cramps and diarrhea. These usually disappear after a few days. Some people dislike the smell of fenugreek.

Blessed thistle (*Cnicus benedictus*): As with fenugreek, there is very little to support its use to increase milk supply. However, it seems to help. We have had some mothers add blessed thistle to fenugreek (or vice versa) and they reported that the two together work better than either one alone.

We have not heard from any of the mothers that they had any side effects from blessed thistle.

Note that blessed thistle is not the same as milk thistle (*Silybum marianum*). Some lactation specialists feel milk thistle does work well, but I have no experience with it.

Malunggay (*Moringa oleifera*): This has been used as a nutritional supplement in the Philippines for many years, and in fact the information suggests that it is very nutritious.

In our clinic we have had limited experience with this, but just as with fenugreek and blessed thistle, most mothers do report improvement in their milk supply.

One company that supplies malunggay suggests taking two capsules three times a day. Side effects seem to be rare.

Other herbs: Many herbs have been suggested to increase milk supply. We tend to recommend no more than two or three because more big capsules can be overwhelming. Other herbs include goat's rue (which seems to be useful for many mothers), raspberry leaf, and marshmallow root. There are still others that we have had no experience with.

Domperidone: This medication is very useful for increasing milk supply, but it needs to be prescribed rationally. Many physicians/midwives/nurse practitioners have very little experience with it. Some will prescribe it without helping the mother to breastfeed. Some will prescribe it for only a very limited time, even though many mothers may need it for weeks or even months. Some will not prescribe it because of the warning in June 2004 put out by the Federal Drug Administration (FDA) in the United States.

The FDA has jurisdiction only in the United States, yet Canadian physicians often use the warning as justification not to prescribe domperidone for breastfeeding mothers (while, of course, continuing to prescribe it for gastroparesis and reflux).

In 2012, Health Canada put out a warning about possible sudden death in older people (average age 75) from domperidone. The warning was ill-advised, poorly written and based on poor science, poorly interpreted. We have used domperidone on many thousands of women and few have experienced anything more than very mild side effects.

Domperidone is considered a safe enough drug that in several European countries it can be bought over the counter without a prescription. These countries include Great Britain, Ireland, the Netherlands and Belgium. However, no drug is 100% safe. Every drug causes changes in the body that may also cause unwanted side effects. Sometimes the side effects are serious. The risks of the drug must be weighed against the benefits. In the vast majority of mothers, increasing the milk supply is of greater benefit than the risks of the medication, which tend to be minor and do not last for more than a few days. (Side effects are explained below.)

Some helpful information about domperidone:

- Domperidone does not cross from the blood into the brain. This is important because, unlike metoclopramide (Reglan, Maxeran) and the major tranquilizers (chlorpromazine, haloperidol), which also increase milk production by increasing prolactin secretion from the pituitary, domperidone does not seem to cause significant psychiatric or neurological side effects.
- In theory, domperidone should not work well in the first three or four weeks after birth, because

it probably works by increasing prolactin levels which are still elevated in the first few weeks. In some cases, however, it seems to work anyway. We start domperidone at a dose of three tablets (30 mg) three times a day. Although lower doses may work, the mother is much more likely to get a response by starting higher. We often go up to four tablets (40 mg) three times a day, and we don't usually go higher than four tablets four times a day. These doses are higher than the company's recommendation, but they are recommending it for reasons other than increasing milk production.

- Domperidone works best in mothers who once had a good milk supply but, for some reason, no longer do. See the chapter "Late-Onset Decreased Milk Supply." It works less well in mothers who never developed a good milk supply, but it almost always does increase it at least somewhat.

- Some mothers get a good response at first and then seem to get less of a response as time goes on. The theory is that domperidone causes a release of stored prolactin from the pituitary, but once this is used up, domperidone no longer has an effect. But this doesn't explain why the decrease in milk supply after initial good response doesn't happen with most mothers who take it. Increasing the dose usually helps, but we rarely recommend more than four tablets four times a day. The fact that upping the dose seems to improve milk supply again suggests that the explanation of the prolactin in the pituitary being depleted does not quite make sense. We have tried reducing the dose for a few days or a week and then increasing the domperidone again. This may work. It is also possible that the body responds to increased prolactin secretion by trying to "get back to normal." Many

of the body's hormonal functions work on the basis of feedback, both positive and negative. Thus, it is just as likely that if a drug makes prolactin secretion go up, the higher levels of prolactin tell the hypothalamus (the source of dopamine, which inhibits the production of prolactin) to make more dopamine and thus decrease the level of prolactin. But again, why does this seem to happen only to some mothers? We don't know.

- Some mothers have claimed that domperidone *reduced* the milk supply. This is distinctly unusual and we rarely if ever hear this from our clinic patients, but I do hear of it in emails. I cannot explain how domperidone might decrease the milk supply. Most of the mothers contacting me about this are both breastfeeding and pumping milk, and they say they are getting less pumped milk since being on domperidone. Is another explanation possible? I think so. If the mother now has more milk, the baby will drink better from the breast (babies respond to milk flow!), with the result that the baby drains the breast better; the mother therefore gets less when she pumps. In any case, pumping is a poor way of judging how much milk a mother is producing. Obviously, if she can pump a lot then she is producing a lot, but it doesn't follow that if she can pump only a little that she is producing only a little. Many mothers whose babies are gaining very well on breastfeeding alone say that they can express or pump only tiny amounts, even if they use a very good pump. We have seen one case in our clinic with a mother whose baby was not latching on. She was pumping a lot of milk, but because the baby wasn't latching on, we suggested she go on domperidone. But after starting the drug, she was able to pump much less milk, though still enough for the baby to gain well on breastmilk alone. How to explain this? I don't know.

- We encourage mothers who go on domperidone not to start weaning off the drug until the baby is well established on solids. A significant number of mothers on domperidone find that decreasing the dosage results in a drop of milk supply. For others, it is not a problem. But if the milk supply does drop, the baby can make up the difference by eating more solids until the mother increases the domperidone again. Often mothers get prescriptions for domperidone for a very limited time period. But most mothers need to be on it for many weeks, even months, to avoid a drop in milk supply, and even then the supply may drop if they stop taking it, especially if they stop "cold turkey." I do not think continuing domperidone for several months is a big concern, because some people who take it for stomach disorders have been on the medication for a decade or more.

- We have some experience now with mothers who took domperidone with one baby but didn't need it for the next. It is possible that with more experience and perhaps better help, the mother's next lactation just went better.

Step 6: If the baby needs supplementation, give it by lactation aid at the breast

It is not always easy to decide when the baby needs supplementation. We try to maintain exclusive breastfeeding if possible. If, by going through steps 1 to 5, we get the baby drinking reasonably well, we may be able to avoid supplementing. It takes clinical judgment to know when supplementation is needed, taking into account a number of factors.

Unfortunately, supplementation is often introduced very early. Too often, by the time we see a mother and baby at the clinic, the baby has

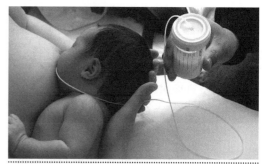

A baby being supplemented with a lactation aid at the breast. The baby is still breastfeeding!

CREDIT: **JACK NEWMAN**

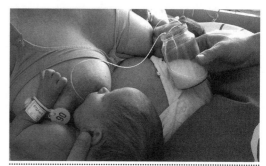

Both at the same time: newborn twins being supplemented at the breast with their mother's colostrum.

CREDIT: **JACK NEWMAN**

been supplemented with formula, usually by bottle, for many days, often many weeks, leading to a significant drop in milk supply. The fact that the baby is being fed large amounts of supplement off the breast means a significant amount of breast stimulation has not been happening. In many cases, the baby will start to refuse the breast if the bottles continue.

Bottles *do* interfere. Not all babies refuse the breast completely after being given bottles, and the mother may say her baby "takes both fine." But do the babies take the breast "fine"? If one looks at how the baby sucks at the breast, in many cases, he is hardly drinking. Essentially, the baby is drinking from the bottle and sucking without drinking from the breast; the more bottles that are given, the worse this gets.

Yes, some babies drink very well at the breast and take the bottle and drink from the bottle and go back to the breast and drink from the breast. But these are the babies of mothers who have a lot of milk; theirs is not the issue discussed in this chapter (dealing with the baby who is not getting enough from the breast). In addition, the babies may do fine for a number of weeks, several months even, and may start having problems only later. Teresa recalls a mother who talked about how pleased she was that her baby took both breast and bottle. When the baby was seven months old, however, the mother told Teresa that he had weaned himself. Babies *do not* wean themselves at seven months!

Another mother contacted me because her four-month-old had been given supplements by bottle from the time he was two weeks old and was soon refusing the breast completely. She had been pumping and giving him milk with bottles ever since. She hoped I could help her start breastfeeding again.

This mother clearly had enough milk—she was feeding her baby exclusively on the milk she could pump—but the advice to "top up" with a bottle had led to the baby refusing the breast within a short period of time.

I received an email from yet another mother about her two-month-old son. The mother said she'd been diagnosed with insufficient glandular tissue. Despite nursing every two hours, the baby was losing weight and having only two or three wet diapers in 24 hours. The mother began taking supplements to increase her milk supply and started pumping her milk and supplementing with formula in a bottle. Her son then refused the breast completely, even though he had been nursing well before. I could cite hundreds of emails along the same line. Suffice it to say that this baby refused the breast because of the use of bottles.

Why is the lactation aid at the breast the best solution for a baby who needs supplementation?

The baby continues to get milk from the breast even while being supplemented. And by being at the breast and getting some more milk from it even while being supplemented, he may increase the mother's milk supply. Feeding the baby when he is not at the breast does not do this, whether the baby is supplemented by bottle, finger feeding, syringe, cup or any other gadget that has been or will be dreamed up. Babies learn to breastfeed by breastfeeding. Babies respond to milk flow. If they get more milk flow when they use their mouth and tongue as they should, the most effective method of using their mouth and tongue will be reinforced. There is good evidence that sucking on a bottle and breastfeeding are completely different processes.

Mothers learn to breastfeed by breastfeeding. Mothers also learn by doing. Bottle-feeding—or any method of supplementing the baby off the breast—is not breastfeeding. When the lactation aid is in place and working as it should, mothers can clearly see that pause that tells them the baby is getting milk. (See the video clips at www.breastfeedinginc .ca showing babies drinking milk from the breast or not.) Once they see this and understand the implications, they can cut through so much of the information out there that is contradictory, confusing and just plain wrong.

The baby refuses the breast. In our clinic, we see babies every day who refuse to latch on whose mothers were told that the bottle won't interfere with breastfeeding. Once the baby won't breastfeed, it becomes very difficult to fix the problem, especially if the mother's milk production is low. Some will say, oh well, the mother can just pump her milk and give it in a bottle. But that is not the same as breastfeeding. Breastfeeding is much more than nutrition, much more than milk. It is a relationship, a special, intimate relationship between a mother and a child. I think that is one reason there is often resistance to breastfeeding: people who may have been deprived of this relationship cannot stand to see the beauty of the mother and child together at the breast, cannot bear to see the love that transfers back and forth. Nothing can replace this relationship. It is difficult for many people in our society to understand this. Our society is enamoured with gadgets and every few months a bottle "which is just like the breast" comes out and is marketed as simulating the breastfeeding relationship. And people fall for it. Even some lactation specialists eat this up. Some lactation consultants tell mothers it's okay now to go to the bottle because the baby is feeding well. The truth is that no bottle duplicates the breastfeeding relationship, no matter how closely the mother holds the baby while bottle-feeding. When supplementation is given at the breast, the baby is still breastfeeding. Perhaps this is not the ideal the mother was looking for, but it's a lot better than bottle-feeding, finger feeding or syringe feeding, even if done close to the breast.

When do you insert the lactation aid?

Except under certain unusual circumstances (such as when the baby will not stay at the breast except for a very short time and will pull off if the lactation aid isn't there) it should *not* be inserted at the beginning of the feeding. However, if the baby spends too much time sucking without drinking, he may fall asleep and not wake up for the other breast, even if still hungry. It is important to feed the baby on *both* sides. The advice to feed on just one side so that the baby gets the "high-fat milk" is absurd. If the baby is not drinking, he is not getting high-fat milk because he is getting no milk at all! So, if the baby is hardly drinking and starts to fall asleep (or pulls at the breast) because the flow is slow, the mother should switch sides and repeat the first steps in the protocol

above. Then she inserts the lactation aid and lets the baby drink as much as he will. (See the video clip "Inserting a Lactation Aid" at www.breastfeedinginc.ca.) If things work as they should, as the baby takes more milk from the breast, he will take less supplement. If the mother starts the lactation aid at the beginning of the feeding, how will she know when she doesn't need it anymore? This way, as his mother's supply increases, the baby naturally weans himself from the supplement and there is no need for a plan on how to stop using the lactation aid.

Lactation Aid Basics

A lactation aid is a device that allows a breastfeeding mother to supplement her baby with expressed breastmilk, glucose water with added colostrum, plain glucose water or, if necessary, formula, without using a bottle.

The lactation aid used at the breast is by far the best way to supplement, *if the supplement is truly necessary*. The lactation aid is better than using a syringe, cup feeding, finger feeding or any other method, since the baby is on the breast and breastfeeding. Babies, like adults, learn by doing. In this case, they learn to breastfeed by breastfeeding. Furthermore, the baby who is supplemented *while latched on to the breast* is also getting breastmilk from the breast.

A lactation aid consists of a container for the supplement—usually a feeding bottle with an enlarged nipple hole—and a long, thin tube leading from this container. Do not cut off the end of the tube as it may make the edges sharp. Manufactured lactation aids are available and are easier to use in some situations, such as with an older baby, when a mother needs to supplement twins, when the lactation aid will be used long term, or whenever difficulty arises using an improvised lactation aid. Though the manufactured lactation aid is not inexpensive, the cost is about equal to two weeks of the usual milk-based formula.

Using a tube with a syringe, with or without a plunger, as some lactation consultants suggest, is more complicated and less effective in helping to improve the baby's breastfeeding skills. Pushing the milk into the baby's mouth with the syringe does not teach the baby how to breastfeed because he gets milk even if he sucks poorly.

How to use a lactation aid

1. Latch the baby on and breastfeed on both sides. On the second side, the breast should be *gently* eased out of the way so that the corner of the baby's mouth is visible, and the tube, held between the index finger and thumb, should be slipped into his mouth so that it enters *straight* toward the back and at the same time slightly upward toward the roof. The tube is well placed when the supplemental fluid works its way down at a rather rapid rate. There is usually no need to fill the tube with supplemental fluid before putting it into the baby's mouth. (Refer to video clip "Inserting lactation aid": http://youtu.be/KPfVK6FAKMY)

2. You can also latch the baby on to the breast and tube at the same time. Adjust the tube so that the end is near the end of your nipple (but not past it) and the rest of it runs alongside your breast. The tube should be placed so that it is at the corner of the baby's mouth when he latches on.

3. You may tape the tube to the breast, though this is not really necessary and not always helpful.

4. It is occasionally helpful to hold the tube in place with your finger, as some babies tend to push it out of position with their tongues.

5. If the lactation aid functions only when the bottle is held higher than the baby's head, something is wrong. Keep the bottle higher only if the doctor or lactation specialist suggests this (as in the case of breast refusal, for example).

6. How often should you supplement? Usually it is best to use the lactation aid at every feeding, after nursing the baby on both breasts first. Some mothers find it easier not to use the lactation aid at night. It is better to give smaller amounts of supplement more frequently (say, 30 ml at each of eight feedings) than larger amounts infrequently (say, 120 ml twice a day).

7. If it takes half an hour for the baby to drink 30 ml of milk from the lactation aid, the tube is probably not well positioned, or the baby is poorly latched on, or both. When the lactation aid is functioning well, it takes 15 to 20 minutes, usually less, for the baby to drink 30 ml (1 oz.) of the supplement.

8. A trick for easier use: wear a shirt with pockets, and put the bottle in the pocket or stick it under your bra strap.

9. If you are unable to manage the lactation aid alone, get help. Even if you can manage the lactation aid twice a day instead of at every feeding, it is still better than not using it at all. Or if you can manage it for only part of the feeding, it's still better than not at all.

10. After using the device, clean the bottle and nipple. Do not boil the tube. It should be emptied, rinsed through with hot water (suck up hot water into the tube from a cup) and then hung up to dry. Soap, though not necessary, may be used if desired, but rinse the tube well. Tubes may become stiff and unsuitable after a few days to a week.

See the website (www.breastfeedinginc.ca) for videos illustrating how to use the lactation aid.

It is not always easy to use a lactation aid at the breast.

While using the lactation aid isn't complicated, mothers do need good instruction. The baby needs to be latched on as well as possible. If he has been on bottles for even a few days, his latch may not be good. While the baby is actively sucking, the mother can slide the tube into the corner of his mouth. The goal is to have the end of the tube at the end of your nipple, so you may want to measure this on your other nipple before inserting it. Some mothers have used a bandaid on their breasts to keep the tube in place.

Learning how to place the tube properly takes practice. Some mothers catch on sooner than others. Sometimes mothers try to keep the baby on the breast for long periods of time before using the lactation aid, but the baby gets sleepy and slips off the breast when the mother tries to insert the tube. It is important to insert the tube on the second side while the baby is still sucking actively, even while he is still drinking.

If you have difficulty inserting the tube while the baby is on the breast, you can take him off, line the tube up with the end of the nipple and latch the baby on to the breast and the tube at the same time.

It is very helpful, at first, to have extra hands (your partner or another family member) to help with the tube. Once you get used to it, the process is quite easy.

More ways to increase milk intake
You can lie down to feed the baby in the evening

Many mothers notice that they have less milk in the evening. In the late afternoon or evening, many babies start to fuss at the breast, pull at it or want to return to it frequently. Worrying that their babies are hungry, some mothers start supplementing them in the evening, especially if they have been convinced by and formula company marketing that the father should give the baby a bottle to give the mother a break.

(Yes, mothers need breaks, but they should happen at times that don't involve feeding. And breastfeeding itself is often restful for mothers, once problems—if there are any—are overcome.) Too often one bottle becomes two bottles, and then three and so on.

Many babies will be calmer if the mother feeds them while lying down rather than sitting up. And since there are few new mothers who are not tired, lying down can be a time of rest; the mother may even fall asleep while the baby suckles. It is during sleep that prolactin levels increase and help produce more milk. That's why mothers notice substantially more milk in the early morning, even if the baby breastfed frequently in the night. This boost in milk production is missed if, for example, the father gives a bottle during the night, as formula ads often suggest. Their marketing experts apparently read the research more than most health professionals.

What about pumping or compressing milk?

I generally discourage mothers from pumping if they are already supplementing with formula. Why?

1. Pumping is expensive to rent or buy the machine.
2. Pumping is tiring and time consuming.
3. Pumping diminishes the mother's enjoyment of breastfeeding.
4. If not done properly, pumping may cause sore nipples.
5. Even when we warn mothers that the amount they pump doesn't indicate how much milk they are producing or can produce, they may look at how little they pump and get discouraged.
6. Some mothers pump between feedings, probably because they get more milk than if they pump immediately after the baby was at the breast. Unfortunately, this results in slower milk flow at the next feeding and a baby who breastfeeds less well.

7. Compression is like pumping, but instead of pumping into a bottle, the mother expresses into the baby.

Many mothers stop breastfeeding altogether because they focus on pumping in order to increase the milk supply. It is much more important to continue breastfeeding than to pump. Many mothers go over to bottles completely because they find it's easier just to pump and bottle-feed than to put the baby to the breast, supplement and pump. The chances of getting to exclusive breastfeeding are greater if the mother follows our protocol, which does not include routine pumping.

How adding solids can help

This is discussed in more detail in the chapter "Late-Onset Decreased Milk Supply," but I mention it here as a light at the end of the tunnel for mothers who don't like using the lactation aid. I suggest that when the baby is around four months old the mother can start adding solids in order stop supplementation with a lactation aid at the breast.

It's not necessary to wait until six months before starting solids. Health Canada, the Canadian Paediatric Society, UNICEF and other groups encourage mothers to breastfeed *exclusively* to six months. However, if the mother is supplementing with formula, she is not exclusively breastfeeding anyway. Most babies can take solids around four months and if the mother is tired of using the lactation aid, starting solids can avoid bottles. Formula (or, preferably, expressed milk) can be added to the solids; the baby doesn't have to drink the supplement. If he eats enough solids, there is no need to add formula. And the baby should be allowed to eat as much as he will eat, as frequently as he will eat, without being forced. (Forcing food into the baby's mouth is *never* good.) The mother does not have to start with commercial cereals; babies at this age can eat banana, avocado, mashed potato, ground beef and chicken, the latter two being much better sources of iron than commercial cereals or formula for that matter. See the chapter "The Breastfed Baby and Solids."

Usually the mother can quickly go from breastfeeding and supplementing with a lactation aid to breastfeeding and feeding solids.

One caution: Babies of four months still like fast flow. If the flow from the breast is slow, the baby may not be patient, especially if he is used to getting fast flow from the lactation aid. Giving the baby some solids just enough that he's not ravenous, before putting him to the breast, might result in his being more patient with the slower flow. If not, it may be necessary to continue with the lactation aid, at least at some feedings. The baby might be happy at the breast in the morning, but not in the evening, for example, so just add food or the lactation aid as needed.

What's wrong with the following?

I received an email from a grandmother whose daughter had given birth to a baby girl who weighed just under six pounds. Breastfeeding appeared to be going well at first, and by day five she had regained three of the six ounces she had lost. (*When a baby is weighed on two different scales we can be fooled. When we learn the full story we will see that it's unlikely this baby really gained the weight back.*) However, by day eight the little girl had lost an ounce. The mother was told to nurse every two hours. (*Putting a baby who is feeding poorly to the breast more frequently rarely works. She needs to be helped to feed more effectively.*) The grandmother went on to explain that the baby was very sleepy and didn't breastfeed effectively. By day 11, she had lost another two ounces, and the doctor recommended she be supplemented by bottle. (*It is quite possible, even likely, that this baby needed to be supplemented, but why with a bottle? A lactation aid at the breast would be a much better way, and the next sentence shows why.*) She was now taking 1.5 to 2 ounces per bottle feeding, but was not interested in breastfeeding.

Too many health professionals take the following approach: "Express your milk and give it to the baby in a bottle so that we know how much he is getting." In some cases the health professional actually believes that the amount the mother expresses is an indication of how much the baby gets at the breast. Not true: a baby latched on well can get more than the mother can express; a baby latched on poorly will get less.

The doctor will calculate whether this is an appropriate amount for a baby of this weight and age. If the baby is getting enough milk, but is not gaining weight, then there may be a need for further investigation. If the baby is getting less than the appropriate amount, then obviously that's why he isn't doing well.

But if the mother is able to express all the milk the baby needs, why aren't we helping her breastfeed (by using How to Increase Breastmilk Intake, p. 102)? On the other hand, if she is not able to express all the milk the baby needs she may be convinced that she cannot produce enough milk. This is not necessarily true.

Finally, after we've done all this, what if the baby won't go back to the breast? We have given up too much in order to gain information that is useless. Our obsession with numbers has dealt another mother's breastfeeding a fatal blow.

Following are a number of situations that we encountered at our clinic. We've changed names and refer to all babies as boys, and have included letter notations (e.g. [a]) so that we can easily refer to specific points.

Situation #1: Disaster narrowly averted

This baby was brought to our clinic when four days old. The problem, according to his mother, Susan, was that the baby would not latch on to the right breast. Susan had sore nipples, but did not consider this a problem, because, as she said, "breastfeeding is supposed to hurt" (a).

The baby was feeding about eight times a day, every three hours. He would spend 15 to 20 minutes on the left side (b). He was calm after the feedings (c). He had had, in the last 24 hours, two black bowel movements and six wet (but only just moist) diapers (d).

Susan was a 31-year-old physician. This was her first pregnancy (e). The pregnancy was unremarkable; labour started spontaneously at 38 weeks and lasted four hours. Susan received no pain medication, and the baby was well at birth.

He weighed 3.07 kg (6 lb, 12 oz.). He was not tried on the breast until a few hours after birth (f).

The hospital stay lasted 24 hours, during which time the baby got sugar water once by cup (g).

At the first visit at the clinic, the baby was moderately jaundiced (h). His weight was 2.64 kg (5 lb, 13 oz.) (i). The rest of the physical examination was normal.

When we observed Susan breastfeeding, we could see that the baby only appeared to latch on to the left side. It was easy to pull him off the breast even though he was sucking and awake. A hungry baby who is latched on will not slip off the breast. So he was not latching on to *either* side.

I helped Susan latch the baby on better and he took both sides, and drank very well. Susan had less pain with the feeding. I suggested she breastfeed the baby on the first side until he would no longer drink, and then use breast compression to keep him drinking. Once he was no longer drinking, she should change sides and repeat the process. The baby breastfed quite well on both sides. Susan realized that he had never really breastfed before—in other words, never actually drank milk at the breast. He was pretending to breastfeed on the left side and couldn't be bothered to pretend on the right side.

I could not follow up the next day, but offered follow-up with one of our lactation consultants. I did arrange to see Susan four days after the initial visit. I phoned her the day after the first visit, leaving a message that if the baby was not drinking to get back to me. I got no message and neither did the lactation consultant.

At the second visit, the baby was latching on to both sides and drinking very well. Susan still had some soreness, but the pain was lessening considerably. The baby's weight was 2.8 kg (6 lb, 3 oz.) (k). He was less jaundiced (l). His bowel movements were now yellow and he was having many every day, some quite large. He was also urinating much more than before.

I heard from Susan again when the baby was three months old. He was still exclusively breastfeeding and gaining weight well. Susan had intended to return to work after six weeks but decided to take the year off and stay with her baby.

Notes on Situation #1

a) "Breastfeeding is supposed to hurt." Not true. Women have been given such poor information and help for so long that the abnormal has come to be seen as the normal. More on this in the chapter "Sore Nipples."

b) The baby was breastfeeding every three hours for 15 to 20 minutes on one side only. This is not necessarily a problem. After all, a mother can feed twins exclusively with two breasts; she can breastfeed one baby exclusively with one breast. But the baby was not actually breastfeeding. This case demonstrates the folly of relying on rules and numbers. It is not how often or how long the baby feeds that matters, but how well he feeds.

c) The baby was calm, but this is not always a good sign: a baby who is not getting enough in the early weeks may be quite lethargic.

d) The information about the bowel movements is worrisome. This was the fourth day and the bowel movements were still black when they should have transitioning to yellow.

e) Although Susan was a physician, that didn't help her identify the real problem or figure out how to breastfeed more effectively.

f) The baby was not tried on the breast until a few hours after birth. That was precisely a few hours too late.

g) The baby was given water by cup. Why? The mother didn't know. Was the nurse concerned about something? If there was a feeding problem, the mother should have been helped with breastfeeding. I am sure that this nurse would protest that she was supportive of breastfeeding because she did not use a bottle. However, if there is a problem, the first thing to do is help the baby latch on well. If a supplement is needed, it should be given with a lactation aid. If the baby was not latching on well on discharge, the mother should have been referred urgently to our clinic or to someone else who could help her (Susan was not referred to anyone). Is it likely that a mother who was able to breastfeed exclusively for at least three months and whose baby was doing just fine did not have enough colostrum?

h) The baby was moderately jaundiced because he was not feeding well. See section on jaundice on pages 81–86.

i) This represents a weight loss of 14%. A reason to supplement? The scale is different, so we cannot compare the weights; in any case, percentage weight loss means nothing. There is no reason to panic; if the baby can start getting milk, he will make up the weight loss. Even supplementation with expressed milk isn't necessary if he starts drinking well (and he did).

j) The baby only appeared to take the breast. This is the most common reason babies become dehydrated. What happens is not "dehydration in breastfed babies" as the media call it. If the baby were breastfeeding, he would not become dehydrated. A baby who only pretends to latch on cannot get milk and becomes lethargic, and then may feed poorly or not at all. A vicious circle ensues.

k) This represents an increase of 160 g (almost 6 oz.) in four days. Yes, the scale was different, as I saw the baby in two different hospitals for the first two visits, but *the way the baby fed at the breast* showed he was getting lots of milk. The change in bowel movements and the obvious increase in urine output support the observation that the baby was breastfeeding well.

l) The jaundice was obviously reduced, good evidence that the problem was insufficient intake. Many physicians would have told the mother to stop breastfeeding and give the baby formula. Because the baby would have been getting food for the first time in his life, the bilirubin would have dropped, which would have reinforced the doctor's *mistaken* notion that the problem was the breastmilk. No! The problem was that the baby was not breastfeeding. Fix the breastfeeding and the bilirubin will come down.

Here, then, is a case of disaster narrowly averted. Another day without help, and the baby might have become so sleepy from dehydration that he might not have woken up enough to latch at all. In that circumstance, I'd have the mother express her milk and finger feed the baby. Once he woke up (maybe after a feeding or two), we would work on latching him on. The first rule in such a situation is *feed the baby.* Unfortunately, the only approach in too many physicians' repertoire is *supplement with formula.*

It was a piece of cake to fix this problem. The mother's milk had probably just come in and when the baby went to the breast (with my help), he got milk and breastfed beautifully. The Canadian Paediatric Society recommends follow-up of babies within the first week after birth to make sure, among other things, that the breastfeeding is going well. However, very few pediatricians observe the mother breastfeeding and depend only on the scale to make sure the baby is feeding well. As I've mentioned before, depending on scales leads to errors, potentially fatal errors, all the time.

This near tragedy could easily have been prevented on that first day in hospital. If someone knowledgeable and experienced had spent just a little time helping the mother with the latching, one more mother would be wondering, "How can anyone have problems with breastfeeding?" In this case, the mother and baby were lucky to find appropriate help quickly. Too many do not.

Situation #2. Weight loss, no need for supplements

This baby was seen at our clinic when 14 days old, referred by a lactation consultant. The problem was weight loss.

This was the first pregnancy for Linda, who was 29. The labour was at term (39 weeks) and the baby was born after seven hours. He weighed 3.61 kg (7 lb, 15 oz.) and was fine.

The baby was tried at the breast within an hour of birth and *apparently* breastfed well (a). The baby was given sugar water by cup because he "wasn't urinating" (b). Linda was with him 24 hours a day, and mother and baby were discharged on day two.

At the first clinic visit, Linda said the baby was breastfeeding six or seven times a day, with one feeding between midnight and 6 a.m. He would stay on the breast for an hour and frequently fall asleep on the breast but cry when he was taken off (c). According to Linda, the baby had quite infrequent bowel movements (about every two or three days), and only three soaked diapers in a day (d).

On examination, the baby looked reasonably well, and no abnormalities were noted. His weight was 3.23 kg (7 lb, 1.5 oz.), 380 g below birth weight (e).

At the breast, he was doing little drinking. I showed Linda how to latch him on better and how to use compression, and he breastfed *very* well.

One week later, Linda returned to the clinic with the baby and said she thought things were better (f). The baby's urine output was much increased, and his bowel movements became larger and more frequent about two days after the first visit (g). His weight was 3.46 kg (7 lb, 10 oz.) or an increase of almost nine ounces in a week. This weight gain was corroborated by the obvious drinking the baby was doing on the breast.

The baby was still breastfeeding exclusively at five months of age and doing well (h).

Notes on Situation #2

a) "Apparently" feeding well—but if the baby needed water, was he really breastfeeding well?

b) Same as note g in case #1 with regards to the cup and sugar water. Probably the baby urinated, but what about the *real* problem? How would this prevent the weight loss later on?

c) There is a difference between being on the breast and breast*feeding*. Babies tend to fall asleep at the breast when the flow of milk is slow, not necessarily because they have had enough to eat.

d) These are definite signs that the baby is not getting enough milk. The mother didn't know this, and that says something about what breastfeeding mothers are taught.

e) But the scale is different, and we do not know exactly how much weight the baby actually lost.

f) Linda was right. Sometimes mothers have difficulty determining whether the baby is doing better, but they can learn how to tell when a baby is feeding well.

g) Once the baby's intake is increased, it may take a couple of days before he has regular bowel movements.

h) Poor weight gain, or weight loss, is *not* due to insufficient milk production, but is a result of the baby not getting the milk that is available.

Situation #3: Weight loss, but again, no supplements to fix the problem

This baby was first seen at our clinic when 15 days old. This was Maria's first pregnancy and the baby was born at 38 weeks gestation. The labour lasted only two hours and although the baby was fine at birth, he was not tried on the breast until three or four hours after (*three or four hours too late*). At that time, as frequently happens, the baby was no longer interested. An opportunity lost to get breastfeeding started well (a). The baby weighed 3.1 kg (6 lb, 13 oz.) at birth.

The baby and mother roomed in 24 hours a day. No supplements were given.

When Maria brought the baby to the clinic, she said that he breastfed all the time and would stay on the breast forever if she did not take him off (b). He slept fours hour at night, however (c). She had sore nipples.

At the first visit to the clinic, the baby weighed 2.885 kg (6 lb, 5 oz.) (d). He was thin and moderately jaundiced. His latch was not ideal, but he was getting some milk. I showed Maria how to latch him on better. The feeding was absolutely painless for the first time. I showed Maria how to know when the baby was getting milk, how to do compression and how to switch him from one breast to the other when he was no longer drinking on the first side.

I felt the baby was drinking well enough that he would not get into trouble over the next week, so we made a follow-up appointment for a week later. Maria returned five days later because she was worried the baby was not getting enough milk. The baby's weight at this point was 2.9 kg (e). I reassured her that the baby was drinking well. One week after the initial visit, the baby weighed 2.95 kg (only 70 g, or a little more than 2 oz., more than seven days before) (f).

One week later (two weeks after the first visit), the baby weighed 3.13 kg (140 g, or slightly less than 5 oz., more than seven days before). In addition to being heavier, the baby was obviously more content, spent less time on the breast, and urinated more. One week later, he weighed 3.43 kg (300 g, or more than 10 oz., more than the week before). He was content and fed about every three hours.

A month later, Maria left a message that the baby was continuing to gain weight at the rate of about an ounce a day.

When the baby was five months old, Maria left a message that, through breastfeeding only, he now weighed 6.1 kg (13 lb, 9 oz.) (g).

Notes on Situation #3

a) Babies are often very eager to breastfeed during the first two hours or so after birth. After the first couple of hours, they may lose interest and sleep, whether they have fed or not. No argument can be made in this case against an immediate attempt at breastfeeding, other than inconvenience to the staff, or outdated, invalid hospital routines. Maria told me she wasn't tired and had no idea why breastfeeding had been delayed.

b) Did this baby really breastfeed all the time? Given his weight loss, he probably wasn't feeding most of the time he was on the breast.

c) Sleeping four hours at night in the first two weeks of life is sometimes a tipoff that things are not going well. Obviously, if the baby is getting plenty of milk and he sleeps four or more hours a night at two weeks, this is fine. On the other hand, sometimes long sleeps at night *may* mean he is not getting enough milk.

d) The scale is different than the hospital's or the pediatrician's, but other things tell us that the baby is not getting enough milk.

e) Only a little heavier than five days beforehand, but it was a different scale. But the baby was drinking better and that's what counts, not the scale.

f) This pattern of the weight "bottoming out" before starting to rise is common when there has been a delay in fixing the breastfeeding problem. But the baby was feeding better and that's what counts.

g) The baby took almost a month to return to his birth weight. The birth weight is not a holy number that must be reached in a certain time or else supplementation is required. Supplementation in this case was avoided by improving the breastfeeding. Note the baby's moderate jaundice, too often diagnosed as breastmilk jaundice, whereas here it might be called "not-enough-breastmilk jaundice." This case is typical. Some babies will not turn around in one week as the baby in Situation #2 did. Because the baby was breastfeeding poorly for two weeks, the mother's milk supply had likely decreased, but luckily better breastfeeding brought her supply up again and the baby could gain well.

Situation #4: How the lactation aid works

Celine, 29 years old, came to the clinic with her first-born son, 13 days old, because he was not latching on. The pregnancy had been unremarkable, but Celine commented that she had had no breast changes during the pregnancy (a). The labour was unremarkable. The baby was tried on the breast immediately after birth and *apparently* latched on well (b). The mother and baby roomed in, no supplements were given during the hospital stay, and they left hospital at 48 hours after birth. The baby's birth weight was 4.09 kg (9 lb).

At the first clinic visit, the baby weighed 4.245 kg (9 lb, 5 oz). He had been supplemented from the third day, because he was refusing the breast. The mother and baby had been seen at another clinic a few days before and the mother was taught finger feeding in order to help the baby get to the breast (c). For about two days before the visit to our clinic, the baby was taking the breast. Nevertheless, Celine was supplementing with 110–150 ml (4–5 oz.) of formula at *each* feeding. Furthermore, she was now experiencing sore nipples (d).

Physical examination of the baby showed he was normal. He was latched on poorly, but once the latch was corrected, he drank fairly well at the breast. We also showed Celine how to apply our Protocol to Increase Breastmilk Intake, including how to use a lactation aid (e).

The baby and mother returned to the clinic a week after the first visit. The baby weighed 4.53 kg (10 lb). He was now taking 110–150 ml (4–5 oz.) of formula over a 24-hour day. Celine complained that he woke more frequently to feed. This is often concerning to mothers, but in fact it is a very good sign. She was no longer sore. The baby breastfed very well and it was obvious he was taking lots of milk, much more than at the first visit. I encouraged Celine to continue working on the latch, the compression and the switching, but not to limit the baby's supplementation as he would take what he wanted.

Here is an excerpt from a letter I received from Celine.

"J. is just turning four months, the last three of which he has been solely breastfeeding. He now weighs over 7.27 kg (16 lb). We are both very well now. I love breastfeeding! I never thought it could be so easy and so rewarding!" (f)

Celine called me when her baby was six months old, still breastfeeding exclusively and gaining well, to ask about starting solids. She also called me when the baby was 18 months old to say a dentist had told her to stop breastfeeding as it might affect the baby's teeth; I told her she should continue. See the chapter "The Normal Duration of Breastfeeding" for more on nursing a toddler.

Notes on Situation #4

a) Mothers are often told that if they don't see breast changes during the pregnancy they will not produce enough milk. This is not our experience. Some mothers who are unable to produce a full milk supply have no changes during pregnancy but some who do have changes also have problems. And some mothers with an abundance of milk report no changes. True insufficient milk supply may be more frequently associated with no changes during the pregnancy, but it should not be assumed that no changes will mean not enough milk.

   Breast changes during the second and later pregnancies tend to be much less dramatic than during the first.

b) He "apparently" latched on well, but I don't really buy it. A baby who "latches on well" and then refuses the breast when the mother becomes engorged, as in this case, probably never latched on at all but really was only allowing the breast into his mouth. When the engorgement occurred (this is usually worse when the baby has not been nursing well) the baby found it hard to do what he was doing before, and actively refused the breast (instead of passively doing it as he had before).

c) See chapter "When the Baby Does Not Yet Take the Breast."

d) This soreness means that the baby is not latching on well. This is also suggested by the fact that he seems to need so much formula supplementation.

e) Some mothers will keep the baby on each breast until he falls asleep. This is not necessary, since if the baby is not drinking well, he is not getting much to eat. Waiting until the baby is asleep or almost asleep makes the feedings longer without necessarily decreasing the amount of supplement he will take. Indeed, the baby may take a while to wake up before he will take the second side, further lengthening the feeding.

   The better the baby latches on, the less the lactation aid will be necessary. And the better he latches on, the easier it is to use the lactation aid. A well-placed tube, with a baby well latched on, will result in the baby taking about 30–60 ml (1–2 oz.) of supplement every 10 to 20 minutes. If it is taking an hour to give the baby 30 ml (1 oz.), something is not right. The mother needs to get help from someone with experience.

f) Stopping the lactation aid usually takes time, sometimes several weeks. Some mothers cannot stop it at all, since once the milk supply is down, it may be impossible to bring it back completely. Some mothers can get off the lactation aid when the baby starts solids, but even then some cannot. Some babies will breastfeed only as long as the flow is rapid, and pull away if flow is too slow.

Situation #5: Premature twins

Ruth's twins were born at 33 weeks gestation. The labour was unremarkable and the babies were born without the mother receiving any medication (in itself fairly remarkable). Ruth had previously breast-fed two other children (not twins) without problems for about seven months. At birth, one twin weighed 2.02 kg (4 lb, 7 oz.); the other, 1.6 kg (3 lb, 8 oz.). The twins had no breathing problems, received no oxygen, and had no jaundice. The babies remained in hospital for five weeks, three weeks in the hospital where they were born (where the problems with breastfeeding began), and two weeks in another (where the problems continued).

The babies received intravenous fluids for the first four days. Then they were given formula, first through a tube into their stomachs, then with bottles. Breastfeeding was not even attempted until several weeks after birth (a). At some point during the babies' stay in the first hospital, Ruth was started on domperidone (b). The babies were discharged from the second hospital being bot-tle fed, mostly formula but also some expressed breastmilk.

At the first visit to our clinic, the babies were almost three months old. They took the left breast a little, but refused the right side completely. Each feeding consisted of expressed milk, about 30 ml (1 oz.), and formula 60 ml (2 oz.). At this first visit, the babies weighed 3.35 kg (7 lb, 6 oz.) and 3.25 kg (7 lb, 2 oz.) (c).

Neither baby would go near the right breast, arching and screaming rather than latching on (d). They *appeared* to take the left side, but in fact, they merely allowed the breast into their mouths. I showed Ruth how to use the lactation aid to give the babies a supplement at the left breast. With the lactation aid they did take the right side a little, but not much. They did take more supplement on the left side.

To increase Ruth's milk supply, I suggested fenugreek and blessed thistle as well as domper-idone.

I asked Ruth to continue working with the lactation aid and the latching at home, and to return with the babies in a week.

The next week things were obviously much better. The babies were taking the left breast and breast*feeding*. They were still getting some bottles, especially at night. They weighed 3.49 kg (7 lb, 11 oz.) and 3.35 kg (7 lb, 6 oz.). This was a reason-able weight gain for both.

Two weeks after the first visit, the babies were now taking the right breast and breastfeeding well on the left side. We forgot to weigh the twins at this visit.

Four weeks after the initial visit, the babies weighed 4.02 kg (8 lb, 13 oz.) and 3.81 kg (8 lb, 6 oz.). At this point they were getting only about 60 ml (2 oz.) of supplemental formula a day. The babies breastfed very well on both sides. The father, who was initially not supportive, believing the babies would be fussier when breastfeeding, was now very supportive because he had seen that the one who was getting formula during the night was always the one who was fussier then.

By the fifth week after the initial visit, the babies were breastfeeding exclusively and gaining weight appropriately. They were still breastfeeding exclusively at six months of age, when I last saw them (e).

Notes on Situation #5

a) These babies were apparently both quite well, and they were fair-sized if premature. There was no reason not to try them at the breast once it was obvious they were not running into immediate problems. Skin-to-skin contact would have helped; the father could have held one of the babies on his bare chest. Perhaps neither baby would have latched on, but they would be learning. Staff in NICUs often argue that the premature baby has to learn how to bottle-feed before he can breastfeed and that it is less stressful for a premature baby to bottle-feed than breastfeed. This is nonsense, pure and simple. Research shows clearly that *breastfeeding is less stressful for the premature baby* than bottle-feeding. Furthermore, there is no need to start bottles, since cup feeding seems to cause fewer problems than the bottle and can be used if the baby is not taking the breast. The mother's supply would have been better if there had been skin-to-skin contact with her babies. Formula should have been used only if the mother was not expressing enough milk. Obviously Ruth could produce plenty of milk.

b) The mother was started on domperidone! This is too typical of the medical approach: don't fix the problem (poor latch or, in this case, no latch); give the mother a drug.

c) This is nowhere near intrauterine growth rate, the supposed reason for giving formula or fortifiers.

d) If this is not nipple confusion, what is it?

e) From virtually exclusive bottle and formula feeding (with some breastmilk) to exclusive breastfeeding in five weeks. These babies were in hospital for five weeks. With a little help, this mother and her babies could have been breastfeeding from the beginning. There is no doubt that Ruth's determination made it happen, but she needed support and practical help. Unfortunately, many health professionals do not believe that breastfeeding twins is practical or possible. With the "help" this mother got in the first few weeks, all too typical, it is not surprising that breastfeeding twins is considered difficult or even impossible.

These five examples are typical. Most problems we see could have been avoided. And while these cases all ended well, it's not always possible to turn around a situation that has gone as badly as the twins'. Everything that has been said here, which is geared to the healthy baby, is also true for the baby who has special problems, such as trisomy 21, or other congenital or medical problems. Indeed, with very few and fairly rare exceptions, babies with problems don't need breastmilk (and breastfeeding, which is *not* the same thing) less, they need it more. Unfortunately, as we saw with the twins, too many health professionals assume that breastfeeding is not in the cards for the sick baby. Many believe formulas are better. This is almost never true.

9 | Late-Onset Decreased Milk Supply

Over the past 20 years we have been noticing that there were mothers whose babies were breastfeeding well for two or three months but then things started to go wrong. Babies who had been content at the breast were no longer content. Babies who had been gaining weight well were no longer gaining weight.

At first, we saw this only occasionally, but now it has become a common problem. Two things have happened to account for this change in what we're seeing. One is that mothers now expect to breastfeed exclusively until the baby is about six months. But until 2005, the Canadian Paediatric Society and Health Canada recommended starting solids at four and six months. Most mothers start solids at four months, so if their milk production decreases it is not as obvious, since the babies made up calories with solids. The other thing is that now many mothers do not accept the family doctor's advice about starting the baby on solids or (even worse) giving him formula; instead, they are seeking help to solve the problem. They often don't see it as a problem of milk supply, but they come because the baby is not happy at the breast, or is not gaining well, or has been diagnosed with "reflux" or "allergy." So we see more of them.

A decreased milk supply does not necessarily mean that the baby won't gain weight well. Even a decreased milk supply may be sufficient for the baby to gain weight; however, several symptoms can point to a decreased duration of rapid milk flow.

What symptoms suggest a late-onset decrease in milk production?

The baby's rate of weight gain decreases or stops, or the baby actually loses weight. Of course, after the first two months it is normal for the rate of growth to slow down. As well, our guidelines about what is normal growth are just that, and the whole baby needs to be taken into account. A baby who is growing slowly but steadily and is happy, energetic and developing normally is not a problem. However, some babies can seem happy or at least calm if they suck on their fingers a lot (or a pacifier) even though they are actually hungry. It is not always easy to decide if the baby is fine, just growing a little slowly, or if he needs more milk. And scales can be wrong! The best way of knowing if the baby is getting too little milk from the breast is to watch a feeding and see if he is drinking well. This is not always easy: a four-month-old is sometimes very distracted when breastfeeding, especially if he is not particularly hungry or if the milk flow is slow.

The baby cries at the breast, pulls at the breast, returns to the breast but is not happy. In the first few months of life, babies tend to fall asleep at the breast when the flow of milk is slow. As they get older they tend to pull at the breast without letting go or pull off the breast when the flow of milk slows down. Of course, all babies are different—some babies always pull at the breast, demanding faster flow even when only a few days old; others always fall asleep when the flow of milk is slow. Some do both at different times. Babies also fall asleep on the breast or pull off the breast when they are full.

As mentioned before, the baby may actually continue to gain weight well even while fussing at the breast. Fussing usually occurs if the mother's milk production is still good, but has decreased. Babies get used to a fast flow, and if they don't get it they may pull away from the breast even when the flow is reasonable.

This behaviour—pulling off the breast, returning to the breast, and pulling at it again—is often diagnosed as reflux or gastroesophageal reflux disease (GERD), and the babies are put on medication. Because the baby is still gaining, the physician doesn't consider that a decrease in milk production could be the problem. Medication hardly ever works, because reflux is not the issue.

As an aside, I should say that reflux and/or GERD (which are not quite the same thing) are *the* diagnoses of the 21st century. Physicians are pleased to have a solution that doesn't involve telling the mother to switch to formula, which was what they used to recommend. Giving formula used to work, because it fixed the problem of not getting a rapid flow of milk at the breast, but at the cost of weaning the baby from the breast—both mother and baby lost. Unfortunately, when the reflux medication doesn't work (and it usually doesn't), formula is the next step.

The parents like the diagnosis of reflux because it says the problem is the baby's; it's not their fault. It isn't their fault, actually; the problem is the way we teach (or rather don't teach) parents how breastfeeding works. If every mother (and every health professional) knew how to recognize when the baby is getting milk from the breast, they would realize that when he is not getting good flow he pulls away.

Speaking of medication for reflux, babies who are happy and gaining weight, often very well, are also often put on medication for reflux simply because they spit up a lot. I used to say that if the baby is content and gaining well, spitting up is just a laundry problem (I believe Dr. William Sears originated the term). In fact, if the baby is calm, drinking well and gaining well, spitting up may actually be a good thing (I owe this insight to Dr. Stephen Buescher, a pediatrician and infectious disease specialist in Virginia). Breastmilk is full of immune factors (not just antibodies, but dozens of factors that interact with each other) that protect the baby from invasion by bacteria and other microorganisms (fungi, viruses, etc.) by forming a protective layer on his mucous membranes (the linings of the gut, respiratory tract and other areas). This protective layer prevents micro-organisms from invading the body through these mucous membranes. A baby who spits up gets extra protection, first when the milk goes down to the stomach, and again when he spits it up. This is another example of how breastfeeding is so different from formula feeding. Spitting up formula, if all else is going well, is probably not bad. Spitting up breastmilk, if all else is going well, is probably good.

Pulling at the breast is also frequently diagnosed as a sign of milk flowing too rapidly. Unfortunately, this diagnosis is sometimes made without watching the baby at the breast to see if he is drinking. Mothers may then be advised to feed the baby on only one breast at each feeding or feed the baby several times at the same breast to increase the hind milk he is getting, which only makes things worse since the milk supply will decrease even more.

Evening crying or colic. The decrease in milk supply may result in the baby crying more and longer, especially in the evening when most mothers seem to have less milk and flow is slower. This evening crying is typical of colic, but colic does not start at two or three months—it typically ends around three months. See the chapter "Colic (The 'C' Word)" for more on this.

The mother develops nipple pain after a period of pain-free breastfeeding. Unfortunately, it is common for mothers to have sore nipples in the first few days, usually due to the newborn baby not latching well, but most pain improves over time. The baby learns that a deeper latch results in more milk and he adjusts his latch. However, if milk production decreases later on, the mother may start to get sore nipples again. One reason is the baby pulling back on the nipple; another is the baby biting or chomping or clamping down on the nipple; and a third is the baby slipping down and sucking only on the nipple. Another major cause of late-onset nipple pain is an infection with *Candida* (yeast or thrush). This is discussed further in the chapter "Sore Nipples."

Nursing strikes. Frequently a nursing strike is due to a decrease in milk production. The mother will say that during the day, the baby hardly takes the breast at all or refuses completely, except for the first feeding in the morning, when milk supply is greatest. The baby will often take the breast during the night, especially if he is bed-sharing, but also if the mother gets up to feed him. For the mother whose milk supply has decreased, this problem may come on suddenly or gradually. The baby may start by refusing one feeding in late afternoon or early evening but will refuse increasingly as the days pass. If the cause of decreased supply is eliminated (see the following section) and/or the mother is put on domperidone, the baby will start to take the breast better.

Allergy to something in the breastmilk. The symptoms we've described are often put down to the baby being allergic to something in the milk.

Although sensitivity to some protein in the mother's milk may result in the baby being fussy and crying a lot, I think it is more likely that the symptoms are due to a decrease in the milk supply. Putting the baby on a hydrolyzed formula may result in dramatic improvement, not because he has allergies, but because he is getting more milk more quickly. The cost of these formulas is significant and the child may be unnecessarily labelled allergic. Before we ask mothers to eliminate various foods from their diets, the baby should be observed at the breast and the history of his feeding evaluated.

Here is an example. A mother contacted me because she was told her baby was allergic to breastmilk. The baby often had blood in his stools. The mother had eliminated dairy from her diet since her son was a month old, but he continued to be fussy and have blood in his stools periodically. The pediatrician recommended switching to hypoallergenic formula. The mother added that she had had an overactive letdown in the beginning and her son would gag and choke when nursing in the first few months but had settled down. Because of this overactive letdown, she gave the baby only one breast per feeding. When I asked her to watch some videos of a baby feeding well at the breast, she realized that her baby was mostly nibbling at the breast and not drinking very much. The amount of blood in the baby's stools was minimal (flecks).

When blood in the stool is present only in minimal amounts, as long as the baby is growing well and content, I don't worry about it. But this baby was *not* content. Why? The mother and pediatrician both believed that his fussiness was due to allergy to breastmilk. But the real reason was that he was not getting milk well from the breast. The mother had limited the baby's feedings to one breast per feeding, which not only restricted his intake of breastmilk but also decreased milk production. Why did the baby get better on the special formula? Because he got more milk and wasn't hungry anymore.

It is not a good idea to feed the baby on just one side in order *to follow a rule*, as many mothers are being taught. The goal is for the baby to get the higher-fat hind milk, but if he is not drinking, he is not getting hind milk (because he's not getting any milk, or hardly any, when he's nibbling). Yes, making sure the baby finishes the first side before offering the second is generally helpful, but if he is not actually *getting milk* there is no point in sucking for long periods of time. The mother should finish one side and if the baby wants more, offer the other.

How does the mother know the baby has finished the first side? Because he is no longer drinking, even with compression (see the video clips and information sheet on compression at www.breastfeedinginc.ca). It's good to wait a minute or two in case the mother gets another let-down, but if the baby is starting to sleep, stops drinking or starts to pull at the breast, it's time to offer the other side.

If the baby lets go of the breast on his own, does it mean that he has finished that side? Not necessarily. Babies often let go of the breast when the flow of milk slows; sometimes when the mother gets a milk ejection reflex the baby, surprised by the sudden rapid flow, pulls off. He can be offered that side again, or go to the other breast.

The baby was sleeping well during the night but is now waking up more frequently. Waking up can be the baby's way of getting more milk when supply has decreased, but there are other reasons a baby may wake up more frequently around four or five months. These include starting to be aware of himself as separate from his mother. This is a scary notion for a young baby, who then seeks the protection and security he may get from the breast. Again,

we need to observe the baby at the breast. If he stays on the breast nibbling for very long periods of time, or, conversely, only very short periods, the reason is likely a decrease in milk supply. Babies react differently, so some will stay on the breast for long periods of time even if they are not getting much from the breast; others will pull off after only a couple of minutes if the flow slows. And the same baby can react differently at different times. If he's not too hungry, he may fall asleep at the breast. If he's hungry, he may pull away.

The length of time a baby is on the breast does not tell us how much milk he is getting. A baby who drinks very well from the breast can be full in a short period of time. A baby who spends an hour on the breast only nibbling may get very little milk. If someone says, "The baby gets all he needs in the first 10 minutes" or "You shouldn't let the baby suck more than 30 minutes on each side," they really don't understand how breastfeeding works.

However, if there is a change in the baby—he's now spending a much longer or much shorter time at the breast—it *may* be a sign of decreased milk production. We have to be careful not to jump to conclusions, though, as babies change over time.

Why would the milk production decrease after two or three months when it was so good at first?

The mother was started on a hormonal birth control method. Although most obstetricians disagree, I believe birth control pills can decrease the mother's milk supply. Too often we hear: "Everything was going very well, then at six weeks I was started on the pill, and within 10 days it was obvious that my milk had dried up." It doesn't happen to every breastfeeding mother, but it happens often enough. The combination birth control pill works by fooling the mother's body into thinking she is pregnant. When breastfeeding mothers become pregnant, their milk production decreases dramatically, because the hormones of pregnancy (including the estrogens and progesterones that are in most birth control pills) inhibit the action of prolactin, the hormone that stimulates the breasts to make milk. The effect of the birth control pill on milk supply may occur with progesterone-only pills as well. The IUD, which releases progesterone, also seems to decrease milk production in some mothers. I wonder how obstetricians know the hormonal methods don't cause problems, since they rarely see mothers after the six week follow-up appointment.

A mother may take birth control pills with one baby and have no difficulties, but may have a problem with a later baby. If she had abundant milk production the first time, going on the pill may not have *seemed* to make a difference, since the baby just kept gaining and was not particularly fussy. But if for some reason, with the next baby the mother has less milk, the pill may cause a significant problem.

Breastfeeding decreases a woman's fertility almost as much as the birth control pill. If the mother is breastfeeding exclusively, if the baby does not use a pacifier, if there are no long periods of time when the baby is not at the breast, including at night, and if the mother has not had a *normal* menstrual period, the chances of her getting pregnant are almost the same as if she were on the birth control pill—about 2%. Even so, many women are wary of relying on breastfeeding to prevent pregnancy; in this case they can use a barrier method in addition to breastfeeding. Even once the baby starts taking solids, as long as the mother has not had a period between 6 and 12 months after the birth, the risk of pregnancy remains about 6%, according to a recent study. (I find it interesting that at the six-week visit

many new mothers are told by their doctors that breastfeeding does not prevent pregnancy so they need to take the pill or have an IUD inserted. But when a woman whose breastfeeding baby is 12 or 14 months old wants to get pregnant and asks her doctor why she's not getting her period, she is likely to be told that she can't conceive as long as she's breastfeeding. Yes, it happens!)

Most doctors don't know that mothers who breastfeed into the second year do not get their periods back until 14 months after birth on average (based on a small study I did many years ago; however, a larger study in Slovakia confirmed my rather unscientific survey). The variation is very wide. I have heard of a mother who got her period five weeks after the birth (even though she was breastfeeding exclusively and the baby was gaining well) and, in one case, 35 months after the birth. Most women become fertile again between one and two years after the birth of the baby.

Incidentally, mothers who do get their periods in the first few months or get pregnant soon after the first child *may* be giving the baby a pacifier or using other methods of keeping him from feeding frequently. They may be exclusively breastfeeding, but not really feeding on demand.

Sometimes mothers blame the decrease in milk supply on an early return of menstrual periods—say, three months after birth. I think it is the other way around: the milk supply decreased, and that caused her period to return.

The mother is pregnant again. This is uncommon for a breastfeeding mother whose baby is younger than six months, but it does happen, and milk production usually decreases significantly during pregnancy. If the baby is older than six months when the mother conceives, he can take the breast, get some milk from it, and eat solids and drink liquids. There is no need for a seven- or eight-month-old to drink formula or use a bottle. A baby this age or older can usually drink from an open cup or have liquids mixed with his solids.

The need for formula to a year or longer is largely the result of formula company marketing, and it is very successful, as many pediatric societies recommend it. But if the baby is eating a wide variety of foods in ample amounts and the mother wants to give him other milk, plain ordinary cow's milk (or soy milk for vegan families) is acceptable. If the parents are concerned about calcium intake, the baby can eat yogurt, cheese or tofu. If the baby is only three or four months old, it is still possible to avoid the bottle so that he does not refuse the breast. The baby can be given formula by spoon or by cup, though some babies or parents find it difficult to use a cup at that age. It can be done, however. I mention formula because it is unlikely the mother can express much while pregnant. If she expressed milk and stored it before she became pregnant, she should use that. Banked breastmilk is an option, although it is expensive and not always easily available.

If the baby is three or four months, in order to avoid the bottle, it might be better to start him on solids mixed with formula. I see it as a better solution than feeding the baby by bottle, because that can lead to rejecting the breast completely, which is worse than starting solids earlier than recommended.

Maternal illness can decrease milk production. Mastitis or blocked ducts are not infrequent causes, but any febrile illness may be a culprit. Fortunately, most maternal illness does not affect milk production. If you do get sick, though, go to bed and rest, with plenty of fluids close by. Bring the baby into bed with you and breastfeed as often

Other medications that may reduce the milk supply

The experience of many mothers suggests that these medications can reduce milk production:

- **Bromocriptine (Parlodel)** and **cabergoline (Dostinex)** definitely do. These two drugs inhibit the production of prolactin and therefore dry up the milk. Cabergoline is safer than bromocriptine, which has apparently caused several deaths due to stroke. Neither should be used to stop milk production after birth if there is even the slightest chance that the mother might change her mind about breastfeeding. She can effectively stop milk production by not putting the baby to the breast and by expressing just enough milk to feel comfortable. Even better, she can put the baby to the breast and reduce the feedings slowly.

- **Antihistamines.** I know of no study that has shown decreased milk supply after taking antihistamines, but mothers report this. Antihistamines are used for relief of symptoms of allergies and colds, often combined with pseudoephedrine (Sudafed).

- **Pseudoephedrine (Sudafed)** has, in one study, been shown to decrease milk production. Local treatments using antihistamines and/or other medications are better than oral medications. Oral medications go through the whole body; local treatments go only where they are needed. The amount that gets into the milk is very small.

- **Antidepressants**. We sometimes hear from a mother that she started taking SSRI antidepressants (for example, Prozac,

Lexapro, etc.) and her milk supply decreased. This is unusual and may be due to other factors. The drug most often mentioned is bupropion (Wellbutrin), which is not related to the SSRI antidepressants. It is also used to help people stop smoking.

Alternatives to oral antihistamines and pseudoephedrine

You can ask your doctor about treating allergies with:

- **Nose drops** containing medications that cause constriction of blood vessels, decrease mucus secretion or those that contain antihistamines can be used to treat nasal congestion and itchiness.
- **Drops containing antihistamines** are used for watery, itchy eyes. The drugs that cause blood vessels to constrict are also found in eye drops and can be helpful as well.
- **Drops or sprays containing corticosteroids** are effective for nasal congestion and itchiness. Corticosteroids or other drugs delivered by inhaler for problems such as wheezing are very effective and these drugs do not affect milk production. Furthermore, these inhaled medications do not get into the mother's bloodstream in any significant amounts and cannot get into the milk. Corticosteroid eye drops should never be used without an ophthalmologist's okay!
- **Cromolyn** does not seem to be used much these days but it is a safe and effective drug for allergy symptoms. It is available for inhalation, orally and in eye and nose drops.

as the baby wants. Don't worry about passing the virus on to the baby—he was already exposed before you even knew you were sick, and now you'll be passing on antibodies and other immune factors in your milk.

The baby is getting more than the occasional bottle. It is best to avoid bottles altogether. Formula company brochures encourage mothers to have their partner feed the baby a bottle in the evening so the mother can rest and her partner and the baby can "bond." Formula companies know what they are doing; one bottle in the evening becomes two bottles and then three, and soon the mother is not able to express enough milk and must start formula. Some mothers have a generous enough milk supply that they can manage in spite of bottle-feeding, but many do not. Don't take a bottle when you go out with the baby—just breastfeed wherever you are. If people are offended, that's their problem. In every jurisdiction in Canada the human rights commissions have always found in favour of mothers who have been told to stop breastfeeding by business owners or security staff. In the United States, many states have enacted laws stating that babies can be breastfed anywhere that mothers are legally allowed to be.

I also encourage mothers to take as long a maternity leave as they can. In the United States, maternity leave is disgracefully short; it is shocking to think that mothers have to leave their newborn babies only six weeks after birth or even sooner if they can't afford an unpaid leave. It is destructive to breastfeeding, but even if the mother is not breastfeeding, it is a horrid thing to do. A maternity leave of less than six months is, in my opinion, indecent. But if the mother has at least six months, she never has to start formula or bottles. See the chapter "Breastfeeding and Mother–Baby Separation."

Parents are trying to stretch out the feedings and/or make the baby sleep through the night. By the time the baby is three or four months, everyone tells the parents he should not be feeding more than every two or three hours and/or that he should be sleeping through the night. One "expert" said all health professionals are now in agreement that breastfeeding on demand is "dangerous." (*Really? Well, here's one who doesn't agree.*) She added that mothers must start a three-hourly breastfeeding routine while in the hospital; if they feed before the three-hour timeline the milk the baby gets is "unmade"! (*What on earth is "unmade milk"?*)

A possible cause of this late-onset decreased supply is that even mothers who are breastfeeding "on demand" are influenced by such nonsense. They breastfeed, and then an hour later, say, the baby starts to show interest again. The mother assumes (because of the endless advice about feeding every three or four hours) that the baby can't possibly be hungry again. She may pick him up, rock him, walk around with him, do whatever she can to calm him. And since he's not ravenous yet, he settles down. She may give him a pacifier or he may find his finger to suck on, and he stops fussing. Half an hour later, he tries to signal his desire to breastfeed again, and she again puts him off. Finally, after around three hours or whatever the mom thinks is "reasonable," the baby is fed.

The overall effect is a gradual decrease in milk production. Babies need to feed when they need to feed. Women have breastfed since the beginning of mammalian life on earth when the baby asked for it, without clocks to limit feedings. In fact, short frequent feedings seem to be the norm for breastfeeding.

What about the mother who says that feeding her baby so often is tiring, or that she's not getting other things done?

Well, we *can* make breastfeeding more efficient. But mothers all over the world and throughout history have breastfed their babies as needed, while often doing very taxing physical labour. Wraps, slings and baby carriers make it all easier, and having a relaxed attitude about breastfeeding helps considerably. A mother can breastfeed while walking around, while reading a book to her toddler, while working on the computer. As for sleeping through the night at four months or so, here's a secret: there are lots of formula-fed babies who are not sleeping through the night at four months. We just don't hear as much about them. There are also exclusively breastfed babies who *are* sleeping through the night at four months. But it is normal and okay for your

---

Keeping your baby close?

All primate mothers, from the most primitive to the most evolved, carry their babies a large part of the day. They also sleep with them. They breastfeed, which is much easier and more convenient and likely to succeed if the baby is in close contact with them. The longer the pregnancy, the bigger the brain, the more helpless the baby, the longer he is breastfed and carried. This approach to feeding and rearing has worked from the beginning of mammalian time on earth. This is how it has always been until recently.

So what happened? By the end of the 19th century, humans were enamoured with science, which seemed to make life so easy. We still are enamoured, despite the many failures of technology. During this time period, we applied science not only to wash our clothes and move around in automobiles and airplanes, but also to raise children.

Breastfeeding was a problem for science. As Lord Kelvin, one of the great scientists of the 19th century, stated: "If you can measure that of what you speak, and can express it by a number, you know something of your subject; but if you cannot measure it, your knowledge is meagre and unsatisfactory." How could you measure how much the breastfed baby got? Bottle feeding was "more scientific" because you could measure this. And how could you measure the effects of childrearing if they were constantly being carried? Observations were difficult as babies moved around. So babies were put into boxes that allowed calm observation. This approach changed the model of what was normal infant feeding and childrearing. In other words, babies fed bottles and kept in cribs became the new normal and anything that varied from this norm was considered not good for the baby. It did not take long for the conclusions of these experiments, as abnormal as the conditions were, to spill over into what pediatricians and other "experts" were advising mothers to do.

By the 1930s, mothers were sternly warned not to pick up their babies except at very specific times. When babies cried, the mothers cried too, but the word from the "experts" was that it was forbidden to pick up or even touch their babies. This would spoil them. One Canadian pediatrician even wrote that picking up a two-week-old who was crying was the first step towards juvenile court.

We have learned a lot since then, but the mentality of spoiling has not disappeared. In the 1960s premature babies lived in boxes, too (incubators). Parents were not allowed to hold them at all and could not even touch them unless they were gowned, masked, capped and gloved as if they were doing surgery. In the last 20 to 30 years we have learned that this is not good for premature babies and that Kangaroo Mother Care is much better for their stability and development. But despite masses of evidence, many special care units for premature babies still have not adopted it.

The same can be said for carrying babies. Forty years ago, experiments compared the effects of movement on the development of baby monkeys. The monkeys were raised in cages in which the "mother" was a non-animate object (an empty bleach bottle) which was either stationary or attached to a rope. The baby monkeys would cling to the bottle whether it moved or not. But the monkeys who were raised in the cages with stationary mothers developed depression, had difficulty interacting with other monkeys, did not like to be touched, and developed the type of stereotypical rocking behaviour which was once frequently seen in children who were deprived of contact. Other pathological behaviour included self-mutilation and chronic self-soothing behaviour such as sucking their toes obsessively. As juveniles and adults, these monkeys demonstrated violent behaviour.

It is interesting that in recent years self-soothing has become a new idea in pediatric advice even though in other mammals it is seen as abnormal. It is said to be a good thing that a child is able to "self-soothe." This is stated particularly in relation to breastfeeding. "Do not breastfeed your baby to sleep," the experts say. "Let him self-soothe." But why? Well, basically because the child who is not nursed to sleep no longer makes demands on the parents, particularly the mother. After all, a baby who breastfeeds to sleep will continue to want to breastfeed to sleep and that is inconvenient.

It is true that babies can be inconvenient. But modern ideas can be very damaging and perhaps we need to rethink them. The fact that in the long run it is easier to breastfeed a baby to sleep, the fact that babies and toddlers love it and often mothers do too is ignored. The idea is to render the child "independent" as if *forcing* independence is a good thing. Forced independence is not true independence; independence that arises from security is.

The self-soothing approach is applied to carrying of babies. "If you carry your baby, he won't be able to self-soothe. He won't be able to do without you. He won't become independent." This is just so much nonsense. Babies were made to be carried and should be carried. They will, as they get older, want to be carried less and less. Eventually they will want to be carried only when they are tired. It will happen more rapidly than you expect. And maybe you will even miss carrying them.

baby to wake up at night. If you keep your baby close to you at night, everyone will get more sleep.

The mother has had an emotional shock. For many years I dismissed this possibility, probably because the situation was uncommon, but a few cases convinced me. In one case a mother breastfed beautifully until her baby and her husband were admitted to the hospital on the same day, the baby with pyloric stenosis and the father with appendicitis. The mother's milk supply dropped through the floor but responded well to domperidone. The few other cases I have seen responded very well to it too.

The mother is trying to do too much. Mothers frequently say that they have decreases in their milk production because they are trying to do too much. Whether this is true or not, it is probably a good thing to get more help from their partners, or extended family, or to allow themselves to let other things go.

The mother is feeding one breast at a feeding, or block feeding. I wrote about this in the first edition of this book, but I think the whole process was misunderstood. I already discussed one-sided feeding earlier in this chapter. One-sided feeding can be used to decrease an oversupply of milk, which can make babies fussy, but we should be careful not to turn advice for a specific problem into hard and fast rules.

If milk production decreases with one-sided feeding, the baby may not be happy with the amount he gets from one breast. He's hungry, but when he cries the mother may assume she needs to limit his feeding even more, and go to several feedings on the same breast (block feeding). If the baby seems hungry after feeding on one side, the mother should offer the other breast. I wish we had never heard of "hind milk" and "foremilk." The concept was useful in ending the strict limits on feeding times (such as 15 minutes each side), but too many people, including some lactation consultants, don't understand the implications.

If a mother feeds the baby just on one breast, at some point he stops drinking and just nibbles. At some feedings, he may drink a lot and be satisfied with just one breast. At other feedings, he may drink a short time only and then nibble. If he's nibbling, he's not getting "hind milk" because he's not getting any milk at all. The mother can compress the breast to increase his drinking (see the chapter "Increasing Breastmilk Intake by the Baby"), but if he is getting sleepy or pulling off, she should offer the other side. Most mothers find they have more milk in the morning than in the evening, so one breast at a feeding might work in the morning, but not in the evening. Some mothers just don't have enough milk for the baby to be satisfied with one breast at any time of the day.

This reason is probably the most common of them all. In the first few weeks, babies tend to fall asleep at the breast when the flow of milk slows down. If the baby is not latched on well, this tends to happen earlier in the feeding, but if the mother has an abundant milk supply he can still gain well. He's depending on the letdowns to get milk. So he'll suck and sleep and suck, getting a bit more milk each time the mother has a letdown. Once the baby is older, however, he may pull away from the breast when the flow slows down, often within minutes of starting the feeding. When this pulling occurs, most mothers put the baby on the other side. But then the same thing happens. The baby is still hungry but may refuse to take the breast and will suck on his fingers instead. By pulling off, he's not getting those extra milk ejection reflexes. He takes less milk, the milk supply decreases, the flow slows down even earlier in the feeding, he takes less—a vicious cycle. Some babies may gain weight well even if they spend only a short period of time on the breast. They may still pull off and suck their hands because they want more sucking (which is pleasurable), but if they are content and weight gain is good, there is no need for concern. The way to prevent all this is to get a good latch from the beginning. Many mothers are told the latch is perfect when, in fact, it is far from it. The latch can still be improved even in the older baby, with good help; however, a baby with a tongue tie will have difficulty latching on well and though he may not have problems at first if the milk supply is abundant, with time the milk supply will decrease. Often, domperidone will increase the milk supply significantly. However, we don't use domperidone during pregnancy; it is unlikely to work and may be unsafe.

So what can be done if we suspect a late-onset decrease in milk supply?

One thing to avoid is giving the baby bottles. Even if it's expressed milk in the bottle, the bottle is the problem. If the mother has had a significant decrease

in milk production, starting bottles can finish off the breastfeeding quickly. If the baby is four months old or so and in urgent need of more nutrients, adding solids would be a better approach than supplementing with bottles. Breastmilk, preferably, or formula, if necessary, can be added to the solids. The baby should be offered, without forcing, as much of the solids as he will eat, as often as he will eat them. We do not recommend commercial cereals as first foods because they are low in calories and nutrients, taste awful and can cause constipation.

However, adding solids is usually not necessary. In most cases the baby is healthy even if he has not gained weight in a month or so because he gained so rapidly before the milk intake diminished.

We try to eliminate any factors interfering with milk supply: stopping birth control pills immediately, for example, or starting to feed the baby from both breasts at each feeding. We treat most mothers with domperidone, because it brings back milk production quickly. Many mothers don't like the idea of taking domperidone and would rather pump, but experience tells us pumping just doesn't work well, perhaps because the problem had been going on for many weeks. It frustrates me that many physicians are eager to prescribe the birth control pill, but when it causes the mother's milk production to decrease, they are reluctant or refuse to prescribe domperidone. We start domperidone at a dose of 30 mg (three tablets) three times a day. Sometimes we go up from there, but generally nine tablets a day suffice and the baby starts gaining weight. If not, we look for other reasons the milk supply has decreased and consider adding solids.

A last word on starting solids earlier than six months in these cases. The Canadian Paediatric Society, Health Canada and most pediatric societies around the world recommend exclusive breastfeeding to six months (but that does not mean exactly

182½ days). Mothers with late-onset decreased milk supply are often told they cannot give solids at five months but must give formula instead if the baby is not gaining well. But in these cases, the baby needs extra calories. If he gets formula, he won't be exclusively breastfeeding anyway. And giving a bottle will often be the final blow to breastfeeding. If we let the baby eat as much high quality food as he wants, he will get the nutrients and calories he needs to gain more weight, and will still get the nutrients, calories and protection from illness from his mother's milk.

10 | Sore Nipples

Myth #1: It is normal for breastfeeding to hurt, at least at first.

Fact: This myth scares some mothers away from even trying to breastfeed, causes considerable pain and suffering for many and often leads to early weaning. It may be *common* for nipples to hurt, but it is not *normal*. It can be prevented and treatment usually works. For the majority of mothers who receive help to start with and who have a baby who latches well, breastfeeding will almost always be painless.

Myth #2: Taking the baby off the breast to give the nipples a "rest" is a good treatment for sore nipples.

Fact: I accept this as a *last* resort, but the problem is that once the baby is off the breast for the time it takes for nipples to heal, he may not take the breast again, having gotten used to the bottle. If he does take the breast, he may not latch well, and the nipple pain will return.

It's just not true that pain is a *necessary* part of breastfeeding, not even in the first few days after birth, when mothers are told that the nipples have to "get used to breastfeeding" or that the nipples must "toughen up." I cannot believe we still talk about toughening up nipples—after all these years!

During the first few days after birth, some mothers will describe a mild discomfort as the baby suckles. It shouldn't be more than that, and it shouldn't be bad enough that she dreads feedings. If the mother has significant pain, something is

wrong. Probably, the baby's latch is not as it should be. Fortunately, many hospital staff and midwives now realize that a poor latch is the usual cause of having nipple pain in the first few days.

Unfortunately, most have not learned how to help improve the latch. Mothers are told, "If it hurts, the latch is not as good as it could be." So far, so good. But then if it still hurts, they are told, "Take the baby off the breast and latch on again." It hurts again, so the mother is told, "Take him off again, and latch him on again . . . and again and again and again . . . as long as it hurts." What is the result? If the mother takes the baby off the breast and relatches the baby five times, she has five times more pain, the nipples are damaged five times, and both she and the baby are frustrated. In fact, many mothers coming to our clinic have said they took the baby off the breast and relatched him 10, 15 and even more times, each time with pain (and each time with more damage to the nipple).

Usually, if the baby latches on and it hurts but the mother doesn't take him off the breast, the pain decreases and may even disappear as the baby feeds. The pain can be made to diminish more quickly by pushing the baby's bottom in closer with the forearm so the latch is more asymmetrical. The mother can also gently pull down the baby's chin so that he has more of the breast in his mouth. These two adjustments can diminish the pain and help the baby get more milk faster, shortening the feeding. The mother should then get help with the latching on the other side or at the next feeding.

Preventing nipple pain

Preventing nipple pain comes down to one thing: getting as good a latch as possible as soon as possible after the baby's birth.

1. If the mother has as few interventions during birth as is consistent with good care, the baby is more likely to latch on better. Of course, sometimes interventions are necessary to decrease the risk of injury or death but when the epidural rate is approaching 100% in many hospitals and Caesarean section rates are regularly 30%, something is not right.

2. Encouraging immediate skin-to-skin contact after the birth and giving the baby the time to find the breast on his own (breast crawl) will usually result in a good latch. Looking for the nipple and areola, squeezing them with his hand, and finally latching on, the baby usually takes the breast well and without causing pain. Narcotics given to the mother during the labour and birth can interfere with this process.

3. Separation of the mother and the baby, delays in starting breastfeeding or feeding by the clock may result in a less-than-adequate latch. Mothers and babies should be together skin to skin as much as possible in the early days after birth. Feeding by schedule increases the likelihood of the breasts becoming engorged, or so painfully "full" that the baby cannot latch on easily or at all. If the baby feeds well at the breast, the mother is much less likely to become engorged.

4. Many babies will spend hours on the breast in the first few days of life, and this is often seen as contributing to sore nipples. But long feedings do not automatically cause pain. The problem is that the baby is latched on poorly and not getting the milk that's available. It is essential to ensure the baby is well latched on and drinking at the breast much of the time, not just sucking without drinking. Making sure the baby is drinking may require the use of breast compression. Breast compression often works quite well during the first few days after birth. However, it may take several cycles of compression to get the colostrum moving (see the video clip of the two-day-old baby at www.breastfeedinginc.ca). By getting more milk out of the breast and into the baby, the risk of engorgement is reduced, and this sets up a "virtuous" cycle as opposed to the too-frequent

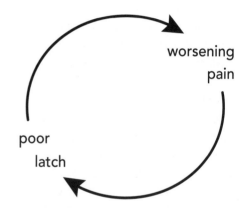

worsening pain

poor latch

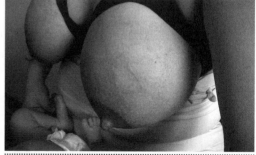

Postpartum engorgement due to fluid from an intravenous. Notice that the baby can latch on only to the nipple, thus not getting milk and, at the same time, causing the mother nipple pain. There is a scab on the nipple.
CREDIT: JACK NEWMAN

vicious cycle: poor latch—engorgement—long and inefficient feeding—worsening pain.

5. If the vicious cycle described above has begun, the nurse may suggest a bottle (or the mother may ask for one) to give the nipples "a rest." But this teaches a baby to suck on a bottle, not to breastfeed. A baby sucks very differently on a bottle than at the breast, and if he gets a reward (milk) from the bottle that he didn't get from the breast, one does not have to be a genius to figure out which he will prefer. The bottle method of sucking will interfere with the baby's latch and result in more pain when he returns to the breast. The point is to *fix the problem,* and the bottle is not a fix. If the mother cannot keep the baby on the breast or fixing the latch still does not result in milk, the lactation aid at the breast is the best solution. It keeps the baby at the breast but shortens the feeding time.

What if the mother gets engorged? Should she use a breast pump?

As mentioned earlier, much of the engorgement that occurs after birth is not due to milk building up in the breast, but to edema, the accumulation of intravenous fluids given during labour and after birth. By using a pump, the mother may actually increase the fluid in the front of her breast and make the situation worse, not better.

So how does one treat engorgement?

Hand expression can soften up the nipples and areolas so that the baby can latch on and get milk. If that doesn't work, we use reverse pressure softening, a technique suggested by Jean Cotterman, an American lactation consultant. In effect, what we are trying to do is push the fluid from the front of the breast backwards so that the nipple and areola are softer and the baby can latch on more easily.

Reverse Pressure Softening
K. Jean Cotterman RNC-E, IBCLC

More health care providers are observing that mothers who receive multiple intrapartum IV's (large amounts of IV fluids during labour and delivery) experience delay in expected postpartum fluid shift. Increased edema during the early postpartum period intensifies engorgement, increases sub-areolar tissue resistance, distorts the nipple and interferes with comfortable, efficient latching.

I want to share an intervention that has proven very helpful in the first seven to fourteen days postpartum. I call it Reverse Pressure Softening. The key is making the areola (the circle) very soft right around the base of the nipple right before every feeding, for better latching. Your baby needs the areola to be soft to get a "good mouthful" of breast beyond the nipple in order to remove more milk and be very gentle to your nipple.

Try this in the early weeks of learning to breastfeed if pain, swelling or fullness cause problems:

- Lie most of the way down on your back when you soften the areola. (This is a great way for your baby and you to learn to breastfeed too).
- Look at the pictures that follow. Choose the easiest way for you to press on the areola.
- Be gentle to avoid pain, but press the circle firmly and steadily in toward your heart, counting slowly to 50. *Count very slowly if very swollen.*
- In the hospital, ask someone to show you. At home, ask for help from a relative or friend
- Soften the areola right before each feeding (or pumping) till latching is always easy.

If you need to pump milk for your baby,

- Always soften the areola first before you pump.
- Use only medium or low vacuum so swelling won't move back into the areola.

- Pause to re-soften the areola once or twice to get more **total** milk out.
- Make pumping sessions short, but frequent (every two to three hours), during the daytime.

Method 1: Two-step method. Use the straight fingers of both hands placed with the knuckles touching the nipple: Count to 50 in each position. **If very swollen, count very slowly.**

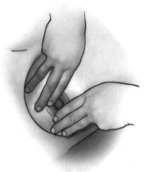

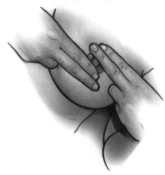

1. Place fingers on each side of the nipple

2. Place fingers above and below the nipple

Method 2: Soft ring method. Cut off the bottom half of an artificial nipple and place on the areola. Press with fingers as in Method 1. Count to 50. **If very swollen, count very slowly.**

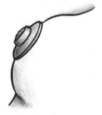

Method 3: One-handed "flower hold." Place curved fingertips where baby's tongue would go. Count to 50. **If very swollen, count very slowly.**

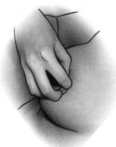

ILLUSTRATIONS: **KYLE COTTERMAN**

What about sucking problems?

Mothers often email me about their babies' weak sucks, which they think are the cause of their breastfeeding problems. Frequently the mothers of babies with "weak suck" also have sore nipples. Other mothers ascribe their nipple pain to the baby's "strong suck." Any abnormal suck can cause sore nipples as well as poor intake of milk.

But are the sucks "weak" or "strong"? The weak suck is due to slow flow or early and continued use of artificial nipples. A strong suck probably means the baby is latched on poorly. Full-term, healthy babies should not have abnormal sucks. If they do, it is usually because of their feeding experiences.

Clearly, though, some babies do have difficulties with sucking normally. Babies with cleft palates cannot suck properly because they cannot form a seal with the breast. Babies with tongue ties don't latch well and can't move their tongues normally, so they don't suck well. But if the flow of milk from the breast is rapid, they don't have "weak" sucks. Babies with neurological problems can also have sucking problems. Neurological problems are often temporary, if, for example, they are due to the drugs the mother received during the labour and birth.

In the first few days, if a baby latches on well, sucks and gets milk, he learns that this is how to breastfeed. I realize there are conditions that make getting off to a good start difficult, but most mothers and babies should be able to get going immediately after birth.

What if the mother gets sore nipples?

Treatment should be started as soon as possible. It is much easier to heal sore nipples starting on day two than on day 22. This is one of the problems with telling mothers that sore nipples are normal for the first two or three weeks; the mothers keep struggling (and suffering). Some will decide they can't take it anymore and stop breastfeeding, or pump and give bottles. Some are devastated when they pass the three- or four-week mark without improvement. Even if the pain ends by then, the mother has gone through weeks of unnecessary pain.

Getting a good latch as soon as possible is the treatment of choice.

Finish the first side before offering the second side. If the baby drinks really well at the first breast, he may not want the second side, giving that nipple a little break. Use breast compression (see videos at www.breastfeedinginc.ca) to help the baby get more milk from the first side. He may want to take the second side, especially in the evening, but a good latch and breast compression will mean he spends less time on the breast. We don't recommend that you limit the baby's time breastfeeding, but if he feeds really well it should happen naturally.

Breast compression can reduce the pain even if the feedings are not less frequent or shorter. Long feedings in themselves don't cause nipple pain, but when the baby changes from mostly drinking to mostly nibbling, the pain returns or worsens. By using compression and increasing the flow of milk to the baby, the pain decreases significantly.

Exposing the nipples to air helps with healing. Breast pads can cause more damage as they get wet; they often stick to the nipples, which hurt even more when the mother tries to remove them. So unless you have vasospasm (Raynaud's phenomenon, see page 144), exposure to the air (even the sun, but not long enough to get sunburned) can help considerably. When you can't expose your nipples to the air, try using a breast shell to protect them. You can add cotton breast pads on the outside of the shell, if needed, to catch any milk that leaks.

The all-purpose nipple ointment (APNO)

We call our nipple ointment "all-purpose," since it contains ingredients that help deal with multiple causes or aggravating factors of sore nipples. Mothers with sore nipples don't have time to try out different treatments, so we have combined various treatments in one ointment. Of course, preventing sore nipples in the first place is the best solution, and adjusting how the baby takes the breast can do more than anything to decrease and eliminate nipple soreness. The APNO contains:

1. Mupirocin 2% ointment. Mupirocin (Bactroban is the trade name) is an antibiotic that is effective against many bacteria, including *Staphylococcus aureus* and MRSA (methicillin-resistant *Staphylococcus aureus*). *Staphylococcus aureus* is commonly found growing in abrasions or cracks in the nipples. Mupirocin apparently has some effect against *Candida albicans* (commonly called thrush or yeast). Treatment of sore nipples with an antibiotic alone sometimes seems to work, but we feel that the antibiotic works best in combination with the other ingredients discussed below. Although it can be taken by mouth, it is so quickly metabolized in the body that it is destroyed before blood levels can be measured. Most of the ointment stays on the skin so that very little is taken in by the baby.
2. Betamethasone 0.1% ointment. Betamethasone is a corticosteroid that decreases inflammation. By decreasing the inflammation, the APNO also decreases the pain the mother feels. Most of the betamethasone in the ointment is absorbed into the skin by the mother, so that the baby takes in very little.
3. Miconazole powder. Miconazole is an antifungal agent very effective against *Candida albicans*.

Because it is added as a powder, the concentration can be increased to 4% or decreased to less than 2%. We feel 2% is the best concentration for most situations. Fluconazole powder to 2% may be substituted for miconazole and so can clotrimazole (Canesten) powder to 2%, but I believe that the latter irritates more than the other drugs in the same family. Miconazole cream or gel cannot be substituted for miconazole powder as the compound will usually separate. If miconazole, fluconazole or clotrimazole are not easily available as powders, it is better to use only the mupirocin and betamethasone ointments mixed together than to add a cream or a gel, or nystatin ointment, for example.

By using a powder, the concentration of the other two ingredients is not as decreased as they would be if another ointment were used for the antifungal agent (for example, nystatin ointment). Thus, in the above preparation the concentration of the betamethasone becomes 0.05% (due to combination with the mupirocin) and the mupirocin concentration is decreased to 1%. Note that nystatin ointment, which we used to use and which decreases the concentration of the other ingredients, is far inferior to miconazole and also tastes bad. I write the prescription this way.

1. Mupirocin ointment 2%: 15 g
2. Betamethasone ointment 0.1%: 15 g
3. To which is added Miconazole powder to a concentration of 2%
    Total: about 30 g combined

If possible, it is best to get the prescription filled at a compounding pharmacy, which is not like most neighbourhood drugstores. A list of compounding pharmacies in Canada, the United States and some other countries can be found at the website www.iacprx.org. Click "For Patients, Pet Owners" in the red box on the left side of the page, then click "Finding a Compounding Pharmacist Near You." The mother will need to sign in. Canadians should make sure to leave a space between the two sets of three characters in the postal code: e.g., M2K 2E1, not M2K2E1.

How to use the ointment:

Apply sparingly after each feeding—just enough to make the nipple and areola shiny. Do not wash it off or wipe it off, even if the baby comes back to the breast earlier than expected.

How long should the ointment be used?

Any drug should be used for the shortest period of time necessary and the same is true for our ointment. If the mother still needs it after two or three weeks, or if the pain returns after she has stopped using it, she should get "hands on" help again to find out why the pain hasn't stopped. The most important step for decreasing nipple pain is still getting the best latch possible. Sometimes a tongue tie that has gone unnoticed is the reason for continued pain.

Some pharmacists tell mothers that the steroid in the ointment will cause thinning of the skin if she uses it for too long. While this is a concern with any steroid applied to the skin, we have not seen this happen, even when mothers have used it for months.

Some other treatments

Cranial sacral therapy. With babies who have had difficult births or who keep slipping off the breast, cranial sacral therapy sometimes seems to help. It is often done by chiropractors or sometimes specialists in infant cranial sacral therapy. Some mothers swear by it. It is a very gentle treatment that has nothing to do with cracking backs. The

main drawback is that if the family does not have insurance it can be expensive.

Surgical dressings. On the recommendation of Montreal's Herzl breastfeeding clinic, we started to treat mothers with significant cracks in their nipples with a surgical dressing called Mepilex. Some mothers find it very helpful, others do not get much relief. The sheets are expensive, but the mother will need to use only small amounts at a time. She cuts a piece that will fit into the crack. Then, on top, she places another piece that will hold the first one in place. She takes off the dressing when she feeds the baby on that side, but as long as it sticks and is not stained with secretions, the same piece can be re-used.

Some approaches I disagree with

1. Taking the baby off the breast to let the nipples "rest" and "recover" from breastfeeding (or, to use an expression I hate, "Take a nipple holiday"). With this approach, the mothers are advised to pump their breasts and usually feed the baby by bottle. This should be a *last* resort only, when the mother has so much pain that she can't face breastfeeding.

But how did the mother get to this point? The mother didn't get the help she needed earlier. When a mother says that she was advised to take her two-day-old baby off the breast, I have to ask, "Was everything else really tried before this suggestion was made?" Somehow I doubt it. What's wrong with taking this approach? Usually the nipples *do* heal and many (though not all) mothers find that pumping is less painful than breastfeeding. The problem is that when the mother tries to put the baby back on the breast, he often refuses or latches worse than ever.

Here is a common story, one I've heard from hundreds, even thousands of mothers: "I experienced cracked, bleeding nipples and yeast infection. I had a prescription for these problems. I was told to use the bottle while the infection went away. Now my baby doesn't want to take the breast and prefers the bottle."

Another mother wrote to me that her nipples had become very sore, so she was advised to use a nipple shield and now was pumping and bottlefeeding exclusively. The baby would take the breast only occasionally, and then only with the nipple shield. She loved breastfeeding, her baby had loved breastfeeding, and she wanted him back at her breast, but had no idea where to start. What could she do?

It isn't easy to get a baby who is used to bottles or nipple shields to take the breast again, and the mother will need skilled help. And if the baby does take the breast with a bottle-feeding type of suck, the pain may come back. The mother may think perhaps she has *Candida* (thrush) even though the problem is the baby's latch.

Furthermore, exclusive pumping often leads to a significant decrease in the milk supply. A baby who feeds *well* on the breast will get more than a mother can pump. So with less breast "emptying," the supply decreases. I often hear from mothers who say that after their nipples have healed, they try to latch the baby back on the breast. Often the baby latches well, but during the feeding he starts crying and flinging his head from side to side as though not satisfied. This sounds very much like Late-Onset Decreased Milk Supply, doesn't it?

One thing the mother can do is take ibuprofen or another pain reliever to help her continue to breastfeed.

Another option would be to have the mother express milk from one breast, then use that expressed milk in a lactation aid while she feeds the baby at the other breast. In this way, the baby should get all the milk he needs while nursing only on one breast,

allowing the other breast to "rest" for a bit. The pain associated with "nibbling" will be avoided, the feeding will go more quickly and the baby's latch and sucking may also improve with the faster flow of milk.

Taking the baby off the breast is often suggested if the mother's nipples bleed from a crack or abrasion. But blood in the milk is not a reason to take the baby off the breast. The issue is the pain the mother feels, not the blood. Blood in the baby's stomach can cause spitting up but is not dangerous. If we can make the mother's pain tolerable, even if the nipples continue to bleed, let's keep the baby on the breast. If the damage is minimized by fixing the way the baby takes the breast, the abrasions/cracks will heal and the bleeding will stop.

2. Taking the baby off the breast and relatching several times until it doesn't hurt. I've already discussed this, pointing out that it doesn't work, causes more pain and leaves both mother and baby frustrated.

3. Starting with the less sore side first. In principle, if the baby is ravenous and "attacks the breast," it may be more bearable to start on the less sore side. When he goes to the second side, no longer as hungry, he may suck more gently. But some babies don't open their mouths as wide when they are less hungry. And, really, the key point is to get a good latch on both breasts.

4. Nipple shields. In my experience, not only does a nipple shield not fix the problem, it creates more problems. Yes, many mothers have less pain, maybe even no pain with the nipple shield, but it still is not the answer. Because the nipple shield very likely decreases the milk supply, the mother often ends up either pumping to maintain the supply and/or starts giving the baby formula. Using the nipple shield plus pumping makes breastfeeding complicated,

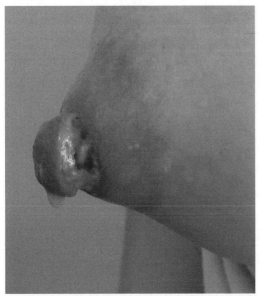

This should never have happened: severe nipple trauma due to poor latch and poor management of the mother's problem. There is a large crack in the nipple. This woman would be a good candidate for the surgical dressing Mepilex.

CREDIT: **JACK NEWMAN**

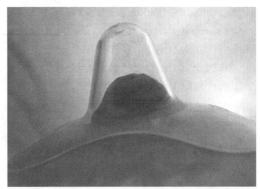

A nipple shield in place. How can the baby draw out the nipple? He will have to depend on the mother's milk-ejection reflex in order to get milk. If she has an abundant milk supply, the baby may gain weight all right. But if she does not, the baby may not get enough. And even if the woman has an abundant supply now, it will decrease with time.

CREDIT: **ANDREA POLOKOVA**

and the more complicated the process, the more likely the mother will stop. We have even heard of women using a lactation aid under the nipple shield to make sure the baby gets enough milk.

But what if the nipple shield is the only thing that helps? If the mother had had *good* help earlier, she would not have reached the point of "needing" the nipple shield. In fact, I think it is better for the mother to express (pump) her milk and give it in a bottle than use a nipple shield. It is less work to do this than to feed with a nipple shield, pump, and supplement with the pumped milk.

Here is just one of many similar cases I have seen: The mother has a nine-week-old baby, and has been to several different clinics for help. Early on, her nipples became very sore and were soon blistered and scabbed. She began using nipple shields and felt they

helped—except that her baby would fall asleep within minutes of being latched on. He'd then wake again within an hour, crying for food. The mother began to pump her milk and feed it to the baby in a bottle, which seemed to work well for a few weeks. But then she developed painful cracks in her nipples from pumping, and at the same time found her milk supply dropping so that she was having to supplement with formula as well. We see similar situations in our clinic frequently and are then in the very difficult position of trying to fix the ravages caused by the nipple shield.

The nipple shield is not even of temporary help sometimes. Here is another email similar to many that I receive. "The lactation consultant also provided me with a nipple shield to use, but the pain was even worse when I used it. It was extreme pain and a burning sensation, and it lasted for a while after feeding, so I stopped using it." Good decision by that mother!

Another mother emailed me to say that she had several cracks on her right nipple that were excruciatingly painful. She seemed to believe that these had developed because the baby was latching on only to the right breast, but that was not true. She had used a shield in the hopes of helping the nipple to heal, only to find that it was even more painful with the shield in place. I assume that the baby didn't latch on to the left breast because there was less milk on that side. On the right side, the baby "sort of" latched on; this poor latch caused the mother significant damage and pain. Feeding on one breast with a *good* latch should not be painful.

See more on nipple shields in the following chapters: "The Preterm and Near-term Baby," "When the Baby Does Not Yet Take the Breast" and "Breastfeeding Devices."

What else can cause nipple pain or make it worse?
Bacterial overgrowth

Often abrasions and sores on the nipple grow bacteria, the most common being *Staphylococcus aureus*. Whether these bacteria are actually causing infection is questionable. Antibacterial creams and ointments have been used in the past to treat sore nipples and seemed to help, at least some of the time. It is for this reason that we include mupirocin as part of our all-purpose nipple ointment. Some breastfeeding clinics advise Polysporin for sore nipples. This ointment contains three different antibiotics but no antifungal agent or corticosteroid. I'm not sure why three different antibiotics are recommended, but I'd be concerned that they might increase the risk of dermatitis (skin inflammation).

Raynaud's phenomenon (vasospasm)

Raynaud's phenomenon may accompany such illnesses as rheumatoid arthritis and lupus erythematosis, although many people exhibit symptoms without having autoimmune disease. It usually involves fingers or toes. When the temperature goes from warm to cold, the blood vessels in the fingers and/or toes go into spasm, blood flow decreases, and the ends become pale or white. The absence of blood results in pain, and when the hands/feet are warmed again, the colour of the affected areas turns red and is often accompanied by a throbbing pain (due to blood pulsating back into the area) or a tingling of pain. Not everyone experiences all the colour changes.

Vasospasm may also affect the nipples/areolas of breastfeeding mothers. The pain of the vasospasm typically occurs after the baby has come off the breast, presumably because even on warm days the inside of the baby's mouth is still warmer than the ambient temperature.

Usually vasospasm occurs as a reaction to other causes of nipple pain, so treatment should begin by fixing the latch. Eliminating the pain during feeding will usually also eliminate the pain due to vasospasm.

Some mothers get vasospasm during pregnancy, others develop it without ever having sore nipples from another cause, while still others become pain-free through other solutions yet continue to suffer from vasospasm. Depending on how much distress the mother is having from the vasospasm, treatment may be indicated. To throw a curve ball into the mix, some mothers have very definite vasospasm with dramatic colour changes yet feel no pain. We do not treat mothers who don't have pain.

An aside: I frequently get emails in which the mother complains of various symptoms, including redness or cracks in the nipples, and yet has no pain. Another example is the baby who has thrush whose mother doesn't have pain. I believe that one should not treat a symptom or sign just because it's there. If the mother has nipples that are bright pink and yet she has no pain, why treat them?

How to treat vasospasm: Treating the mother for nipple pain during feeding will often prevent pain due to vasospasm. However, for some, the pain of vasospasm is very distressing and sometimes more severe than the pain during the feeding. There are mothers who complain of no pain during a feeding yet when the baby comes off the breast, the nipples are flattened on one side like a new lipstick. This suggests that the baby's latch is not good so that even if the mother does not have pain, the blood vessels in the nipple and the areola may become irritated and go into spasm in response to the cooler air.

If the pain of vasospasm is significant and adjusting the baby's latch and the use of the all-purpose nipple ointment (APNO) is not helping, here are some other treatments:

- Avoid exposing the nipples to air after the baby has come off the breast. Edith Kernerman, IBCLC, of the International Breastfeeding Centre in Toronto, has found it often helps to massage the nipples immediately after a feeding, either with some pure olive oil warmed by rubbing it between the fingers, or with the APNO. The pectoral muscle massage treatment used for mammary constriction syndrome can also help (see the section on MCS on page 146).
- Vitamin B6. We have recommended vitamin B6 to mothers with vasospasm for at least 15 years and have found that it works very well in *some* mothers. We usually recommend 200 mg a day as a single dose for four days and 25 to 50 mg a day as a single dose from then on. If the vasospasm returns after lowering the dose, we recommend resuming the higher dose and every so often trying to lower it or stop it altogether. Although some suggest that vitamin B6 can reduce milk supply, I have not seen this even when mothers took 200 mg a day for many weeks. In our clinic we recommend vitamin B6 multi complex, although this combination of B vitamins has not been shown to be any better than the vitamin B6 alone.

- Nifedipine. This drug is in the family of calcium channel blockers, which prevent uptake of calcium by the muscles around blood vessels, causing them to relax. Nifedipine is used primarily to treat high blood pressure, angina and some types of irregular heartbeat. Very little gets into the milk. Although there is a possibility that a mother who normally has low blood pressure might experience too severe a drop, this has not been a problem for our patients.

  The usual dose of nifedipine we use is a 30 mg slow-release tablet once a day for two weeks or so. This dose usually works and can normally be stopped within two to three weeks. Most mothers, if the latch is fixed and the APNO is effective, will also be able to stop the nifedipine without a return of the vasospasm. For some mothers, the pain returns and a second course of nifedipine is needed. Few require more prolonged treatment, though every so often we hear from a mother who needs nifedipine for long periods of time, sometimes as long as they are breastfeeding. I believe it is better to continue with nifedipine for several months than to have a mother suffer or stop breastfeeding. Occasionally we have used larger doses of nifedipine (30 mg twice a day) with success.

  There are other drugs similar to nifedipine. For example, verapamil and diltiazem, also calcium channel blockers, could also be used if for some reason nifedipine doesn't work. Another family of drugs called ACE inhibitors could also be used. Two examples are enalapril and benazepril.

- Nitroglycerine paste. We no longer recommend this for vasospasm. Although it is quite effective, it's easy to put too much on the nipples. The drug is rapidly absorbed and nitroglycerine can cause severe headache, sometimes leading to worse pain than the pain from the vasospasm.

Mammary constriction syndrome (This section written by Edith Kernerman, IBCLC)

This newly described syndrome is related to vasospasm. Many breastfeeding mothers complain of breast pain. We know from much clinical experience and a recent study done at the International Breastfeeding Centre that almost all of these complaints are due to how the baby latches on. The latching difficulties include positioning and tongue tie, which can lead to a secondary problem of vasoconstriction in the breast and nipples.

Vasoconstriction is the tightening of blood vessels, leading to decreased blood flow and oxygen to a particular area. Because of difficulties the mother may have had during pregnancy, labour, or after birth, she may have tightness in her shoulders and chest that causes her pectoral (chest) muscles to press on the blood vessels that lead to her breasts and nipples, causing a lack of blood flow and oxygen, leading to pain. This pain may be throbbing or constant, deep or superficial, itchy, tingling, aching or knife-like, burning or freezing, shooting, sharp or dull, or a combination of any of the above. Also, if a latch feels painful, the mother may tighten her shoulders, clench her teeth, etc., causing the cycle triggering pain to begin again. Many mothers describe the pain as so debilitating they must lie down after a feeding. Others quit breastfeeding altogether. We had often thought these symptoms were a sign of yeast (*Candida*) and in many cases this type of pain may still be due to it. However, we now frequently attribute these symptoms to what we have named mammary constriction syndrome (MCS), a cluster of symptoms caused by the process described above. Vasoconstriction may also trigger vasospasm of the nipples, causing them to change colour or blanch,

and may cause a cold or hot burning sensation, as with Raynaud's syndrome.

How to treat MCS: We use a technique called pectoral muscle massage that is very easy for the mother to do herself. It involves rubbing the chest muscles (*not* the breast) on the affected side quite vigorously—using firm pressure and quick hand movements—for about 45 to 60 seconds, with a flat hand. There are four places to massage: 1) above the breast against the chest wall; 2) between the breasts, just to the side of the breast bone; 3) under the breast, against the rib cage; 4) on the side of the body, beside the breast, against the rib cage. Treating one of these four areas is likely to relieve the pain. Women suffering from MCS should try to avoid hunching over the baby and/or carrying heavy objects, including car seats. We recommend massage therapy to help ease tension in the upper torso. Many mothers have success doing gentle pectoral muscle stretching just before a feeding. One technique is to stand in a doorway with forearms and elbows against the door frame. Lean forward without bending the knees and hold for 30 seconds. Then go back to the vertical position, straighten the arms so just the hands are against the door frame (and high up) and lean forward again. Hold for 30 seconds.

Dermatological conditions

There are several dermatological conditions that can affect the nipples and areolas; the three ingredients in our all-purpose nipple ointment (APNO) should cover all these possibilities. The corticosteroid will help decrease the inflammation of most dermatological conditions. Sometimes eczema or contact dermatitis is aggravated by bacterial infection (especially *Staphylococcus aureus*) or perhaps *Candida* (yeast, thrush), which is why the other two ingredients are included.

If the skin condition is present before birth, it should be treated before the baby is born.

Atopic dermatitis (eczema). Eczema is a fairly common condition, often starting in infancy. It is manifested by dry, scaly, itchy skin, the areas affected varying according to age. Itching is often the most distressing symptom. If the eczema affects the nipples, the mother will sometimes have pain without itching. The pain tends to start within a few weeks of the baby's birth and, as with a *Candida* infection, it often begins after a period of pain-free breastfeeding. The mother describes the pain as burning and itching. However, eczema differs in that the nipples and areolas are usually dry, scaly and have a whitish sheen but the affected area may ooze as well. Nipples infected with Candida may show few changes or may look bright pink.

If the pain is due to eczema, a simple steroid ointment rather than the all-purpose nipple ointment may be enough. It should be applied sparingly after each feeding rather than three or four times a day. However, because of the frequent presence of *Staphylococcus aureus* complicating eczema, I normally recommend the APNO even if I believe the soreness is due to eczema.

It should be noted that *long-term* use of corticosteroids on eczema can actually make it worse. In that case, stopping any steroid ointment is a necessity.

Contact dermatitis. This condition is related to eczema. Anything one puts on the skin may cause contact dermatitis—jewellery, for example. Creams and ointments (including those to treat sore nipples) can also cause it. This is one reason why it is best to put only what is necessary on the nipples and areolas. Our APNO can be said to break this principle by using three ingredients when one might be enough, but the three work together rapidly to help with the

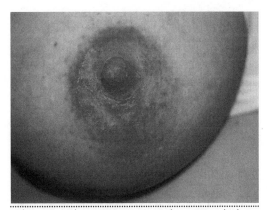

Either atopic dermatitis or contact dermatitis, which affect skin in essentially the same ways. Changes in the nipple are due either to eczema or to contact with an ointment the mother was using.
CREDIT: JACK NEWMAN

most common causes of nipple pain. New mothers' pain is often severe and there may not be time to try out different single-ingredient ointments.

Psoriasis. Psoriasis can also appear on the nipples. It is often there before the baby is born and should be treated before birth. A steroid ointment alone will often be very helpful. Psoriasis is often treated with oral medications. Some of these, such as methotrexate, are thought to be contraindicated during breastfeeding.

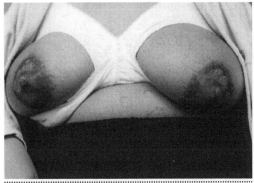

Psoriasis of the areola. There is another lesion of psoriasis on the woman's stomach, at the right edge of the photo.
CREDIT: JACK NEWMAN

As mentioned in the chapter "Breastfeeding While on Medication," methotrexate used for weeks or months is a problem, but there are alternatives such as azathioprine.

Nipple blisters or "blebs"

Sometimes mothers develop a white or yellowish bubble on the end of the nipple that blocks one of the nipple pores and causes significant pain when the baby nurses. Occasionally mothers get blisters on the nipples in the first few days after birth, but these are somewhat different. The typical blister or bleb shows up weeks after the baby is born, when breastfeeding seems to be going fine. There is often no obvious cause. They are often painful. If they are not, there is really no reason to do anything about them.

There appears to be a relationship between these blebs and blocked ducts, but it is not clear. Sometimes a mother develops a blocked duct and a bleb in the area where the duct from that area empties; for example, she will have a blister on the upper inner side of the nipple and a plugged duct on the upper inner side of the breast. But many women have blocked ducts without getting blebs, or vice versa. Some will get a blocked duct first and develop the nipple bleb later.

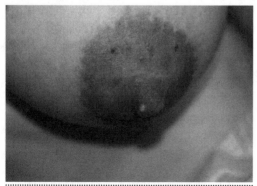

A nipple blister. Only a drop of blood came out when the nipple was punctured, but the blister healed afterwards.

CREDIT: JACK NEWMAN

Is the nipple blister due to *Candida* (thrush, yeast)? Maybe, but there is no proof. My theory is that the blisters occur in areas of previous damage, where the milk is not flowing well. Skin can't grow over a duct if the milk is flowing quickly through it several times a day, but it could if the milk is not flowing for some reason. A blocked duct can diminish milk flow, explaining why a blister sometimes appears two or three days later.

Or, if a baby is breastfeeding inefficiently (perhaps because of the introduction of bottles or pacifiers), he may not "drain" certain areas of the breast well, so a blister forms on the nipple. As a result of the baby's inefficient feeding as well as the blockage from the blister, a plugged duct then forms in the same area.

What about blisters without blocked ducts? There are connections between ducts, so that if one is blocked at the nipple, milk may be able to drain out another way, preventing a blocked duct from developing. Finally, a blocked duct can occur without the presence of a blister. The blockage of the milk drainage can occur anywhere along the duct, not necessarily at the opening of the duct at the breast.

As the baby nurses, he pulls more milk into the blister, putting pressure on it and therefore causing pain. The mother may actually have more pain toward the end of the feeding. Sometimes the nipple hurts when the baby latches on, then the pain diminishes for a while and increases again as the blister enlarges.

We usually suggest opening a blister to allow drainage of the milk. The mother can do this herself by piercing the skin with a needle. There is no need to dig around; simply opening up the blister is enough. It's easier to do this right after the baby has breastfed because the blister will be larger. If the mother hand-expresses, thickened milk like toothpaste may come out. It's good to squeeze out as much

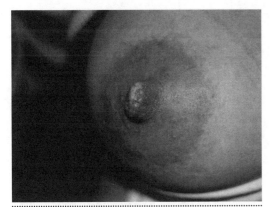

I'm not sure what this was, but the mother was experiencing considerable pain. Opening the area with a needle allowed us to express a fair quantity of milk with the consistency of toothpaste. The mother's pain resolved.

CREDIT: JACK NEWMAN

of this thickened milk as possible. While the blister will be less painful at this point, it will still hurt (just as an ordinary blister still hurts after it has broken).

At the clinic, I have the mother breastfeed first so I can improve the latch, hoping to prevent future blisters. Once the baby comes off the breast, I clean the nipple with a little soap and water and use a sterile needle to pierce the blister. Sometimes a drop of blood appears—not a problem. I then have the mother express some thickened milk; if none comes out after a good try, the attempt should be abandoned.

Once the blister has been opened I prescribe the all-purpose nipple ointment (APNO) to treat the pain and decrease the inflammation to prevent the blister from returning. If *Candida* is involved, the APNO will treat it. The ointment should be applied after each feeding for about a week or 10 days. If the blister has not reappeared by this time, it probably won't.

Many mothers have a painful flat white area on the nipple rather than a blister, but if there is no bubble, *do not* try to open it. Instead, adjust the latch and use the APNO.

A decrease in milk production as a cause of sore nipples

Many babies older than eight weeks will react to a decrease in milk flow from the breast in one of three ways: by pulling at the breast, coming off the breast repeatedly or slipping down onto the nipple (see the video called "Jiggling and Pulling" at www.breastfeedinginc.ca); all three may cause nipple pain. The solution is to increase the mother's milk production.

A special situation occurs when the mother is pregnant again. Pregnancy decreases the mother's milk production, leading to pain. However, pregnant mothers also get nipple and breast soreness because of the pregnancy itself; for some women, nipple soreness is the first sign of pregnancy. Most women find that it helps to remind the baby to latch on well, as many older babies or toddlers can get quite nonchalant about how they latch on.

Candida albicans *as a cause of sore nipples*

Many feel that *Candida albicans*, a fungus that sometimes causes illness in humans, cannot cause nipple

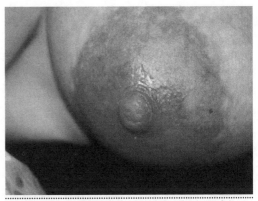

The typical appearance of a *Candida* infection of the nipple. The areola is shiny, and its pink hue suggests inflammation. This woman responded to treatment: an adjusted latch, all-purpose nipple ointment and gentian violet.

CREDIT: JACK NEWMAN

pain because it is difficult for it to grow on nipples. I think it can cause nipple soreness, and here's why:

My son, who was our third baby, developed thrush when he was about six weeks old. My wife, who up to that time had never had nipple pain, developed soreness at almost the exact same time. Treating her and the baby with gentian violet cured them both very rapidly. Based on this experience, I started treating mothers and babies with gentian violet if the baby had thrush and the mother had sore nipples. Pain relief for the mother was almost 100% treated with gentian violet only. Yes, gentian violet also kills some bacteria, and perhaps this decreased the pain, but given the association with the baby's thrush, which is not caused by bacteria, I was convinced that at least sometimes *Candida albicans* causes nipple pain.

As time went on, I realized that some nipple pain could be associated with *Candida albicans* without the baby having signs of thrush. Again, treatment seemed to confirm this.

However, I noticed that some mothers with nipple pain seemingly due to *Candida albicans* infection did not get better if treated with gentian violet alone. Was the fungus becoming resistant to gentian violet? Or was the problem not *Candida albicans*?

I now think that some of the causes of late-onset sore nipples, which I didn't know about at the time, were probably present. I also hear of yeast infection commonly diagnosed in any mother whose sore nipples are not improved by fixing the latch. I think the problem is that the latch has not really been "fixed." If you read the descriptions in this book and watch the video that shows how we teach latching on, you will notice that we teach it differently. I believe our approach works better much of the time. The asymmetry of the latch is very important. Many mothers are told their latch is perfect when, in fact, the nipple is sitting in the middle of the baby's mouth. It's not surprising that these mothers still have pain.

We now treat *Candida albicans* infection in the mother with a combination of the best latch possible and our all-purpose nipple ointment. This will work most of the time, even if the nipple pain is not caused by *Candida*. Admittedly the APNO treats several problems at once. If I am convinced the problem is *Candida albicans*, I will add grapefruit seed extract (GSE) and possibly gentian violet to the ointment, and will often give the mother grapefruit seed extract taken orally as well.

Some mothers have pain in the breast as well as the nipple, or pain only in the breast (see the information on mammary constriction syndrome on page 145). The evidence that *Candida albicans* in the ducts or breast causes pain is skimpy, but mothers do often improve with oral antifungal medication (fluconazole; Diflucan). There are rare case reports of *Candida albicans* growing in breast abscesses, so there is a possibility that such infections can occur. See the chapter "Sore Breasts."

Because pain from the nipple may radiate into the breast, breast pain may not originate in the breast itself. For this reason we do not treat nipple and breast pain with oral medication alone. If the mother has sore nipples, it is necessary to treat the nipples aggressively first and add fluconazole only if treatment is unsuccessful. What is aggressive treatment of the nipples? 1. Fix the latch as much as possible. 2. Use all-purpose nipple ointment, gentian violet and grapefruit seed extract, the latter both on the nipples and by mouth, as in the *Candida* Protocol (go to www.breastfeedinginc.ca and click on Online Info, followed by Information—English, or see page 153).

Diagnosing *Candida albicans*

Some mothers do get nipple pain due to infection with *Candida albicans*. Sharp observers have noted that pain due to *Candida* was often different from the pain caused by a poor latch.

- The pain of a poor latch is usually worse when the baby begins feeding, and decreases as the feeding continues. With a *Candida* infection, the mother usually describes pain throughout the feeding, often continuing after the feeding is over.
- The pain associated with a poor latch is often limited to the nipple and areola, but radiation into the breast is certainly possible. In the case of a *Candida* infection, the pain often radiates into the back or shoulder. The mother often describes a "shooting" pain in the breast as well.
- The pain of a poor latch is often described as "knife-like" or "stabbing." In the case of a *Candida* infection, the mother often describes the pain as "burning."

None of these symptoms is definitive, and a mother could have both a poor latch and a *Candida* infection.

Furthermore, sore nipples from a poor latch usually develop soon after the baby's birth. By contrast, *Candida* infections frequently begin after a period of pain-free nursing. However, as mentioned earler, other causes of sore nipples may begin after a period of pain-free nursing (eczema, nipple blister, late-onset decrease in milk supply, etc.).

Other factors may suggest the possibility of a *Candida* infection:

1. Recent use of antibiotics by the mother and/or the baby. Mothers who have Caesarean sections almost always get a dose of antibiotics during the procedure. Often the mother doesn't realize this and may say she hasn't had any antibiotics. Of course, even if neither mother nor baby received antibiotics, the problem could still be *Candida*.
2. The baby has thrush or a diaper rash. Again, the baby may have *Candida* and the mother may not, or vice versa, but it should be kept in mind.

3. The fact that the mother has a vaginal infection. This does not mean that her nipple pain is due to *Candida*. On the other hand, the absence of other sites of infection does not mean that the mother does not have a *Candida* infection of her nipples.

How does Candida albicans develop?

If you are diagnosed with *Candida* you may wonder how and why you got it. We all have *Candida* on our bodies normally; what we call a *Candida* infection is an overgrowth of this fungus.

The hormones of pregnancy increase the risk of infections with *Candida*, as does taking birth control pills. Diabetes increases the risk, as does taking antibiotics. Trauma to the nipples can allow *Candida albicans* to proliferate and invade. Preventing nipple soreness due to *Candida albicans* starts with a good latch from day one. The use of pacifiers and bottles can lead to a poor latch and increase the risk of *Candida*.

Treatment of sore nipples due to Candida albicans

There are many methods of treating a *Candida* infection of the nipples, but it is becoming resistant to many of the frequently used medications. Here's our approach:

Gentian violet

Gentian violet is an old treatment for *Candida albicans*. It should be given only as a 1% solution. In some areas, especially in the United States, pharmacies carry only 2% gentian violet. This is too high a concentration; it should be further diluted.

Gentian violet has some important advantages:

- A prescription is unnecessary as it is sold over the counter.
- It often works, and works quickly.

- It is an easy way to treat both the baby and the mother at the same time.
- It is inexpensive.

There are, however, some concerns about using gentian violet:

- It is messy, and although it does not stain permanently, clothing may require a few washes to get it out completely.
- On rare occasions, usually when gentian violet has been used improperly, babies have developed ulcers in their mouths. Stopping the gentian violet allowed the ulcers to heal within 24 hours. However, the worry about ulcers is exaggerated; I have seen it in only three or four babies out of hundreds for whom I have suggested this treatment.
- Some mothers and physicians are concerned because gentian violet is dissolved in 10% alcohol. However, the amount the baby gets is tiny, only a drop or two each day and usually for only a few days, and most of that is not swallowed.
- Preparations of gentian violet sold in pharmacies are usually labelled as toxic. All drugs are toxic. Side effects of gentian violet, in my experience, are very uncommon and disappear quickly once the treatment is stopped.
- There is also concern that gentian violet may increase the risk of cancer. This is based on a study done in mice where the mice were fed huge amounts of gentian violet every day. Based on this sort of study, I would have no concern about my baby receiving gentian violet. Indeed, as mentioned earlier, one of my children did take it and it cured his thrush and my wife's pain within a day or two. At the end of the three-day treatment, the level of liquid in the bottle did not seem to have gone down—that's how little is needed.

Using gentian violet

1. The liquid makes everything it touches purple. So undress your baby down to his diaper, undress yourself from the waist up, and put an old, dark-coloured towel on your lap.
2. Take a clean cotton swab, dip it into the gentian violet, and paint the inside of the baby's mouth.
3. When the baby's mouth is purple, put him onto the breast.
4. At the end of the feeding, the baby's mouth will still be purple, and your nipples and areola should be, too. If they aren't, get another cotton swab, dip it in the gentian violet and paint them. Do this once a day for three or four days, up to a maximum of seven days. You should have a considerable decrease in pain after a few hours of the first application. When the symptoms are gone, stop the treatment. If you do not feel better after seven days, *Candida* may not actually be the problem.
5. Any artificial nipples that the baby takes, including pacifiers, should also be treated with gentian violet or boiled once a day. Better still, don't use artificial nipples.
6. The reason we recommend stopping treatment after seven days is that if gentian violet has not helped by then, it probably won't work at all.

Using all-purpose nipple ointment (APNO)

I suggest mothers combine the gentian violet treatment with the all-purpose nipple ointment. Use the gentian violet once a day for three or four days, or up to a week. After all the other feedings, apply the APNO sparingly. Don't wash or wipe it off (even just before the next feeding).

The ointment contains antifungal medication. It also has a steroid that decreases inflammation, which causes much of the pain. It is true that steroids can sometimes encourage the growth of *Candida*, but the combination works. The antibiotic may help even with a fungal infection, since *Candida albicans* often lives in harmony with certain bacteria, and the presence of these bacteria contributes to the conditions it requires to multiply and cause infection.

If this combination relieves the pain, stop the gentian violet after three or four days and slowly decrease the use of the APNO over a week or so. If your nipples still hurt, stop the gentian violet, continue the APNO and check back with your doctor or lactation specialist. If there is partial relief of the pain, gentian violet can be continued up to a week. If it has not worked in that time, it probably won't work at all.

The APNO could be used alone for *Candida albicans* of the nipple, but it does not treat the baby's mouth as gentian violet does.

Nowadays we often suggest grapefruit seed extract (GSE); we recommend mothers take it by mouth and use the liquid form directly on the nipples. We suggest a diluted solution (5 to 15 drops in 30 ml or an ounce of water, starting with the lower concentration) painted directly onto the nipples and areolas, followed by the APNO after each feeding, except the one when gentian violet is used. Using grapefruit seed extract orally, either alone or in conjunction with fluconazole, helps with breast pain associated with *Candida albicans*. The oral dose of GSE is two 125 mg capsules three or four times a day. It can be continued after fluconazole has been stopped to prevent relapses. GSE slows the metabolism of fluconazole, giving higher blood levels.

Other treatments

Acidophilus capsules and/or other probiotics have been used to treat or prevent infections with *Candida albicans*. It is difficult to know how well they work. Some mothers swear by it, but others have not found it useful. I would not recommend acidophilus as the only treatment, but it can be used in addition to others. The main problem with probiotics is their cost.

Compresses of vinegar or bicarbonate of soda (baking soda) on the nipple have also been used to treat *Candida* infection with some success. These compresses change the acidity of the environment where the fungus is living, interfering with its growth. But the compresses can also wash away essential oils from the skin. Many mothers have had significant relief, though.

Nystatin is frequently used to treat thrush. I have not found it to be particularly useful and I would not suggest mothers use it as the only treatment. I think that most *Candida albicans* are resistant to it.

Yeast diets (eliminating all yeast, dairy, sugar and wheat) may work. I don't know of any evidence to prove the effectiveness of these diets, but some mothers find them helpful. They are very restrictive and so a burden to follow.

Eliminating *Candida albicans* from the mother's environment isn't practical. The fact is that the fungus is with us all the time. It is impossible to get rid of. The main thing is to re-establish a normal relationship with it.

What about frozen pumped milk collected while the mother has a *Candida* infection? While freezing the milk doesn't kill the *Candida*, the antifungal factors in breastmilk keep the fungus in a form that does not cause problems for the baby. Don't throw away the milk.

To sum up, my usual recommendation for treating *Candida albicans*, also known as the Candida Protocol, is as follows:

- Gentian violet applied once a day for four to seven days. If the pain is gone after four days, stop. If it has lessened, but not completely gone, continue up to seven days. If it has not lessened at all after four days, stop the gentian violet and get more help.

- The all-purpose nipple ointment as described earlier in this chapter, used until pain-free, then the frequency gradually decreased over a week or so. If the pain continues, and it is reasonably certain that the problem is *Candida albicans*, add the following:
- Grapefruit seed extract orally and/or topically. The oral dose of GSE is two 125 mg capsules three or four times a day.
- Fluconazole orally (400 mg at first and then 100 mg twice daily) until *pain-free for a full week*. Fluconazole should be *added* to the nipple treatment, *not used alone*. The nipple ointment should be continued and the gentian violet can be repeated. If fluconazole is too expensive, ketoconazole can be used (400 mg the first day, then 200 mg twice daily for the same period of time). If the *Candida* is resistant to this treatment (ketoconazole does not enter the milk very well), itraconazole can be tried, same dose and time period as fluconazole, although *Candida* is generally less sensitive to itraconazole than to fluconazole. Fluconazole is apparently now available as a generic product and therefore less expensive.
- For deep breast pain, ibuprofen (200 to 400 mg every four hours) can be used until the other treatments take effect. The maximum daily dose is 1,200 mg.

Tongue tie (ankyloglossia) as a cause of sore nipples

While some physicians still don't understand or accept how tongue tie can cause sore nipples and ineffective feeding, there is considerable research showing it does, and that releasing the tongue tie decreases pain and improves breastfeeding. Even

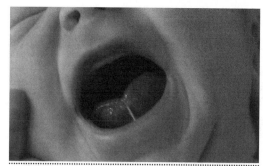

A typical tongue tie, which anyone can diagnose. The mother had sore nipples, and the baby had difficulty getting milk from the breast. Releasing the tongue tie made a big difference.

CREDIT: **JACK NEWMAN**

those physicians who are familiar with this issue may not know that there are varieties of tongue-tie. Some, as in the photo above, are very obvious. The tongue is obviously "tied" to the bottom of the baby's mouth. The result? The baby can't use his tongue effectively and is not able to breastfeed well.

However, some tongue ties are not easily diagnosed by looking. In general, when I see babies and mothers for breastfeeding problems, I sweep my index finger under the baby's tongue, from one side of the mouth to the other. If I come across an obstacle and feel that the mobility of the tongue is limited,

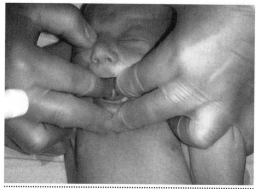

A less-obvious tongue tie. When a finger is swept under the tongue, an obstacle prevents easy movement. The tongue looks normal until upward tension is applied.

CREDIT: **JACK NEWMAN**

then I consider the baby has a tongue tie. Many say that if the baby can get his tongue over the gum line, there is no tongue tie, but I have a tongue tie and I can certainly get my tongue past my teeth and gum line. What matters is whether the baby can use his tongue *properly*.

Between 5% and 10% of babies are tongue-tied, and sometimes the trait runs in families, so if you have one baby with this issue, you may have more.

Some mothers have babies with obvious tongue ties, yet they don't have sore nipples and the baby gains weight well. These mothers obviously have a lot of milk, so they can manage. However, that doesn't mean all mothers and babies will do fine. And I worry that even with those babies who seem fine, the mother's milk production will decrease with time so that the baby may not gain well after three or four months on breastfeeding alone (see the chapter "Late-Onset Decreased Milk Supply").

The solution for a tongue tie is to release it. It's a simple, easily learned procedure that any physician can do in his or her office. It takes a second and the improvement in breastfeeding is often immediate and dramatic, with the baby drinking better and the mother's pain diminishing considerably. However, because of muscle memory, there may be no change for several days, even a week or more, until the baby learns to use his tongue better.

Sometimes improvement for several days is followed by worsening of the mother's symptoms. In these cases, we often find that the tongue tie has re-attached, at least partially. We have initiated a number of "exercises" to prevent the re-attachment, but even when parents are diligent in doing these exercises, re-attachment sometimes occurs. Sometimes the re-attachment is minor, but other times we find it's as if the tongue tie was never released. We have re-released tongue ties up to three times, but if attachment occurs again we desist because it's painful for the baby and distressing for the parents. And if the tie re-attached thrice, who's to say it won't happen again? See www.breastfeedinginc.ca for a video of a tongue tie being released.

11 | Sore Breasts

Myth #1: It is normal for mothers to have painfully engorged, hard breasts by three or four days after birth.
Fact: Painful engorgement is common, but it is not normal and should not occur. It is preventable by avoiding intravenous infusions during labour, birth and after the birth, and by good breastfeeding management after the baby is born. Sometimes IVs are necessary, and in those cases the quantity of fluids the mother receives should be kept as low as possible.

Myth #2: Pain in the breast indicates an infection requiring antibiotics.
Fact: Mothers can have pain in the breast for many reasons and few cases require antibiotics.

Myth #3: If a mother has a breast infection (mastitis) she must stop breastfeeding, at least temporarily.
Fact: Continuing breastfeeding helps drain the breast and results in more rapid healing. Breastfeeding helps protect the baby from getting sick from the bacterium; interrupting breastfeeding increases the baby's chances of getting sick. Medication (antibiotics) used to treat mastitis does not require the mother to interrupt breastfeeding (see the chapter "Breastfeeding While on Medication").

Myth #4: A breast abscess requires a mother to stop breastfeeding.
Fact: Current treatment methods do not require the mother to interrupt breastfeeding even on the side where the abscess occurred.

Engorgement on the third or fourth day after birth

Many new mothers and health care providers believe that it is normal for women to have painful, swollen breasts on the third or fourth day after giving birth. If there is no engorgement, they assume the mothers are not producing enough milk. This is simply not true. It is a problem if the mother gets painfully engorged and an even bigger problem if the baby cannot get latched on to the hard swollen breast.

I hear from several new mothers every week that their babies were breastfeeding "fine" during the first few days and then would not latch on when the milk "came in" and they became engorged. I believe that if that happens, the baby probably never took the breast well; I suspect he allowed the breast into his mouth and made sucking motions but never really latched on and got milk from the breast. The baby was "pretending" to breastfeed. When the breasts became quite swollen as a result of the inadequate breastfeeding in the first few days, the baby could no longer "pretend" to breastfeed.

Intravenous fluids given to the mother during labour contribute to this swelling of the breasts after the birth. To a much lesser extent, fluid normally shifts from the bloodstream to the space around the body cells after a baby is born, but by itself this should not be the cause of a severe engorgement. However, when there is already a problem caused by inadequate breastfeeding and intravenous fluids, this normal fluid shift adds to it.

In other words, it's normal for mothers to feel full, even uncomfortable, for a couple of days when the milk volume increases, but engorgement so bad that it is very painful and that the baby can't latch on is not normal and is *preventable*.

Separation of the mother and baby, swaddling him so that he sleeps instead of breastfeeding, using a pacifier to delay feedings, giving him unnecessary supplements, using bottles, and staff who make discouraging remarks (e.g., "You don't have the right equipment") and more contribute to the engorgement many mothers experience.

Breastfeeding in the first few days

Colostrum, the milk produced in the first few days, is chock-full of antibodies and several dozen other immune components that interact and protect the baby, plus high concentrations of long-chained polyunsaturated fatty acids (PUFAs). Colostrum also has a fair amount of vitamin K, which helps prevent some bleeding problems in the baby (preventing bleeding problems is the reason vitamin K is given to the baby at birth). The amount of protein in colostrum is greater than that in mature milk and colostrum maintains the baby's blood glucose (sugar) and treats low blood glucose better than formula (see the chapter "The First Few Days"). Colostrum is a very special fluid. We should sing its praises instead of saying "It's only colostrum." More importantly, we should make sure that the baby gets it! And the best way for him to get it is directly from the breast.

A baby doesn't need lots of colostrum. Sometimes mothers worry because a bottle-fed baby gets a lot more milk in the first few days than a breastfed baby, even if he is breastfeeding well. The reality is that the formula-fed baby is being *overfed*. Mothers also worry because their babies want to be on the breast for long periods of time and often are not satisfied if we hold them to the "10 to 20 minutes per side" rule. But that rule was based on bottle-feeding. Breastfeeding is very different and the baby should feed for as long as he wants at each session. Breastfeeding is a wonderful source of comfort and reassurance to the newborn, who has just been through an overwhelming experience. It's natural that he'll want to spend lots of time nestled skin to skin with his mother, breastfeeding.

What if the mother becomes painfully engorged?

Getting the baby to latch on and drink well from the breast and feed on demand is the primary approach both to preventing painful engorgement and treating it. Some things can hinder this without the mother even realizing it. I have a series of three videos at http://youtube.com/user/IBCToronto showing an overdressed baby completely asleep being undressed, waking up and feeding. If that baby hadn't been undressed he probably would have slept much longer. The same thing can happen if babies are swaddled or bundled up as they often are in the hospital. The babies are kept very warm and can't move much, so they don't wake when they are hungry. This can lead to engorgement because the baby isn't breastfeeding often enough or well enough. If he can take the breast and drink, the situation will improve over the next few days without any need for interventions. But the baby must *drink!* If the baby can't take the breast or doesn't drink, it may be necessary to decrease the swelling in other ways so that he can latch on and do so.

Hand expression of milk

Often, by expressing a little milk the mother can soften up the nipple and areola enough for the baby to latch on. Hand expression is better because at this point a pump can actually pull more fluid into the nipple and areola and make the swelling worse.

Reverse pressure softening

This is a technique described by Jean Cotterman, IBCLC, that has been used with success to help get rid of excess fluid in the nipples and areolas so the baby can latch on. If your ankles are swollen and you press your finger into one of them, a depression will remain for a few minutes. Reverse pressure softening uses this same technique to push fluid back from the nipple and areola. I have heard the process called "tulip" in some European countries because of the way some lactation specialists teach the technique; they use the fingers of one hand bunched together, like a partially opened tulip, to make a circle around the areola.

For the mother it may be easier to use two hands rather than one, pressing with the fingers of one hand horizontally above the nipple and the fingers of the other hand below the nipple. The procedure is done just before attempting to put the baby to the breast. Jean Cotterman recommends that pressure be put on the areola for a full 60 seconds or more. Once the areola is less swollen, the baby should be put onto the breast immediately, since fluid is likely to re-accumulate quickly. It may be necessary to repeat

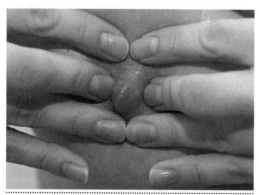

Finger position for reverse-pressure softening.
CREDIT: **TOMAS SZALLER**

the procedure for all feedings over the next few days. (Refer to pages 137–38 or check the YouTube site.)

Cabbage leaves

I believe there is some truth to the idea that cabbage leaves reduce engorgement. I have not seen scientific proof, but many mothers tell me they've had considerable relief with cabbage leaves. Some lactation specialists believe that prolonged use of cabbage leaves can decrease the milk supply, but this would also be difficult to prove since prolonged engorgement can also decrease the milk supply.

Here's what is recommended: Take a green cabbage, remove the outer leaves and discard them. Then take a few of the inner leaves and place them on the breast after feeding, inside your bra. The curved shape helps them fit nicely. Some suggest crushing the leaves with a rolling pin to help them fit the shape of the breast. Actually, there is no agreed upon protocol for using cabbage leaves. Some lactation specialists suggest using them after each feeding and keeping them on for 20 minutes or so. Some suggest keeping them on until they wilt, or until you need to feed your baby. Some suggest using them only three or four times a day. Experiment and see what works for you.

More on dealing with engorgement:

1. Getting help with latching the baby on is important, because the better he latches, the better he will get the milk and the faster the engorgement will decrease.

2. Medication for pain can be helpful. Something like ibuprofen or ketorolac or some other nonsteroidal anti-inflammatory drug (NSAID) works because this family of drugs decreases inflammation as well as pain. No NSAID requires a mother to interrupt breastfeeding. Acetaminophen can also help with pain, but it does not decrease inflammation. There are concerns about codeine,

but if it is necessary, and used only for a few days, it is acceptable. There is no need to interrupt breastfeeding if taking codeine, but watch that the baby is not too sleepy (and stop codeine immediately if he seems unusually sleepy). See more on codeine in the chapter "Breastfeeding While on Medication." If other approaches were used, codeine would rarely be necessary, even for severe engorgement. Furthermore, babies can be sleepy from not breastfeeding well; see the chapter "The First Few Days."

3. If the baby is taking the breast, breast compression keeps him drinking and getting more milk. See the video clip of the two-day-old baby at www. breastfeedinginc.ca. As it shows, it took several breast compressions by the mother before the milk started flowing; compression worked, even though she was not doing it exactly as we suggest. Also see the video titled "Breast compression helps even with poor latch."

4. After the baby feeds, express your milk by hand. Some health professionals say not to express milk because it will increase the supply, but it's not the milk that is causing the major part of the engorgement, but rather other fluid. If you can express some milk, you'll have less engorgement and less pain, and you can give the milk to your baby with a cup or spoon if he won't take the breast.

5. Cold compresses applied to your breasts after feedings may decrease the engorgement.

Blocked Ducts

A tender, painful, firm and in some cases, large lump in the breast is often a blocked duct. Sometimes, a decrease in milk flow results in the baby being fussy at the breast. Usually, though, much of the milk is able to flow out using other branches of the milk ducts.

A blocked duct will usually improve within 24 to 48 hours even without treatment. But it's hard to tell the difference at times between a severely blocked duct and mastitis. It might not matter, as we can treat both in the same way.

Blocked ducts are fairly common. What causes them? Well, they seem to be more common in women with abundant milk supplies, women who pump and women who use nipple shields. A mother will say that she took the baby out for the day in a baby carrier that fit rather snugly against her chest, and by the end of the day she had a blocked duct in the area where the carrier put pressure. Another mother might have the same problem after buying a new bra that was a bit too tight. As well, many women develop blocked ducts without any obvious cause. Sometimes women will say they went to bed feeling fine, but the baby slept longer than usual, and they woke up with a blocked duct.

An abundant milk supply *plus* a baby who doesn't latch well result in partial "emptying" of the breast. (Of course, a breast is never "empty" since the milk is being made continuously, but in this situation the baby leaves more milk in the breast than might be desirable.) That leftover milk can sit in the breast and thicken, blocking the duct. One step to prevent this is to get the best latch possible. Another is to "finish" one breast before offering the second. Breast compression helps "finish" the first side; the baby just nibbling at the breast does not (see the videos).

What can be done to clear a blocked duct more quickly?

1. Don't hesitate to take something for pain. Nonsteroidal anti-inflammatory drugs such as ibuprofen and ketorolac are probably best because they also decrease inflammation. Ibuprofen is often easiest because it is available without prescription (in generic form, or under

brand names Advil or Motrin). Acetaminophen (e.g. Tylenol) can also be used but it does not decrease inflammation. The baby should continue breastfeeding on the affected side. If it hurts too much to put the baby to that breast, take some pain medication and feed the baby as soon as the pain starts to diminish. The baby helps drain that blocked duct. Some have suggested that the baby's chin should be closest to the area that is swollen and painful, which leads to some strange breastfeeding positions. I am skeptical about this, but some find it helps.

2. While the baby is breastfeeding, compressing the area of the blocked duct may help the block clear more quickly. Use steady pressure, as much as you can *reasonably* tolerate. I have been able to help a mother get rid of a blocked duct in minutes using this technique. The baby helps by drawing on the breast and the mother helps by putting pressure on the blocked duct.

3. If you have a milk blister or bleb associated with the blocked duct, it may be worthwhile opening the blister with a sterile needle and squeezing out any toothpaste-like material. Often this results in immediate unblocking of the duct. It is important to apply the all-purpose nipple ointment (APNO) on the area afterwards to prevent infection and a return of the blister. Continue the APNO after each feeding for about a week. If there is no obvious fluid in the white blister or bleb, or if there is merely an area of flat whiteness on the nipple, it is a bad idea to try to open or stick needles into the area.

4. Many mothers find it helps to put hot compresses or a heating pad over a plugged duct or nipple bleb.

5. Cabbage leaves should not be used for a blocked duct.

What if there is no improvement in three or four days? It is good to be patient. As mentioned earlier, most blocked ducts resolve on their own within 24 to 48 hours. Sometimes they take a little longer. However, a mother with a blocked duct that lasts for a week or two should be seen by her doctor (see below).

Ultrasound treatments seem to work, but since most blocked ducts resolve on their own, it is not easy to prove that the ultrasound helps. It takes practice and experience to do this type of treatment properly and many physiotherapists have never heard of treating blocked ducts with ultrasound. If the block always occurs in the same place, a treatment might help prevent further blocks.

The dose of the ultrasound is two watts/cm^2 continuous for five minutes once a day for up to two days. Many ultrasound therapists feel this is a large dose, but I am not aware of any mothers receiving this treatment having any problems with it. Mothers do feel heat while the treatment is being applied but that is all. If the mother has mastitis, physiotherapists may hesitate to use ultrasound, believing it may spread infection.

Usually one treatment is all that is necessary to resolve a blocked duct; sometimes a second treatment is needed. If two treatments have not worked, ultrasound is probably not useful. If the blocked duct has remained unchanged for many days, the lump should be evaluated to make sure it's not something else.

Some mothers say using an electric toothbrush, pressing the vibrating handle end against the lower part of the blocked duct, works. It's worth a try, as long as it doesn't hurt.

Recurrent blocked ducts

Prevention and treatment for recurrent blocked ducts is the same as for a single blocked duct:

1. Ensure the best latch possible.

2. "Finish" the first breast using breast compression before offering the second. Once the baby is no longer drinking much, even with compression (or if the baby is falling asleep or pulling off), offer the second side.

3. Constricting clothing may increase the risk of blocked ducts, so avoid tight bras or other clothing that put pressure on the breast and baby carriers that cut into the breast. Wearing a bra to bed can be particularly problematic.

4. Lecithin refers to a group of phospholipids that are found in many foods, including egg yolk and soybeans; it is sold as a food supplement in pharmacies and health food stores. It may help to prevent recurrent blocked ducts. We usually recommend 1,200 mg three or four times a day, but some mothers take twice this amount. It comes in capsule form and also as a liquid. We usually recommend the capsule form, since it is easier to swallow.

5. Oil of evening primrose can be used as well. We have only very rarely recommended it. I don't know if it works or not. It contains a high percentage of linoleic acid, a fatty acid. It has been used for many years for the treatment of undiagnosed breast pain and menstrual irregularities without any proof that it actually works. Some mothers found it helped with their recurrent blocked ducts.

Candida albicans *as a cause of recurrent blocked ducts*

It is my impression that some cases of recurrent blocked ducts are associated with *Candida albicans*, if not caused by it, and if we treat *Candida*, the mother stops getting blocked ducts. I have heard that grapefruit seed extract and/or fluconazole taken orally prevents recurrences in some mothers.

Persistent blocked duct

What if the blocked duct just does not go away? What if it lasts for two weeks or more? Sometimes this happens, and as long as the lump is getting smaller, even if slowly, it's fine. What if the blocked duct just stays the same size, even if it's not painful any longer? It may not be a blocked duct, but something else: it could be a milk cyst, created when milk collects within the duct or behind some obstruction to the milk flow, forming a lump in the breast. These milk cysts (also called galactoceles) are not usually painful or tender unless they grow quickly. Milk cysts are *harmless* and almost never get in the way of breastfeeding. In only one case did I see a milk cyst that occurred in a spot that prevented the baby from latching on to the breast on that side. I make the diagnosis of a milk cyst by aspirating the milk that is present in the lump. Once the diagnosis is made, the galactocele should be left alone. Surgery of any type is contraindicated except in extraordinary situations. The milk cyst will disappear once the mother stops breastfeeding, but its presence is *not* a reason to stop.

I have seen a number of women with persistent blocked ducts for months who had no diagnosis even after a biopsy. We don't know the cause but there was no long-term problem.

It could be an abscess. This word may sound alarming, but an abscess is actually the body's stratagem to deal with an infection. The body walls off the infection and prevents it from spreading. Though an abscess is usually painful, sometimes it is not. See more on breast abscess below.

Any lump that is not getting smaller after a couple of weeks should be evaluated by a doctor. If necessary, seek out a breastfeeding-friendly surgeon. Many surgeons are not, and too many mothers are told they must wean the baby immediately to have tests such as a mammogram done. This is simply not true. Aside from a history and a physical examination (very important, but many surgeons have virtually no experience examining a lactating breast), the following can be done:

- Ultrasound (for diagnosis).
- Mammogram. Mammograms of a lactating breast are more difficult to read, but can nevertheless provide useful information.
- CT or MRI scan. These studies are being used more and more to diagnose breast lumps and are replacing mammograms in many situations. There is no need to interrupt breastfeeding even for a minute after a CT or MRI scan even if the mother received contrast. See the chapter "Breastfeeding While on Medication."
- Needle aspiration if there seems to be liquid in the mass.
- Fine needle biopsy.
- Core biopsy.
- Open biopsy (should be avoided if possible).

Fistula formation

Open and core biopsies can sometimes result in fistula formation. A fistula is a persistent connection between the breast and the skin that results in milk constantly leaking, which can be very annoying. I have not been able to find any information on how often these fistulas form after surgery on the lactating breast, but they certainly do not form every time. With a core biopsy, it should be a rare complication. An important factor in preventing a fistula is to continue breastfeeding on that breast. If the mother doesn't, the milk is likely to find the path of least resistance to flow, which may be this relatively large opening. Often a fistula becomes apparent after the sutures are taken out, so perhaps in the case of the lactating breast, sutures or staples should be left in much longer than usual. Skin glue

can be used in addition to sutures or staples when closing the wound.

Should a fistula occur, it can dry up on its own without stopping breastfeeding on that side. If the mother does not want to stop breastfeeding on that side and can tolerate the leaking, there is no harm in leaving the fistula. If it is a problem, stopping breastfeeding on that breast *only* is an option.

How to stop on only one side? Don't take medicine to dry up the milk, because that will affect both sides. If you feed on just one side, that side will increase its production while the other side will dry up. You may experience some discomfort on the side you're not feeding from. You can take medication for pain, but if you use cabbage leaves on that side to reduce the engorgement, and express small amounts of milk (or let the baby feed on that side once or twice a day) it will be more comfortable. Some women have dried up on one side unintentionally just by using that breast less and less. Since a fistula is not an emergency, you might even dry up on one side very gradually (by decreasing feedings from that breast over two to three weeks). The other side will also have more time to increase production. If that doesn't happen and you still want to stop feeding on the side of the fistula, binding just the affected breast with a cloth bandage will result in it drying up.

Usually the unaffected breast will increase production in response to the baby's increased feeding and compensate for the lack of milk intake from the breast that has dried up. If not, see the chapter "Increasing Breastmilk Intake by the Baby."

Mastitis

As with almost all breastfeeding difficulties, the risk of mastitis can be diminished by getting the best start from day one. This means:

1.   Immediate skin-to-skin contact after the birth

of the baby, allowing time for him to latch on all by himself.

2. If necessary, good hands-on help to achieve the best latch possible soon after the birth of the baby.

3. "Finishing" the first side before offering the second.

Mastitis is the medical term for an infection in the breast tissue. The mother has the same symptoms as she would with a blocked duct, but more severe. In addition to a painful lump, the area of the breast overlying the lump is often hot, red and swollen. The lump is usually more tender than a blocked duct. But the difference is a matter of degree; it can be difficult to differentiate a mild mastitis from a more severe blocked duct.

If there is no fever, it's more likely to be a blocked duct, but you can have mastitis without fever. If there is enough inflammation around the blocked duct, fever may occur, but fever does not always mean infection. The redness of the breast with mastitis is often more dramatic than that of the breast with a blocked duct. But if the mastitis is deep in the breast, there may not be much redness.

However, I do not believe that mastitis or a blocked duct occur without a lump in the breast. Sometimes breastfeeding mothers have been diagnosed with mastitis because they have a fever and flu-like symptoms. If there is no painful lump in the breast, the flu is the most likely problem

Okay, mastitis: now what?

1. If symptoms are present for more than 24 hours without improvement, I recommend antibiotics (24 hours is an arbitrary measure). The antibiotics should be directed against the bacterium *Staphylococcus aureus*, which is by far the most common causing mastitis. This means that ordinary penicillin and amoxicillin are not appropriate. Erythromycin is also not particularly good because it takes longer to be effective. I usually prescribe cephalexin, 500 mg four times a day for 10 days, but the decision on antibiotics should be based on the sensitivity of *Staphylococcus aureus* in the area where the mother lives, or, if she's been in hospital recently, the sensitivity of the strain found in that hospital. In Toronto, virtually all the *Staphylococcus aureus* isolated from breast abscesses we have drained were sensitive to cephalexin. Dr. Thomas Hale says that in Texas, where he lives, *Staphylococcus aureus* is not often sensitive to cephalexin. In recent years, even the usual antibiotics (cloxacillin, flucloxacillin, cephalexin, clindamycin, ciprofloxacillin, for example) against *Staphylococcus aureus* are sometimes not effective, since more methicillin-resistant *Staphylococcus aureus* (MRSA) are being found in patients with various infections, including mastitis and breast abscess. The drug of choice for MRSA is vancomycin. It is not effective for breast infections when taken by mouth, so it is given intravenously. Other drugs that may work for MRSA are cotrimoxazole, doxycycline and minocycline. None of these drugs require the mother to interrupt breastfeeding. The best way to decrease the prevalence of "superbugs" such as MRSA is not to use antibiotics when they are not necessary, so even when a mother has a definite mastitis, we can and should try to avoid them. Using antibiotics more wisely will also decrease the incidence of *Candida* infections in breastfeeding mothers.

2. If the mother has symptoms for fewer than 24 hours, I will usually give her a prescription for an antibiotic but suggest she wait before starting

to take it. Again, 24 hours is arbitrary. What if it has been 23 hours? We have to take the whole picture into account.

3. If the mother has symptoms for fewer than 24 hours but the symptoms are worsening (more pain, enlargement of the hardened area), she should start taking antibiotics. If she's had symptoms for more than 24 hours without improvement, she should start antibiotics.

4. If the symptoms of mastitis are definitely diminishing, there is probably no need for antibiotics. The fever usually disappears after 24 to 48 hours and the lump starts to decrease by two to three days and is gone or at least much smaller by seven to 10 days. The pain diminishes much more quickly, usually by four days or so. Some redness may remain for a week or so.

5. Heat helps fight off infection. Applying a heating pad to the affected area can help, but with the pain of mastitis, the mother may not notice if the heat is excessive and can actually damage the skin of the breast. Using a washcloth which has been held under hot water and then wrung out avoids any risk of overdoing it.

6. Fever also helps fight off infection, but fever is very uncomfortable, so a drug that both lowers the fever and decreases the inflammation makes sense. Ibuprofen is preferable to acetaminophen.

7. The mother should rest in bed with the baby, drink if thirsty, and eat if she feels like it. Relatives and friends should bring food and help with older children. Rest is important!

In my experience, at least 50% of mothers with mastitis or blocked ducts get better without antibiotics.

Should the mother continue breastfeeding if she has mastitis?

It is discouraging that we still have to address this question. There is no doubt that it is best for both mother and baby to continue breastfeeding on the affected side. By extracting milk and decreasing swelling and congestion, it helps clear up the infection more rapidly. A pump does not do this as well as a baby and it makes no sense to pump instead of having the baby directly on the breast unless the pain is too great. But then, why would pumping be less painful? Usually, if the baby breastfeeds on the infected breast, the mother is more comfortable.

It is unlikely the baby will get sick, since he was already exposed to the bacteria before the mother's symptoms became apparent. Mothers and babies share germs; this is a good thing, and the immune factors in breastmilk help prevent the baby from getting sick. The best protection for the baby is to continue breastfeeding. This is true even if a bacterial culture shows the mother's infection is due to MRSA (methicillin-resistant *Staphylococcus aureus*). Many health care providers have an exaggerated fear of MRSA. True, it is difficult to treat and therefore nasty, but that's even more reason to keep the baby breastfeeding. The treatment options are limited, because the baby has already been exposed to the bacteria. What will protect him? Continued breastfeeding. The immune factors in the milk will help keep the baby from getting sick or help fight off the infection if he does.

Sometimes the mother's pain is so severe that she cannot put the baby to the breast. This calls for antibiotics immediately. The mother should start feeling better fairly soon and be able to resume breastfeeding on that side. Meanwhile, the baby continues breastfeeding on the unaffected side.

Sometimes a mother can feel so ill with mastitis

that she does not have much energy. She should take the baby to bed with her and keep feeding, with help from family and friends to handle diaper changes and other baby care. This also calls for antibiotics started immediately. Usually the mother will start feeling better, within 24 to 48 hours.

The swelling inside the breast can diminish the flow of milk to the baby, making him unhappy and perhaps reluctant to feed. If the baby is unable to get milk from the breast it may be necessary to express the milk on the infected side; sometimes this is not possible due to pain or compression of the ducts. However, with effective treatment the mother should soon be able to put the baby to the breast and he will drink as the swelling diminishes.

"Subclinical mastitis"

This diagnosis is usually made in dairy cattle and is based primarily on the number of neutrophils present in the milk. A neutrophil is a white cell normally present in the blood; when the numbers increase, this suggests, *but does not prove,* the presence of bacterial infection. When the count in a cow's milk is higher than normal, the cow is said to have subclinical mastitis and the milk is not used for human consumption. This is a safety measure only, I am told, and does not mean the milk is unsafe. Pasteurization would kill the bacteria, but not any toxin that the bacterium might have produced. Toxins can cause severe illness.

In recent years the diagnosis has been made in humans as well, in connection with HIV infection. There are studies that show that if an HIV-positive mother has "subclinical mastitis," the risk of passing HIV to the baby is increased. Of course, there may be something about the presence of HIV in the mother that increases the numbers of neutrophils in her milk and the elevated count may not mean that there is some sort of infection in the breast itself.

It is not always appropriate or useful to take information about dairy cattle and apply this information to humans. Dairy cows are usually milked only twice a day, morning and evening, so that there are long periods between milkings. The "emptying of the udder" occurs less frequently than if the calf were allowed to feed freely from the udder. Cows also live in crowded conditions and often lie in their own dung.

Except in the *possible* association with an increased risk of passing HIV to the baby, the significance of "subclinical mastitis," if such an entity exists, escapes me. "Subclinical" means "no symptoms," and it makes no sense to me to test a mother with no symptoms, let alone give her antibiotics because her neutrophils are higher than average.

Breast abscess

Breast abscess was mentioned briefly earlier. An abscess is a pocket of pus formed in an infected area because the body can not completely fight off the infection on its own. It is the body's way of preventing infection from spreading. In other words, formation of an abscess is a protective mechanism.

Without any medical intervention, an abscess will usually work its way to a surface and drain, which cures it. An abscess in the brain is serious, even potentially fatal. But while a breast abscess can be painful, it is not usually dangerous.

The typical story of a breast abscess

Occasionally, mastitis will proceed to a breast abscess in a very short period of time, often as rapidly 24 to 48 hours. In such cases, even early use of antibiotics would not have prevented the abscess.

Most of the time, an abscess forms when there is a long delay in treatment or when treatment is ineffective. The following is a typical course of breast abscess we see in our clinic:

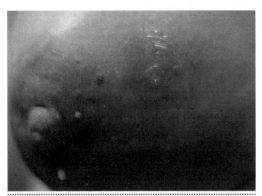

A breast abscess, located in approximately the centre of this photo. It is about to burst on its own. The milk does not contain pus.

CREDIT: **JACK NEWMAN**

- A breastfeeding mother develops the signs and symptoms of mastitis. She is treated with an antibiotic, but advised to interrupt breastfeeding either on the affected side (to avoid passing infection to the baby) or both sides (because of the antibiotic). This advice is incorrect.
- Symptoms decrease but do not disappear completely.
- When antibiotics are discontinued, the symptoms worsen within a day or two. Another antibiotic is prescribed and the cycle is repeated. The tender or painful lump remains in the breast. Thus, any mother with mastitis who has not had complete resolution within five to seven days after starting antibiotics (or has not at least had significant improvement in that time) should see her physician again to make sure an abscess has not developed. If the physician does not believe an abscess has formed, a different antibiotic should be prescribed. Continued breastfeeding plays an important part in helping to resolve either mastitis or an abscess.

How to diagnose an abscess

Usually the mother will have a history of mastitis, and a lump in the breast which is painful if squeezed but not *necessarily* painful when not touched. Sometimes it feels as though there is fluid in the lump. The skin may look very red or not. And sometimes the lump is not painful even when touched. If I suspect an abscess, or if I am unsure what the diagnosis is but believe the lump contains fluid, I will aspirate it with a needle and syringe. It is a bit tricky because you don't always know where to put the needle; as well, sometimes the pus is very thick and hard to get out.

If aspiration yields pus, the mother has an abscess. I continue aspirating as much as possible because, at least temporarily, the mother gets relief from pain.

If aspiration yields milk, the mother has a milk cyst (galactocele). I usually stop aspirating the lump at that point, since milk cysts will almost always refill quickly. If the cyst is not interfering with breastfeeding, it's better to leave it alone. A milk cyst will dry up when the mother is no longer breastfeeding, but this is not a reason to stop.

On one occasion, aspiration yielded a clear yellow fluid (serum). The laboratory sent back an urgent report of cancerous cells in the fluid. The lump, which the doctor had diagnosed as a blocked duct, was actually breast cancer. I want to emphasize that this was ONE case out of several thousand aspirations of breast lumps that I have performed.

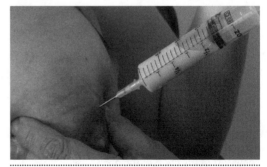

We diagnose a breast abscess by aspirating a suspicious area. The fluid aspirated is pus.

CREDIT: JACK NEWMAN

How to treat an abscess

In 2004 a study was published showing that the approach described below was superior to incision and drainage. We had started using the same approach some time before this article was published, with the help of the radiologists at North York General Hospital in Toronto.

1. The abscess is located and "mapped" with ultrasound.
2. A catheter is placed in the abscess, as far as possible from the nipple and areola, and left there.
3. The mother is encouraged to continue feeding on both breasts.
4. Antibiotic treatment is continued until the catheter is taken out.
5. The catheter is withdrawn when there is no further drainage from the abscess. This can be done by a nurse who visits the mother at home.

In the 10 or more years since we have used this approach, more than 100 mothers with breast abscesses have come to our clinic. All were treated in this way, all continued feeding without interruption on both breasts, and among all these mothers

We refer women with breast abscesses to intervention radiologists, who locate the abscess with ultrasound and place a catheter to drain the abscess. Surgical drainage is no longer recommended. Mothers do not need to stop breastfeeding on the side of the abscess.
CREDIT: JACK NEWMAN

only one had a fistula, which healed without special treatment in a few weeks. Only one had a recurrence of the abscess, which also healed after repeating the treatment. This approach is far superior to incision and drainage. Why?

1. Too many surgeons open the abscess with an incision that is much too close to the nipple and areola. In fact, many prefer using a peri-areolar incision (around the line between the brown part of the breast and the rest of it). This is apparently done for "aesthetic" reasons, but it doesn't always turn out to be an "invisible scar." A peri-areolar incision increases the risk of a fistula, makes it impossible for the mother to put the baby to that breast (because of pain) and compromises milk production, not only for this baby but also for any future baby.
2. The recurrence rate with this surgery is approximately 7%. The procedure we now recommend has a recurrence rate of much less than 1%.
3. Often mothers are admitted to the hospital and given a general anaesthetic for the incision and drainage. Ultrasound localization and placement of a catheter is done on an outpatient basis with local anaesthetic.
4. Pain from an incision and drainage is more severe and lasts longer than pain from ultrasound and catheter drainage (most mothers describe the pain as minimal).
5. Radiologists tend to be much more breastfeeding-friendly than most surgeons. After I pointed out to the radiologists who see our patients that the mother did not have to interrupt breastfeeding on the side of the abscess, they changed their advice. I have often had very strong resistance from surgeons who felt that the mother should stop breastfeeding on both sides.

Is a second abscess more likely with the next baby?

I don't believe so. I have not seen any evidence supporting this idea, and we have never seen a mother at our clinic who developed an abscess in two consecutive lactations.

Candida albicans as a cause of sore breasts

Although there is no doubt in my mind that *Candida albicans* can cause sore nipples, whether it can cause pain in the breasts is a very contentious issue. I think that breast tissue can become infected with *Candida albicans*. There are rare case reports of mastitis and even abscesses apparently caused by *Candida albicans*. These reports come mostly from tropical areas where the environmental context is very different from what we see in temperate climates. There is also evidence of *Candida albicans* infection in mammary glands in goats and cows. So it is not completely unheard of.

On the other hand, it is very difficult to grow *Candida albicans* from human milk or find any markers for *Candida albicans* in it. Many lactation experts believe this rules out any possibility of *Candida albicans* causing breast pain.

Yet breast pain often responds very well to treatment for *Candida albicans*. However, pain in the breast could actually be radiating from the nipple. Many mothers are being treated for *Candida albicans* when they don't have it. If the mother took antibiotics, if the baby has thrush, or even if "we tried everything else," she may be treated for *Candida* but not actually have it.

Many lactation specialists will say that breast pain without a lump is actually caused by a low-grade infection with *Staphylococcus aureus* or *Staphylococcus epidermidis*. But why would a healthy person get *Staphylococcus epidermidis*, which affects virtually only immune-compromised individuals?

Furthermore, *Staphylococcus epidermidis* normally lives on the skin, so cultures of milk "proving" it's the cause of the pain may actually be a contaminant of the culture. As for *Staphylococcus aureus*, it is more likely to cause serious infections, not low-grade ones. On the other hand, impetigo (a common skin infection in children) is a low-grade infection with *Staphylococcus aureus*, so I don't rule out this possibility. We don't know exactly what is going on.

Here are some possible signs of *Candida* infection:

- The pain usually begins late in the feeding or after the feeding. The pain is usually worse in the evenings (perhaps because you are more fatigued).
- The pain is generally of a shooting or burning nature.
- The pain is often felt throughout the breast and sometimes in the back and shoulders.
- The pain may last for minutes or even hours.
- The pain may begin early after the baby is born or months later.

As mentioned earlier, recurrent blocked ducts may be associated with *Candida albicans* infections.

Treatment for breast pain due to Candida albicans

The treatment for breast pain due to *Candida albicans* is the same as for nipple pain. Too many mothers receive immediate treatment with fluconazole (Diflucan) if they have pain in the breasts. If the mother has sore nipples it is important to treat them aggressively first and add fluconazole only if treatment is unsuccessful. Treatment of nipple pain is discussed in the chapter "Sore Nipples."

If the mother has breast pain only, oral grapefruit seed extract can often help. It can be taken for weeks or months if necessary. Fluconazole is undoubtedly more effective and can be used instead of or in addition to grapefruit seed extract. Grapefruit in any form can increase blood levels of fluconazole.

When we treat with fluconazole, we start with a dose of 400 mg the first day, then 100 mg twice a day the next day. This is a large dose, but we find it works. Smaller doses (100 mg or 150 mg a day) sometimes work, but a single dose of 150 mg (which is what women receive for vaginal infections with *Candida albicans*) does not. Improvement often begins within a day or two but is occasionally delayed by as much as 10 days. If the mother has had no relief at all by 10 days of treatment, she probably won't have any improvement with fluconazole.

We like to see mothers pain-free for at least a week before stopping treatment in order to prevent relapses. In unusual cases we've treated mothers for six to eight weeks or even longer. Mostly mothers find that pain decreases early into treatment, but it does take at least a couple of weeks to be pain-free.

Pain relievers, especially those that also provide anti-inflammatory effects (NSAIDs such as ibuprofen), should be an integral part of treating breast pain.

Other causes of sore breasts

Raynaud's phenomenon or vasospasm can also cause breast pain. The diagnosis is made by observing colour change in the nipple, usually after the feeding is over. Mammary constriction can also cause pain. See the chapter "Sore Nipples."

Breast trauma can cause pain that lasts for days or weeks. Breastfeeding should be continued if at all possible and the pain treated with NSAIDs such as ibuprofen.

Other breast and nipple conditions
"Rusty pipe" syndrome (bleeding from within the breast)

Women may have painless bleeding from their breasts late in pregnancy or during the first week or so after the birth. The bleeding may be due to enlargement of the blood vessels and increase in the number of blood vessels in the breast. It is not surprising that sometimes blood vessels leak a little blood into a duct, and it then comes out of the nipple. It is not dangerous for the mother or the baby. Sometimes when a baby swallows blood he may spit it up because it irritates his stomach, but it really does him no harm. The bleeding usually disappears by 7 to 10 days after birth. Breastfeeding must not be interrupted.

Occasionally a mother has blood in her milk at a later stage. She may not be aware of this unless she expresses her milk. Sometimes the bleeding is great enough that the baby has blood in his bowel movements, but not usually.

If the mother continues to have bleeding more than seven days after the birth, or if bleeding starts at a later time, she should see her doctor. She should continue breastfeeding.

Paget's disease of the nipple

Paget's disease is a rash that looks like eczema but is due to an underlying cancer of the breast. It is quite uncommon in women of childbearing age but it *can* occur.

Paget's disease is easily mistaken for eczema because of the flaking skin and itching. Most mothers with eczema get it on both breasts, though, while Paget's disease usually involves only one. If treatment with a steroid ointment does not result in rapid resolution (within a week) of the problem, the mother should see her doctor. The diagnosis is made by biopsy of the nipple. This does not mean the mother should stop breastfeeding on that side—she cannot transfer cancer to the baby by breastfeeding.

Inflammatory carcinoma of the breast

This type of cancer can occur at any age but it is uncommon. It is a particularly aggressive type of breast cancer and sometimes the mastitis-like symptoms can come on over a day or two. The breast may

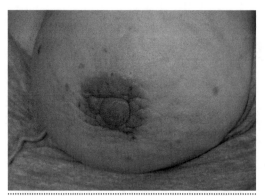

Breast cancer. Note the *peau d'orange* (orange peel) appearance of the breast. If a woman experiences this kind of engorgement later than immediately postpartum and the engorgement does not quickly resolve, she should see her doctor immediately.

CREDIT: JACK NEWMAN

swell rapidly and be quite red. A hint that this is different from typical mastitis is that the skin may have a *peau d'orange* (orange peel) appearance. Sometimes the nipple is retracted as well. (See photo above.)

Breast lumps

Most breastfeeding mothers have various lumpy areas of the breast. These areas of fullness often move around and are occasionally a little tender but are not painful. Mothers may worry about these, but any lump that is getting smaller is almost certainly nothing to worry about. A lump that is persistent, however, should be investigated. A new lump that is not getting smaller after two or three weeks is reason enough to seek a medical opinion. Luckily, most lumps in the breast are benign, but it is better to be sure.

A reminder: almost no investigation of the breast (ultrasound, mammogram, CT scan, MRI scan, needle biopsy, core biopsy, etc.) requires a

mother to stop or interrupt breastfeeding. If there is urgency in making a diagnosis, waiting for the mother's milk to dry up is not rational, since it may take several weeks. Even if there is a reason to stop on the side with the lump, the baby can and should continue breastfeeding on the other side.

Most women will never experience the problems described in this chapter. Nevertheless, it's best to be aware of the symptoms and learn what can be done about these problems.

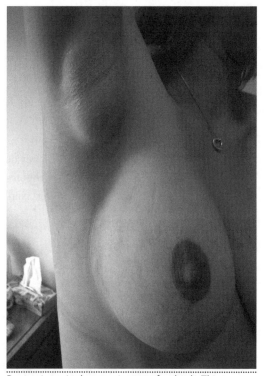

Breast tissue in the armpit soon after birth. This is not breast cancer or mastitis. The swelling decreased during the first few weeks after birth.

CREDIT: JACK NEWMAN

12 Colic (The "C" Word)

Myth #1: If a breastfed baby cries a lot despite gaining well, his mother's milk doesn't agree with him and he should be given hypoallergenic formula instead.
Fact: It's just as important to avoid the risks of formula feeding with a colicky baby as it is with one who is not colicky. True colic gets better with time, and often improving breastfeeding techniques will help.

Myth #2: Reflux is a common cause of babies crying that requires medication.
Fact: Most babies who are diagnosed as having reflux actually don't have it at all; the crying is usually due to breastfeeding issues which can be managed with good help and without medication.

Myth #3: The most common cause of "excessive crying" in exclusively breastfed babies who are gaining weight well is something in the mother's diet that is bothering babies.
Fact: Though proteins from the mother's diet pass into the breastmilk and can cause some babies distress, it's mostly a good thing. The mother's milk also contains specific antibodies and sensitized white cells that target the protein, so breastfeeding probably decreases the baby's chances of becoming intolerant to it.

Colic is a common reason why mothers stop breastfeeding unnecessarily. This is unfortunate because much can be done to decrease the crying. Even if nothing is done, colic typically gets better around three months and often starts to improve after six weeks. That six-week mark is the height of the baby's fussiness and crying. The parents are tired, they've been dealing with an inconsolably miserable baby for three or four weeks now, and everyone is suggesting formula. So they switch, and what happens? The baby starts to improve, just when colic starts to improve anyway. The parents may think it was the formula that caused the improvement, but it would have happened anyway.

What is colic anyway?

Nobody knows for sure. Gas has often been blamed for infant colic. It makes sense in a way. Mothers often talk to doctors about hearing gurgling in the babies' abdomens when they cry. Physicians in the old days often X-rayed the baby's abdomen to show the parents that the intestines were full of air or gas. But babies who cry a lot also probably swallow a lot of air, so it may be that the crying comes first and the air-filled intestines are a result.

Typical colic and theories about its cause

Although we don't really know what colic is, typical colic has been defined by the "rule of threes." It starts at about three weeks, the baby cries for about three hours a day, the crying occurs on at least three days a week and it lasts until the baby is about three months old. Typically, the crying occurs in the evening.

It doesn't make sense to me that this could be caused by gas. If so, why only in the evening? And why does it improve at three months?

Another old theory is that the baby's gut is not mature enough yet to handle food. But getting adequate nourishment is crucial to the survival of the newborn, so why would the gut not be adequately developed to handle nourishment? Breastfed babies are less likely to have colic, perhaps because growth factors in breastmilk stimulate the development of the gut and the enzymes that digest food. So the formula-fed baby might, indeed, have an immature gut.

Overfeeding has been suggested for many years as a cause of colic. It is one reason pediatricians used to advise keeping babies to a four-hour schedule. If the baby fed less frequently, he would have less colic. Why would anyone make a baby who usually feeds about every two hours wait longer to eat? He'll cry most of that time—is it better if he cries from hunger than from "colic"? It also doesn't fit with the typical evening crying spells, because many mothers say they have less milk in the evening, and some studies show lower fat levels in evening milk compared to morning milk. So it makes no sense that the crying would be related to overfeeding when it happens at the time of day when overfeeding is least likely.

Finally, some say tension in the baby's environment is transmitted to him and he responds by crying. To support this theory it is often noted that colic is more common in firstborns. But I would suggest that any household where a baby cried three hours in the evening is likely to be a tense environment!

On the other hand, colic is much less common in resource-poor nations, where babies are carried much of the time, breastfeed on demand, and sleep next to their mothers.

Could crying be due to something else?

Of course. Young babies often cry when they are hungry. Even if a baby is gaining weight well, it may be that if feedings are being limited to one side at a feeding (or 15 minutes per side), he would be calm if he drank even a little more.

Some "colicky" babies do not gain well. Here's a situation where early intervention would have helped: The mother contacted me when her son was nine weeks old. At birth, he weighed 8 lb, 3 oz., but he lost 16 ounces in the first week. At one month, he was still not back to his birth weight. *If the baby was weighed on the same scale, he gained less than 450 g (16 oz.) in 3 weeks. If the slow weight gain had been confirmed by observation of breastfeeding, the mother should have been helped to improve the breastfeeding.* "Now at nine weeks he weighs 8 lb, 7 oz. (3.84 kg), was gaining about 2–3 oz. (57–86 g) a week. His head and length are both at the 25th percentile." *Whether two to three ounces a week is adequate is debatable. I believe that slow but steady weight gain is acceptable if the baby is content and otherwise normal. However, if the baby who is gaining very slowly is crying a lot, as seems likely from the email (see below), it's not colic. It's hunger.*

"I exclusively breastfed for the first four weeks, then added in the occasional bottle of formula when we realized his weight was low." *The occasional bottle, whatever that means, may not be enough to overcome the baby's hunger. The baby's inadequate intake of breastmilk should have been addressed otherwise. See the chapter "Increasing Breastmilk Intake by the Baby."*

"At that point he showed signs of colic and we were referred to a pediatrician." *The pediatrician may not know much about breastfeeding, so he may tell the mother to supplement more (with formula) or wean completely without even observing the baby at the breast. Even if this baby needs supplementation—and it is very clear that he does, given that he is barely over his birthweight at more than two months—it should be done at the breast with a lactation aid, in order to salvage the breastfeeding. One thing is sure. This baby cries because he is hungry.*

Medical problems

Sometimes a medical problem causes the crying. If a baby drinks a lot and yet remains hungry and is not gaining weight, a medical issue may be preventing the baby from absorbing the milk he's getting. A baby who changes suddenly and starts crying may have an infection in the urinary tract. Often the baby will have foul-smelling urine. The parents may notice that he cries only when he passes urine.

This and other possible medical issues should be considered before assuming the problem is colic.

The role of prebiotics, probiotics and the baby's gut flora

In recent years, a new explanation for colic has become popular: the baby doesn't have enough of certain lactobacilli (bacteria normally found in large amounts in the breastfed baby's intestines). Many studies in recent years seem to "prove" that this abnormally low concentration of lactobacilli can cause babies to be colicky, and suggest that giving probiotics (various forms of lactobacilli) will prevent or decrease the symptoms of colic.

I am skeptical. First of all, breastmilk itself stimulates the growth of probiotics in the baby's gut. More is not always better and is unlikely to help. It really just gives a boost to formula company marketing by pushing the notion that their formulas are better for babies. As an example, a physician who works for a formula company (Nutricia, a particularly aggressive marketer of formula) published an apparently peer-reviewed article in a highly respected journal, *The Archives of Diseases of Childhood*, purporting to show that prebiotics in their formula decrease the risk of atopic dermatitis (eczema). Eczema is not colic, but another condition that formula makers have claimed probiotics help with. One study proves little, especially when done by the company that makes the formula and presented in a publication that shows a baby being bottle-fed on its cover. In a page that discusses what's "hot" in this issue, the editor writes: "Although breast-feeding remains the single most important 'intervention' to prevent the development of atopy, many infants are not breast-fed." Breastfeeding, an intervention? Here is a pediatrician who does not accept that breastfeeding is the normal physiological way of feeding babies and toddlers. Furthermore, the editor states categorically that no follow-up trials are necessary because the study is so well designed. This is a stunning comment. *Any* study, no matter how well designed, needs to be repeated for verification because there are many ways that a study can produce unintentionally inaccurate results. This issue of the journal contains three full-page advertisements for formulas, all by the same company that the author of the study does research for, and all the ads point out that the formula contains prebiotics! There are no ads from other formula makers.

In other words, there is no actual proof that pre- and probiotics, given to babies either in formula or separately, will help with colic.

Skin-to-skin contact

On the other hand, there is good evidence that immediate skin-to-skin contact after birth, for more than a token few minutes, helps to prevent colic. Skin-to-skin contact reduces the baby's stress and encourages a solid start to breastfeeding. When breastfeeding works as it should, the baby does not develop the symptoms that are so often described as colic, allergy to breastmilk and reflux, all of which can be prevented. More than that: skin-to-skin contact encourages the mother to fall in love with her baby so she is more willing to hold him, carry him, take him to bed with her and find creative ways in which to help him when he cries.

Do exclusively breastfed babies get "real" colic?

Probably they do. But frequently what gets called colic is due to problematic breastfeeding "techniques," such as keeping the baby on just one breast per feeding as a rule rather than offering the second breast even though the baby is still hungry, or feeding on a schedule.

Canadian researcher Dr. Ron Barr has studied babies around the world, and he found that in every country and every culture, some babies were "colicky" and cried more than others. His conclusion is that some infants are simply more sensitive than others, and as they mature, the fussiness goes away.

But he also found that in tribal societies, where the mothers keep their babies close—usually actually on their bodies—day and night, babies cry as frequently but for much shorter periods of time. In those societies, mothers respond to the crying within a few seconds (by offering the breast, picking the baby up, cuddling him, etc.). In North America, however, Barr found that mothers often took 10 minutes or longer to respond to their babies' cries. That's enough time for a baby to get quite worked up, and then it takes a long time for him to calm down.

Based on the way women in tribal societies responded to their colicky babies—immediately offering the breast and keeping the baby close at all times—Barr thinks there may be an evolutionary reason for colic: these babies tended to be fed more often during the three months that colic lasted, which helped to establish and maintain a good milk supply. Unfortunately, in Western societies, where babies are expected to stick to a schedule and are not kept close to their mothers, colicky babies don't get this same response.

I believe that many cases of "colic" are actually babies who cry in the evenings because their mothers' milk production is lower at that time of day. If you suspect this might be the case with your baby, follow these guidelines:

1. Do what you can to increase the baby's intake of milk at *every* feeding. This would include getting

the best latch possible, using compression to keep the baby drinking when he slows down, and offering the second side even if the baby doesn't seem to want it. Don't force the second breast, but offer it. Many babies will take it even if they don't immediately seem hungry. If the baby takes the second breast, follow the same approach as with the first breast. If you give the baby a little more milk at each feeding during the day, he may not be as hungry in the evening.

2. If you've been told to keep the baby on just one breast per feeding so he gets more hind milk, consider this: if the baby is not drinking milk from the breast, he's not getting hind milk! By keeping the baby on only one breast at each feeding, the milk supply decreases and what may have been a baby who was fussy because he was getting "too much low-fat milk" turns into a baby who is fussy because he's not getting enough milk. In our clinic we often see mothers who had overabundant milk supplies that have decreased significantly. Even if the baby is still gaining well, he may not like the slow flow of milk he is getting on just one breast.

3. If the "colicky" baby is soothed by being at the breast (as many are), it can help the mother to get comfortable, perhaps put on some music or a movie or have a book to read, and breastfeed lying down. Fussy babies often breastfeed better when mother and baby are lying down. The baby may be on the breast much of the evening; maybe this is not so bad. It will likely increase milk production if "lowish" milk production has been part of the problem. And the mother gets a rest! Better than walking the baby around the house all evening.

It's better to avoid giving a bottle in the evening, even a bottle of expressed milk. Here's an experience one mother described that shows why this can be a problem. Her daughter seemed to latch very well and had a strong suck. About the third day after her birth, the hospital nurse had the mother supplement with formula using a lactation aid at the breast. The baby had been sleeping only about an hour between feedings prior to this; now she started going two or three hours between feedings. The mother continued with the lactation aid for the next two weeks, and had two consultations at a breastfeeding clinic (*not ours, I hasten to mention!*). At the second consultation she was told to start giving the baby a bottle at night to make things easier. Instead it seemed to have made the baby even fussier at the breast.

Should formula be tried as a solution?

When a breastfed baby is colicky, mothers are frequently advised to stop breastfeeding and give the baby formula, sometimes "special formulas" specifically designed to help with colic. I think formula works in only two situations: if the baby is hungry (although then there are other things that can be done, as explained earlier), or if the parents think that a baby who is fed should then fall asleep, by himself, and not wake up again until it is time for another feeding. It's easier to overfeed the baby with a bottle of formula, so he may fall asleep on his own and will sleep longer, but at what cost? Is it worth stopping breastfeeding? I would say no, having been through colic with one of our children. We were never sorry we saw it through, as difficult as it was. The risks of formula feeding are not lessened because the formula is specially designed for babies with colic. Perhaps there are even *more* risks than with regular formulas because many of these products have not been around for long and we have little experience with them. For example, soy formulas' estrogenic effects may interfere with babies' normal hormonal balance of babies. Baby girls on soy formula have been reported to develop breasts, likely due to these estrogenic effects. What do we know about hydrolyzed

formulas, which have been around for even less time and have been used with relatively few babies?

Often changing to formula does not even work. The baby goes on regular or special formulas in sequence and is still colicky. In the meantime, breastfeeding is lost.

Even if formula seems to work, the problem may have been that the baby just wanted more milk. Now that he is getting more he becomes calm and happy. This is seen as proof that the problem was breastfeeding or breastmilk. Keep this in mind as you read on.

What else can cause a breastfed baby to be fussy?

One of the common reasons babies are colicky is that mothers have been convinced that catering too much to the baby's needs will result in their being spoiled. This English nanny approach to raising babies is good for the nanny, but it is not good for the baby. I think it is significant that most of these English nannies don't have children of their own.

Babies cry for many reasons—it is the only way they have to communicate their needs. Many people believe that if you pick up or otherwise respond to a baby who cries, he will cry more and more; if you ignore his cries, he'll stop. But research has shown just the opposite. The babies who are responded to most quickly and consistently cry *less* by the time they are a year old. Even more importantly, they tend to talk earlier and make more efforts to communicate, apparently because they have learned they will be listened to.

Even if ignoring the baby made him cry less, would this actually be desirable? If one ignores the baby, if no one pays attention to an older child's needs, he will eventually stop asking. And so will the teenager. How many parents complain that their teenager won't talk to them? Well, if the parents never listened, why should the teenager talk to them?

Another cause of non-colic crying is feeding the baby by the clock. This has been popularized by some religious writers (such as Gary Ezzo) who have no understanding of how breastfeeding works or how babies develop. Some babies have become seriously malnourished as a result of following these rules, and the American Academy of Pediatrics has issued a warning against this approach. The authors say they are "baby wise," but they are actually anything but wise: there is real potential danger to babies when their mothers believe the misinformation in these books. Another point is that babies cry to go back to the breast when they want to suck even though they are not hungry anymore. Babies breastfeed for reasons other than just milk. Putting them to the breast often resolves their crying.

Another cause of colicky behaviour is that parents today are often strongly urged never to allow the baby to fall asleep at the breast. So here's what happens: the baby is breastfeeding and happily dozing off. Then his mother notices and abruptly takes him off the breast. Naturally, he wakes up and cries. I cannot understand why anyone would tell mothers not to let the baby fall asleep at the breast. It's not a bad habit; it's the natural way for mammal babies to go to sleep. The baby won't do it forever. I think mothers who follow this approach are missing out on a lot. The feeling of accomplishment and pride the mother feels and is so evident on her face when she looks at her sleeping baby tells the whole story. And the baby won't cry.

Pulling at the breast

Babies pull at the breast, pull off the breast, fuss or cry at the breast and get angry for several reasons:

a. The flow is too slow for them (this is the most common reason).
b. The flow is too rapid for them. In this case the baby may actually choke, cough or sputter at the

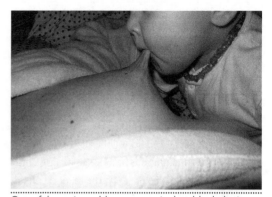

One of the main problems we see in the older baby is pulling at the breast. This behaviour is often wrongly blamed on colic, reflux, self-weaning and many other things, but the real reason is likely a decrease in milk flow.
CREDIT: **ANDREA POLOKOVA**

breast as well. However, if the flow is too slow it can also cause choking.

c. The baby is full but wants to continue to suck, and the milk is flowing faster than he wants.
d. The baby is reacting to something in the milk (i.e., something the mother has eaten or drunk).
e. The baby is on nursing strike (this is discussed in the chapter "Late-Onset Decreased Milk Supply").
f. The baby is experiencing reflux. This "diagnosis" is made far too often.
g. A combination of a and b (too fast early in the feeding, too slow later).

Anyone, especially the mother, can figure out which of the first three things is happening by watching the baby breastfeed. If he is nibbling, it's probably a case of "I want more milk, faster." If he is drinking really well and possibly sputtering and choking, it's probably b or c. If the baby is full, the pulling usually occurs several minutes into the feeding when he is still drinking very well. Often, after initial rapid drinking, the baby is content to nibble and not get much milk, but if the mother has another letdown, the baby will start to get upset again.

Foreign proteins in the milk

Proteins from various foods in the mother's diet can enter into the milk. Several studies have shown that when mothers eliminate certain proteins the baby is less colicky. The most common offender is cow's milk protein.

I think people take this approach too quickly. The first step should be to fix the breastfeeding; only then should you look at eliminating food or drink from the mother's diet. I find it interesting that adult humans do not normally absorb whole or partially digested protein into their blood under usual circumstances, yet breastfeeding mothers do. Why is this? We can assume that the baby needs to receive some of these proteins, at least in small quantities. If these proteins enter into the milk in tiny amounts, along with specific antibodies and perhaps sensitized white cells, the whole process may protect against the baby's becoming intolerant to these proteins. The fact that this doesn't happen with every baby (because some have a reaction to the protein) is not an argument to routinely take out all sorts of foods from mothers' diets. It's not a good idea to eliminate milk products, for example, from your diet "just in case," or even if you had a previous baby with an allergy to cow's milk.

At least one study has shown that all mothers in the study group and the control group had cow's milk protein in their milk, but the babies were colicky only if the mother had lower concentrations of antibody directed against the cow's milk protein.

Even physicians confuse cow's milk protein intolerance with lactose intolerance. Many mothers of colicky babies have been told to go off dairy products so that the baby doesn't get lactose in the mother's milk. But the mother's milk will contain the same amount of lactose whether she is drinking and eating dairy products or not. The issue, if there is sensitivity, is the cow's milk protein, not the lactose.

In addition to crying, what symptoms might the baby exhibit if he is sensitive to something in the mother's milk?

1. Green, frothy, explosive bowel movements. As mentioned earlier, this *in itself* is nothing to be concerned about if the baby is also generally content, and gaining weight well. This is true even if the bowel movement is mixed with mucous.
2. Because the bowel movements are often quite irritating, many babies will develop diaper rash. This is not a reason to stop breastfeeding.
3. Blood in the bowel movements.

See also the section on blood in the bowel movements in the chapter "Sick Babies, Special Babies."

So what to do?

Eliminate foods from your diet, but only one kind at a time. There are any number of foods that may cause symptoms; in fact, any food that contains protein (any dairy products, as well as wheat, peanuts, eggs, soy and seafood) could cause allergy.

Teresa's daughter, Lisa, was very fussy and colicky as a new baby, but she improved almost immediately when Teresa stopped consuming any dairy products (and it took some careful label-reading to make sure she eliminated all of them). Lisa is an adult now and is still allergic to cow's milk.

If you want to eliminate foods, I would eliminate one at a time, starting with dairy products. Some mothers really like their dairy products; in that case, perhaps starting with another food group would be easier. Dairy products do seem to be the most common offenders. The mother should stay off the group of foods for at least three weeks to make sure it was not the cause of the baby's crying. If there is no improvement from eliminating the first food, the mother should reintroduce it and eliminate another food group for at least three weeks.

Mothers' Stories

Bronwyn

Bronwyn brought her six-week-old baby to the clinic. Bronwyn said that Ashley cried almost all the time while awake, which was most of the day and night. She breastfed well, and seemed comforted by breastfeeding.

On examination, the baby appeared normal, although slightly jaundiced, which is normal in an exclusively breastfeeding, well-gaining baby. She weighed 4 kg (8 lb, 12 oz.), after a birth weight of 2.7 kg (6 lb, 2 oz.). The urine was normal.

I was not sure what to suggest. I had just started the breastfeeding clinic, and this was the first baby with this sort of problem. Not having any other ideas, and having heard of the possibility of milk protein causing colic, I suggested Bronwyn go off milk products. Within 24 to 48 hours, Ashley was calm, an almost "perfect" baby.

When Ashley was about six months old, Bronwyn called to let me know what had happened. After a few weeks, she had wondered if the change in Ashley was just a coincidence. Bronwyn was missing her dairy products. So she had a glass of milk. The baby did not start crying, but the next day there was visible blood in her bowel movements. This lasted perhaps a day, and then there was no more visible blood. Bronwyn reported that she did this several times over the four or five months since she and Ashley had been at the clinic. As Bronwyn said, "I could turn the blood in her poops on and off like a tap, just by having a glass of milk."

Some suggest caffeine in the mother's diet will make the baby being fussy. Giving up caffeine might be tough for those hooked on coffee. Infants do not eliminate caffeine as rapidly as adults, so it may take at least three days for a three-month-old baby to get rid of all the caffeine in his body. A newborn may take much longer.

Pancreatic enzymes

If none of these approaches work, the mother can try taking pancreatic enzymes. These can be bought in a pharmacy by prescription, or without a prescription in health food stores, and are used to help people who cannot digest their food. The products sold in pharmacies are said to be more reliable. Take one capsule at every meal to start with. You can increase the dose to two capsules at every meal and one with any snack. The enzymes presumably break down the proteins that are bothering the baby.

If that doesn't work, you could give the enzymes directly to the baby, dissolved in a little breastmilk

and in a lactation aid at the breast. The baby then gets partially digested breastmilk with the protein broken down. It's hydrolyzed breastmilk, much better than hydrolyzed formula.

The enzymes are probably best given at the very beginning of the feeding, with ointment applied to the nipple and areola to protect them. If, for some reason, you are giving breastmilk in a bottle, the pancreatic enzymes can be added to the bottle.

When a baby isn't latching on well, and isn't getting much milk, you may find that expressing milk and giving it in a bottle makes the baby less colicky. Why? Because now he's getting more milk! Fixing the breastfeeding is a better way to go.

Reflux esophagitis and GERD (gastroesophageal reflux disease)

These two diagnoses are now being made more frequently than ever before. Reflux esophagitis and GERD refer to a situation in which the stomach contents flow up into the esophagus (the tube leading from the mouth to the stomach) and cause the baby pain. As a result, the baby may cry (not surprisingly), fight the breast or even refuse to continue breastfeeding. Feedings are frequently short because the baby drinks only long enough to take the edge off his hunger and then pulls away from the breast. Inflammation of the esophagus may be significant.

Eosinophilic esophagitis is related to reflux esophagitis and GERD, but little is known about it. It is sometimes thought to be caused by allergies. The symptoms of reflux, GERD and eosinophilic esophagitis are very similar to those of a decrease in milk supply and milk flow. The decrease in milk supply is probably *far more common* a cause of the baby's symptoms than reflux (I will use reflux as an all-inclusive term). See the chapter "Late-Onset Decreased Milk Supply."

Spitting up without crying, arching or fighting the breast should not be defined as reflux. A baby who is content, gaining weight well and drinking well from the breast but who also spits up, even a lot and frequently, does not have reflux and does not require treatment. When the baby drinks *a lot* of milk at a feeding, spitting up is common. It's not a problem. In fact it is a good thing because it probably increases the resistance of his mouth and esophagus to infection.

Reflux is often diagnosed in babies who drink for a short time and then fight the breast, arch, cry, return to the breast, but pull away again. I think most of these babies are actually reacting to a slowdown in milk flow and don't have reflux at all, even if they are also spitting up. See the chapter "Late-Onset Decreased Milk Supply."

It concerns me that many babies are being diagnosed with reflux and put on medication. In order to confirm the diagnosis, you need to biopsy the esophagus while putting a scope down the baby's throat and esophagus. Many parents don't like that idea and I don't blame them. Often then, a trial of medication is offered instead. But the medication does not fix the problem of slow milk flow, which is a more likely reason why the baby fights the breast.

Sometimes mothers whose babies are both breastfed and bottle-fed say the baby is calm when bottle-fed, even if it is breastmilk in the bottle, but fights the breast because he has reflux when breastfeeding. If the baby had true reflux, his symptoms would be the same whether fed by breast or bottle. If the baby calmly takes the bottle but cries when breastfeeding, it is more likely that he is unhappy at the breast because of slow flow or nipple confusion.

Many parents see that the baby spits up when breastfed but not when bottle-fed and feel guilty. (Remember, spitting up breastmilk may, in itself, be good.) Parents see anti-reflux formula advertised and think perhaps it will help. The first approach should not be medication or formula-feeding, but rather fixing the breastfeeding. See the chapter "Late-Onset Decreased Milk Supply."

"Oversupply" or "Overactive Letdown (Milk Ejection Reflex)"

The terms "oversupply" and "overactive letdown reflex" should be dropped; I think they are misleading. Indeed, I would say that in most cases, the more milk the mother has, the better. We did use these terms and discuss this topic in the first edition of the book, but I think much of what we said was misunderstood.

It is true that some mothers have such an abundant milk supply that the baby cannot control the flow and may cough and sputter at the breast. Some of these babies are quite unhappy at the breast because they are always struggling with the abundance of milk and get frustrated because they can't suck just for comfort.

With these mothers, one approach that Teresa has used is to nurse the baby, then pump or hand-express both breasts to extract as much milk as possible. When both breasts are "empty," the mother begins what is known as block feeding, where each time the baby shows interest in the next two or three hours, he's returned to the same breast. Then she feeds on the opposite breast for the next two or three hours. Usually, after doing this for 24 hours, she can return to feeding on both breasts at each feeding and her supply becomes more manageable. Occasionally, she has to repeat the emptying and a day of block feeding. This method was shared by Caroline GA van Veldhuizen-Staas in the *International Breastfeeding Journal* in 2007. Though Teresa has had some success with this method, I am skeptical about it. I don't like making breastfeeding complicated. Given that a trial of only 24 hours is supposed to work, though, I suppose this is not something I should reject out of hand.

But generally, a baby who has a good latch can control the flow of milk and is not bothered by rapid flow. Often, getting a good latch from the beginning is all that is necessary.

It also happens that when a mother has an abundant milk supply the baby, used to a fast flow, may fuss at the breast as it slows down during a feeding. He's still hungry, and he wants the milk to come faster! Some mothers switch sides at that point, and this generally works until the flow slows down again. Getting the best latch possible will allow the baby to control the flow much better. When it is fast, he will not choke or sputter or cry because he can control it. When it is slower, he can increase the flow by stimulating a letdown reflex. The mother can help when the flow is slow by using breast compression.

To figure out what is going on, it helps to know when the baby is drinking a lot (fast flow) and when he isn't (slow flow). Without knowing this, the mother may not realize why the baby is fussing.

Keeping the baby on one breast only during a feeding (block feeding) can make the problem worse by decreasing milk production.

Breast compression will also drain the breast more completely, so that the baby gets more high-fat milk and his stomach will empty more slowly. This brings us to the issue of lactose intolerance.

Lactose intolerance

In 1989, Woolridge and Fisher published an article in a British medical journal suggesting that much of what we call colic actually is a baby's reaction to timed feedings. Because timed feedings (for example, 10 or 15 minutes on each side) resulted in partial emptying of the breast and the baby got mostly low-fat milk, his stomach emptied quickly. Fat slows emptying of food from the stomach. Because so much milk goes from stomach to small intestine in a very short period of time, young babies, who have a relatively low concentration of lactase (the enzyme that breaks down lactose) in their intestine, are not able to metabolize so much lactose in such a short period of time. As a result, without really being lactose intolerant, the babies demonstrated the typical symptoms: periods of crying; explosive, watery, often green bowel movements; and diaper rash. To repeat, these babies were not truly lactose intolerant.

The bizarre notion that babies should be trained to feed at certain times and for a set period of time at the breast resulted in this so-called colic. By allowing a baby to stay on the breast until he pulls off by himself, he will get better.

However, a baby is not necessarily getting milk just because he's sucking at the breast. Thus, leaving him on one breast until he falls asleep or comes off himself is not going to help the colic if he's not drinking much of the time. Of course, the formula companies jumped on this before the ink was dry. Within weeks, it seems, lactose-free formulas were on the market to help mothers with their colicky babies. In some cases, mothers found they "worked"—because in fact the baby had been hungry, so when he got more milk (even though it was formula), he was happier.

Unfortunately, too many physicians still recommend lactose-free formula or newer special formulas for colic. Time alone will cure most cases of colic. Any sort of formula is clearly inferior to breastmilk, and breastfeeding is much more than breastmilk. So how can we deal with "lactose intolerance"?

1. Help the mother get the best latch possible (see the video clips at www.breastfeedinginc.ca).
2. Teach the mother how to recognize whether the baby is *drinking* from the breast or not (see video clips at www.breastfeedinginc.ca).
3. If the baby is drinking only occasionally, encourage the mother to start using compression (before he gets too sleepy) to keep him drinking, not just sucking at the breast.
4. If the baby is not drinking even with compressions, switch to the other side before he gets really sleepy.
5. If the baby wants the other breast, repeat the stepsabove.
6. If the baby is not interested in drinking, fine.
7. Patience is essential. If the baby is gaining well and drinking well, this too will pass. It's worth continuing to breastfeed and not putting the baby on formula.

Many babies have been diagnosed as lactose intolerant simply because they have green bowel movements. If the baby is content, drinking well and gaining weight well, then green bowel movements are of no significance. If the baby is not content or not drinking well, the problem is not the colour of the bowel movements.

In *some* situations where the baby is colicky from getting too much milk too quickly, and fixing the latch and finishing one side before offering the other breast does not work, it may be worthwhile to try giving one breast at a feeding or even two feedings in a row. The mother needs to be aware that this may cause her milk production to decrease, and that the baby may fuss because he's not getting as much milk as he wants—even if he is still gaining weight well.

What about using a pacifier to calm the baby?

Pacifiers are too often used to quiet a baby when in fact he needs to go to the breast; often the pacifier becomes the first solution whenever the baby is fussy. Some babies are full but still want to suck, and a pacifier might seem like a good idea. Putting the baby back on the breast that is the least full may work, but if he resists and the mother is sure he drank well at the breast, she might let the baby suck on her finger while still cuddling the baby close to her. The mother's body, and the mother's breast, are the best comforts for a baby. Could the baby suck on one of Dad's fingers, too? Sure, but most small babies do have a preference for being close to their mother's body because it is more familiar to them.

After all is said and done

Too many babies are taken off the breast for colic. Too many babies are diagnosed as having an allergy to breastmilk, reflux and lactose intolerance when they have nothing of the sort. See first if the breastfeeding can be improved, keeping in mind that some babies, even breastfed ones, just have colic. If the baby is still fussy, try the following:

1. Holding, carrying and skin-to-skin contact. The father, cousin or grandparent can carry the baby,

and the mother can get a little rest. Ron Barr's techniques for dealing with colic are contact, carry, walk and talk. In other words, keep the baby close, carry him in arms or in a carrier, walk around with him (movement helps calm babies) and talk to him (make soothing sounds or sing, perhaps). Barr found that babies carried in slings or soft baby carriers were much less likely to cry for long periods of time—in fact, carrying cut the total crying time in half. It helps to carry the baby throughout the day rather than just starting in the evening when he is already a bit stressed out.

2. Infant massage. Babies love massage. It calms and soothes them just as carrying them and talking with them. No special training is needed.

3. Cranio-sacral therapy. This is reputed to work for colicky babies. The cost of this treatment is sometimes covered by health plans.

Accepting the situation

It may not be easy, but sometimes the only thing to do is accept the situation. Colic won't last forever; most cases start to improve by six weeks and end around three months. Ask for help: maybe grandparents or partners will be willing to take a turn with the baby and do some of the carrying and soothing while the mother has a break.

Others should help with housework and older children so the mother can lie down and relax as she breastfeeds the baby throughout the evening. The mother and baby may fall asleep this way, which is not a bad thing. The mother should make sure the sleeping place is safe.

A glass of wine won't hurt and it may help. (Yes, it's okay, and mothers don't need to put breastfeeding on hold for two hours for every ounce of alcohol—see the chapter "Breastfeeding While on Medication.") I'm not suggesting the mother get drunk, but a glass or two may help her relax.

I frequently tell mothers that colicky breastfed babies get straight A's in school. I have no proof of this, but I think it's true, probably because they get so much attention at a crucial developmental stage in their lives. This is not to say that calm babies cannot get straight A's in school too, especially if they are breastfed.

You can feel proud of yourself as a parent when you get through the colicky stage and are still breastfeeding. Your baby will have learned he can count on you when things are tough. This is no small feat.

13 | When the Baby Does Not Yet Take the Breast

Myth #1: If a baby does not latch on in the first few days, he probably never will and it's better not to keep trying as it frustrates the mother and the baby.

Fact: Babies who do not seem to be able to latch on at first will often latch on easily when the mother's milk "comes in." If not then, with good help and persistence, the baby will almost always learn to take the breast later. To quote from Johann Wolfgang von Goethe:

> All that depends on habit.
> So from its mother's breasts a child
> At first, reluctant, takes its food,
> But soon to seek them is beguiled.
> Thus, at the breasts of Wisdom clinging,
> Thou'lt find each day a greater rapture bringing.

In other words, even in the early 19th century, before modern obstetrics and modern "help" with breastfeeding, babies often took their time getting started at breastfeeding.

Myth #2: The usual reason babies don't latch on is that the mother has flat or inverted nipples.

Fact: We tend to believe that if a mother's nipple does not look like a bottle nipple, it is flat. True inverted nipples are rare; in 28 years I have seen only a very few. What most people call inverted nipples are nipples that are "infolded," meaning they look inverted, but actually come out easily when suction is applied to them.

Myth #3: Nipple shields are a good way to get the baby to latch on.

Fact: Nipples shields do more harm than good. A baby latched on to a nipple shield is not latched on at all, and the mother's milk supply will often decrease. We find that babies who have been using a nipple shield for more than a few days are the most difficult ones to get latched on.

Why would babies not be able to latch on to the breast?

Probably the most common reason is that we don't give them enough time. In many hospitals, babies are given bottles of formula if they haven't latched on to the breast and fed by three hours after birth, partly for fear of violating the rule that babies *must* feed every three hours, and partly for an unfounded fear that the baby will develop hypoglycemia (low blood sugar). Experienced midwives who assist at home births reinforce Goethe's observations: some babies latch on immediately and feed frequently during the first few days. Some babies feed immediately after birth and then are not interested in feeding again for several hours, sometimes as long as 24 hours. Some will not show interest in feeding in the first couple of hours after birth or for several hours afterwards. All these variations are normal and are seen in perfectly healthy babies who go on to breastfeed well and exclusively.

The rule that babies must breastfeed every three hours from birth on often leads inexperienced or unskilled helpers to push the baby into the breast when he is not interested in breastfeeding. Sometimes this leads babies to develop an aversion to the breast. Then, since the baby didn't feed, the conclusion is that he needs a bottle of formula. Adding formula, especially by bottle, complicates the problem even more.

Once artificial nipples are added to the mix, the situation often deteriorates. Is it necessary to use artificial nipples to feed a baby who is not latching on? Almost never. See the chapter "Breastfeeding Devices."

Obstetrical practices during labour and birth are also responsible for many babies not being able to latch on immediately. See the chapter "How Birth Affects Breastfeeding." Separation of the mother and the baby is another very important reason why babies don't latch on. Skin-to-skin contact immediately after birth and rooming in are important for the baby to latch on. There is no reason, for example, that a healthy baby should be taken to the special care unit simply because the mother has had a Caesarean section. There is no reason for a baby to be in observation simply because he passed meconium, even thick meconium, before being born. If the baby is well at birth, he will almost always be okay and hours of observation are not necessary. Furthermore, following the approach for hypoglycemia in the chapter "Early Concerns" will prevent even the babies at risk for low blood sugar from needing the special care unit. Babies in special care often get bottles because the mother is not there to feed them.

The mother is urged to let the baby go to the nursery because she needs to rest and recover from the birth, especially if she has had a Caesarean section. But there is no evidence that mothers who are separated from their babies are better rested; in fact, mothers are less stressed and get more sleep when they are with their babies. The pleasure that most mothers experience holding and stroking their babies and putting them to the breast often make fatigue magically disappear.

We've mentioned earlier that research showed that when mothers allowed their babies to go to the hospital nursery at night, it was not because they didn't want them with them—it was because they felt *the nurses* wanted the babies to be in the nursery.

Some babies are more reluctant to latch on when they are not skin to skin while the mothers are attempting to breastfeed them. Undressing the baby to his diaper and the mother from waist up can make all the difference.

Starting nipple shields in the first few days can turn a baby who is latching on into one who isn't.

Sometimes a series of events causes a baby not to latch on, a typical series being: separation after birth, followed by the baby being sleepy, having higher bilirubin levels and being under bilirubin lights.

If your baby does not take the breast immediately, you might feel disheartened and frustrated. It's an emotional time, right after giving birth, and it can feel like your baby is rejecting you. This is just a temporary problem that can almost always be fixed with some help, time and patience. Often it is not just one factor, but two or more that stop the baby from taking the breast. Breastfeeding really is worth overcoming whatever challenges arise.

So, the baby is a day old and has not yet latched on.

Trying to force the baby onto the breast is worse than useless. It isn't going to work. If the baby resists the breast, trying to force him onto it is either going to make him angry or go limp. Neither helps with latching on.

Babies are not complicated. If they get what they want, they are happy. If the baby goes to the breast and gets milk, he will usually stay there.

Should you go on herbs to increase the milk

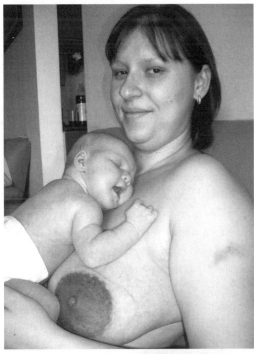
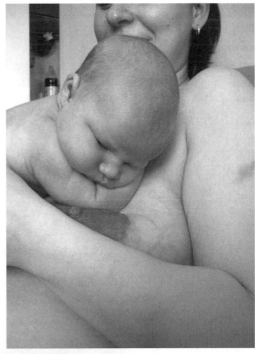
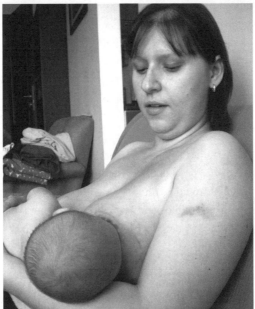

One approach to a reluctant feeder: start with the baby in skin-to-skin contact (*top left*), let him fall naturally towards the breast (*top right*) and then allow him to latch on (*bottom*). (See http://youtu.be/nrYHeQdYWBK.)

CREDIT: ANDREA POLOKOVA

.his stage? With more flow, the baby is more
latch on. If the baby still doesn't latch on,
.y be able to express more milk so that formula
leeded. We have used fenugreek and blessed
.le for many years in our clinic, and mothers who
: them within a few days of birth of the baby seem
/ get a better response than the mothers who use
.hem two or three weeks after birth. Recently we
have occasionally used malunggay with good results.

An angry baby may not take the breast even
if he is ravenous. This is one reason that keeping
babies in the nursery separated from the mother is
not a good idea. The nurse isn't likely to notice the
baby's early cues that he's hungry. Chances are the
baby will be brought to the mother only when he's
crying and upset, which does not help to get breastfeeding started.

Skin-to-skin contact can calm down an upset
baby and once the baby is calm, he may take the breast.
In fact, some babies kept in this position (see photos
on page 185) will often start looking for the breast and
latch on all by themselves. See the video clips "Baby
28 hrs old, Baby-Led Mother-Guided Latching" and
"Baby-Led Mother-Guided Started Upright Left Breast,
Latches" at www.breastfeedinginc.ca.

So what now?

First of all, *do not panic*. A full-term healthy newborn is not at risk of dehydration in 24 or 36 hours.
In fact, if the mother received an intravenous infusion, the baby will have received extra fluids and
may be *overhydrated*. A full-term, healthy newborn
is also not going to get low blood sugar if he has
not fed yet; furthermore, keeping the baby skin to
skin will help maintain his blood sugar. Jaundice
may become a problem because the baby needs
to get breastmilk in order to prevent the jaundice
from rising too high, but it's not usually a concern at
24 hours after birth.

It is a good idea, though, to start to hand-express
colostrum. You can give the baby this colostrum, and
expressing now will help assure a good milk supply.
Express every couple of hours until the baby begins
feeding at the breast. The colostrum can be fed to
the baby with a spoon, a small cup or by finger feeding. Hand expression in the early days is often much
more effective in getting some colostrum than even
the most up-to-date, modern pumps, which generally
only convince mothers that they don't have any milk.
When milk quantities are small, pumps don't seem
to be able to get it out; if they do, the milk gets lost in
the tubing and can't be fed to the baby. If you don't
know how to hand-express, ask for help. It is not
true (as some mothers are told) that if the baby hasn't
latched on by day three (or any other arbitrary day),
he never will. In fact, once the milk comes in, many
babies will latch on easily, especially if the mother
gets skilled help.

Using a nipple shield before the mother's milk
comes in should absolutely not be done. Once the
milk comes in, the baby often latches on. If the baby
is on a nipple shield, the mother may delay getting
help when the milk comes in because she thinks the
problem is solved. It's not, and in many cases, the
milk supply decreases with time.

I have been told by some lactation consultants
that they use a nipple shield because they are concerned that a mother who can't get her baby to latch
on without it will quit breastfeeding. I think the
mother needs not a nipple shield but better information and good help. She needs to know that it
is likely the baby will latch on soon, once her milk
increases. I'm also against using a nipple shield with
a baby who won't latch after the milk has come in.
Even though some mothers have breastfed successfully for many months with a nipple shield (because
they had lots of milk and even if the nipple shield
caused a decrease in the milk supply, the baby still

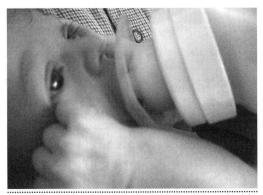

A baby being fed with a bottle through a nipple shield.

CREDIT: **JACK NEWMAN**

got enough), it is still a barrier between the mother and the baby. Mothers who want to get rid of the shield find that when the baby is so used to it, it can be hard to get him to latch directly on the breast. For too many mothers, though, a nipple shield means a decrease in milk supply, so soon they are supplementing with bottles of formula. And getting the baby off the shield and onto the breast once milk production is down can be very difficult. *The single most important factor in getting the baby to latch on is the mother's development of an abundant milk supply.*

The photo above shows a baby being fed through a nipple shield from a bottle. The idea of using a nipple shield is sold to mothers as if nipple shields were just like breastfeeding. So this baby who was not latching on is being fed by bottle through a nipple shield so he can "learn to breastfeed."

Here is an email I received from a mother who was given a nipple shield by a nurse in hospital. "You know, I have done everything right (natural birth, for which I travelled outside Slovakia, skin-to-skin contact) and then a nurse comes in and says she would help me with breastfeeding because my nipples are not long enough and gives me a nipple shield. Then for seven weeks I believed she had saved my breastfeeding, except now my baby squirms and fusses at

the breast and I have had blocked ducts three times already. I have started supplementing with formula and using bottles. I really want to breastfeed."

If the baby is on a nipple shield in hospital, you must not be sent home without an early definite appointment, within a day or two of discharge, with someone skilled in helping babies latch on. If an appointment isn't made for you, make one yourself as soon as you can.

Finger feeding

We use finger feeding to help prepare a baby to take the breast. Finger feeding calms a baby if he is upset, and wakes up a baby who is "too sleepy." Babies seem to use the same motion with their tongues when they suck on a finger as they do at the breast, so finger feeding may help teach the baby to suck. We suggest that the mother (or father, family member or friend) finger feed the baby for a minute or so until he is calm and awake and then try him on the breast. I have been told that giving a bottle for a minute or two does the same thing, but I don't agree. Yes, the bottle will calm the baby, but it won't teach him how to suck as he would at the breast.

Here is how we teach finger feeding:

Finger feeding is best learned by watching and doing. See also the video clip "Finger Feeding to Latch" at www.breastfeedinginc.ca.

1. Wash your hands well. It is better if your fingernail is short, but not necessary. Get comfortably seated with your baby. Have the baby on your lap, half seated, facing you, with one hand behind his shoulders and neck to support him. You want to be able to keep your finger flat in his mouth.

2. Take a feeding tube (#5 French, 91 cm or 36 inches long), and a container with a lid with

a hole, filled with expressed breast milk or supplement. Pass the feeding tube through the enlarged hole into the container.

3. Hold the tube so that it sits on the soft part of your index or middle finger (some people use their thumbs, but this is trickier). The end of the tube should line up no farther than the end of your finger. It is easiest to grip the tube where it makes a gentle curve between your thumb and middle finger and position your index finger under the tube. If this is done properly, there is no need to tape the tube to the finger.

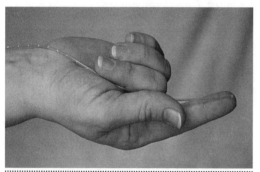

Holding a feeding tube to be used for finger feeding. There's no need to tape the finger.

CREDIT: **ANDREA POLOKOVA**

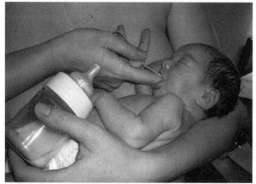

In this example of finger feeding, the mother's finger is pointing too much towards the roof of the baby's mouth; the finger should be flatter. This is easier if the baby is facing the mother. Using a thumb rather than an index finger works better in this position.

CREDIT: **ANDREA POLOKOVA**

4. With the finger and the tube, tickle the baby's upper lip lightly until he opens his mouth enough to allow your finger to enter. If the baby is very sleepy but needs to be fed, the finger may be gently insinuated into his mouth. You can pull the baby's lower lip out if necessary with *gentle* downward pressure on his chin. Generally, the baby will begin to suck even if asleep and will wake up when he gets milk.

5. Insert your finger with the tube so that the soft part of your finger is up. Try to keep your finger as flat as possible so the baby's tongue is flat and forward. Usually the baby will begin sucking on the finger and allow it to enter quite far. The baby will not usually gag on the finger unless he is not hungry or he is very used to bottles. After all, the breast goes in quite far! A baby older than six weeks may not tolerate a finger deep in his mouth, but most younger babies don't seem to mind.

The technique is working if the baby is drinking. If feeding is very slow, you can raise the container above the baby's head, but usually this is not necessary. Keep your finger straight, flattening the baby's tongue, and try not to point it toward the top of his mouth or press on the roof of his mouth. I don't recommend using a syringe to push milk into the baby's mouth. The idea is not to feed the baby, but to teach him to suck properly and prepare him to take the breast.

What about nipples?

As I've said, I don't believe flat nipples exist, and true inverted nipples are rare. I'd also point out that babies don't "nipple-feed" (or shouldn't!). They breastfeed; the shape and size of the nipple is much less important than getting a good mouthful of breast. But it is true that some nipple shapes and lengths can make getting the baby to latch on more difficult; I emphasize "more difficult," not *impossible*. Mothers' breasts change and babies change with time, and what is not possible today may be possible on day 3 or day 15 or later. Patience is often necessary. Nipples and breasts may even change dramatically for the better if the mother received large amounts of fluids during the labour, once her body has rid itself of the excess fluid.

So-called inverted nipples

Most health professionals would call a nipple that doesn't protrude but rather sinks down into the areola and forms a dimple an inverted nipple. I call it infolded. These nipples can make getting the baby to latch on more difficult, but not impossible by any means. In some cases, as the baby latches on and applies pressure, the nipple retracts further, slipping away so that he cannot grasp the breast. What I would call a true inverted nipple has a ring of fibrous tissue around it, with the nipple folded in on itself in the middle of the ring. This is a much more difficult problem to deal with, but it is rare.

Infolded nipples can sometimes be pulled out (everted) with a device shown in the photo below. These devices are available now in some breastfeeding clinics or can be made from an ordinary 12 or 20 cc syringe by cutting off the end that holds the needle, taking the plunger out and putting it into the newly made hole on the other side of the syringe (so that the ragged cut edge is not in contact with the areola, which would be painful).

The photo above shows an infolded nipple. The mother did not breastfeed her first three babies because she was unable to latch them on. I was able to help her fourth baby latch on at five or six hours after the birth. In the middle photo, I am compressing the breast to increase the flow of milk into the baby's mouth and thus encourage him to stay on the breast.

The bottom photo shows a nipple everter pulling out an inverted nipple. The fact that it does

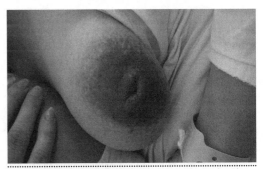

This mother has an infolded, not inverted, nipple. She didn't try to breastfeed her first three babies because she was told she had inverted nipples and breastfeeding would be impossible.

CREDIT: **JACK NEWMAN**

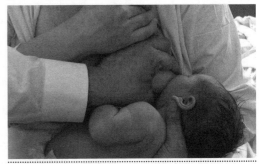

When the same woman received hands-on help, her fouth baby latched on at five hours old and was breastfed normally.

CREDIT: **ANDREA POLOKOVA**

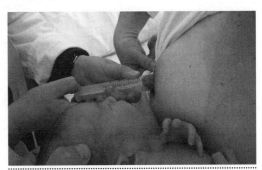

A "nipple everter" easily and painlessly pulls out an infolded nipple, taking only a small amount of milk from the breast.

CREDIT: **ANDREA POLOKOVA**

come out shows it is really not inverted but infolded. Note that the syringe takes out only about 2 cc of milk (colostrum). This is better than using a pump because while the pump may pull the nipple out, it may also remove a lot of milk, so the baby gets less.

Flat nipples

Often postpartum nurses tell mothers they have flat nipples, but what they may be seeing is edema (swelling caused by fluid) of the nipple and areola, caused by the large amounts of fluid most women are given during labour. This may not be the usual appearance of the nipple; in many cases these women actually have normal nipples and breastfeed happily.

Very large or very long nipples

Very large or very long nipples may be more of a problem than flat or infolded ones. The baby may not be able to take in enough of the breast, and he will have to depend on the mother's milk ejection reflexes to get milk. If she has an abundant milk supply, this may work. If she does not, the baby may not gain well. This is similar to what happens with a nipple shield. The baby may also refuse to latch on.

It may take weeks for the baby's mouth to grow enough to be able to latch on well, but time and patience can make things work. The baby in the photo above took four weeks to latch on. Before that, he would allow the nipple into his mouth, but up to the white line. This prevented him from getting much milk and he slipped off the breast easily.

By supplementing him at the breast with a lactation aid, he was able to get milk, and by four weeks he was able to latch on and drink without the lactation aid. Once the baby was feeding well, the mother's milk supply increased and she did not need to supplement.

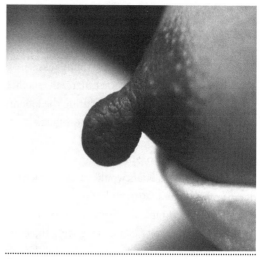

CREDIT: JACK NEWMAN

Breasts

Engorgement

While painful engorgement of the breasts about three or four days after the birth is common, it should not be. If the baby latches well, is fed in response to his cues, feeds well and no artificial nipples are used, this engorgement shouldn't happen. Severe, painful engorgement on day three or four is at least partly due to ineffective breastfeeding. Overhydration with intravenous fluids is part of the problem, but getting the baby latched on well and nursing well would make a big difference. See the photo below of the breast swollen with fluid (note

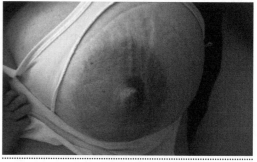

CREDIT: JACK NEWMAN

the indentations from a breast shell) that would not allow the baby to latch on.

Large breasts

Sometimes women with very large breasts have difficulties because they find it awkward to get the baby positioned and to support their breasts at the same time. Women with very large breasts often have flat nipples as well.

A sling made of any soft absorbent material can help the mother support the breast. It's also possible to lay the baby on a table that supports both baby and breast, as in the photo below. The mother's breasts are actually larger than they seem in the photo. The mother is using a lactation aid at the breast to supplement the baby who has been refusing the breast and has been fed only by bottle for several weeks. By supplementing the baby at the breast, milk flow continues rapidly and the baby stays on the breast.

The laid-back position often works because the mother doesn't need to support the baby; she can use her hand to support her breast more comfortably and effectively and provide the baby with a little guidance as he latches on himself. Side-lying is another good position where the mother's hands are freer.

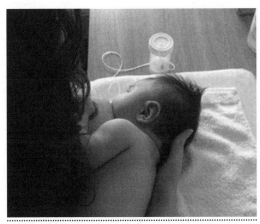

CREDIT: JACK NEWMAN

Issues related to the baby that make latching on difficult

Some babies have difficulties latching on because of medical problems. In some cases latching on may not be possible.

If a baby has special needs or is ill, too many health professionals will say breastfeeding is not possible. In some cases it is true, but we are learning all the time. Many mothers with no formal training in breastfeeding have found solutions to help their babies. The mother who found a way to give breastmilk to her baby with a chylothorax is one example. See the chapter "Sick Babies, Special Babies."

Even if the baby can't or won't breastfeed, it is still worthwhile for the mother to express her milk and feed the baby with a bottle. A cup is better, but few mothers are willing to cup-feed long term. We have seen babies latch on for the first time two months, three months, four months or more after birth. One baby latched on for the first time at the age of nine months.

At nine months, it should be easy to stop all bottles, and stopping bottles will encourage the baby to take the breast. Babies like to suck, and if the baby is kept skin to skin with the mother and the breast is the only option for sucking, he may latch on. Instead of giving bottles, the mother can mix her milk with any solids the baby might eat. The baby should eat as much as he wants, as frequently as he wants, without forcing. At nine months the baby should also be able to drink from an open cup (a sippy cup is essentially a bottle). Skin-to-skin contact using a baby carrier if necessary, is helpful and should continue as much as possible. During naps and at night, safe sleeping side by side (see the chapter "Sleep: Yours and Your Baby's"), the baby in a diaper only and the mother undressed from the waist up, may induce the baby to latch (especially if he doesn't do so when fully awake). Finally, it may be useful to increase the milk supply, usually with domperidone; more milk means a faster flow from the breast and the baby is more likely to latch on.

Lethargic babies

Some newborns are lethargic at birth, usually due to medication given to the mother during the labour and birth. Improvement usually occurs fairly quickly as the medication leaves the baby's body or is broken down by liver enzymes. However, some drugs are metabolized much more slowly in newborns than in adults and the period of decreased responsiveness can last many days or even a week or more. For this reason it is best to avoid narcotics during labour and birth. If the baby is quite unresponsive at birth because of the effect of narcotics, there is medication that can reverse this.

Some babies, however, are less responsive for a longer period of time for reasons unrelated to medication. Babies with trisomy 21 (Down syndrome), babies who were deprived of oxygen in the uterus or during birth, or babies with abnormalities of the brain can have much longer periods of neurological depression than babies who are lethargic because of medication. Still, some of these babies will latch on right away, and others will do so in time. Most will latch on eventually, if we are patient. Babies with trisomy 21 can usually latch on once their hypotonia (floppiness) resolves or at least decreases during the first month. Babies who have had asphyxia (lack of oxygen) can have very serious problems, depending on how badly and how long they were deprived of oxygen. They may have few very mild symptoms or very serious injuries to their brains, hearts and kidneys, which can make treatment complicated and can interfere with getting breastfeeding started. However, these babies often improve considerably and with time, patience, encouragement and skilled help, they may get breastfeeding.

Cleft palate, cleft lip and tongue tie are discussed elsewhere, the first two in the chapter "Sick Babies, Special Babies" and the third in the chapter "Sore Nipples."

One problem I haven't yet mentioned is Pierre Robin Syndrome, in which the baby has a very small mandible (lower jaw) and a tongue that is positioned further back in the mouth than usual, with a tendency to fall backwards and obstruct the airway. The majority of these babies also have a cleft palate. A cleft palate is usually the major problem in getting the baby to latch on, but the position of the tongue is also likely a part of the problem. Some lactation consultants feel that simply having a small mandible causes difficulty in getting latched on. I don't agree. By using an asymmetric latch, almost any baby can get onto the breast if the only problem is a small chin.

The baby in the photo below has a very small chin. But he latched on just fine.

What to do when the baby does not take the breast

Probably the most important thing the mother, her family and any helper needs is patience, but being patient isn't easy. I think nipple shields are used so often because whoever is helping the mother

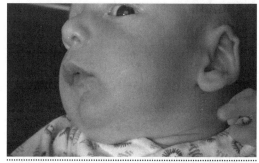

This baby has a small chin, which is said to interfere with latching. But with good help, he latched on without difficulty.

CREDIT: **JACK NEWMAN**

doesn't have the patience to wait for the baby to be ready. Not every problem has to be fixed the first day. Given time, many babies will come around and breastfeeding will happen.

One reason babies resist the breast is that inexperienced and unskilled people try to force them into the breast. This is not going to work; it will only make the baby angry or resistant. It helps to bring the baby onto the breast *briskly*—but if the baby resists, it is important not to keep him pushed into the breast. Let him move away from the breast, then try again if he's not too upset. If he is distressed, take a little time to calm him down. The mother can hold him skin to skin, walk with him, gently jiggle him up and down. The baby may throw himself toward the breast and may even latch on when he is calm and skin to skin with the mother. We have had mothers bounce on a big exercise ball with the baby in their arms; often the baby calms down and latches on. If the baby remains upset, finger feeding will often calm him and give him a little to drink. Glucose water (5%) can be used in the first few days if colostrum is not easily available. Expressed milk should be used if it's available, but if not, formula may be needed for a baby older than three or four days.

We use finger feeding only to calm the baby and get him sucking as if he were on the breast. If that does not work, feeding the baby a little breastmilk or formula with a cup or, if necessary, a bottle may work; as soon as the baby is calm, we put him to the breast. If the baby doesn't latch on the first day, there is no need to panic.

Thirty or forty years ago, babies were routinely not fed during the first 24 hours because it was believed that their stomachs and intestines were not ready. This makes no sense. Why would a baby born at term not be ready to take oral nourishment? Possibly the idea came from the observations that babies overfed with formula during the first day were fussy and often spat up a lot. But a breastfed baby gets small amounts, and growth factors in breastmilk help the gut mature more quickly. However, the point is that these babies survived just fine despite not being fed. Babies whose mothers got intravenous fluids during labour and birth are born with extra fluid on board and may have even more leeway.

If there is concern that the baby hasn't breastfed yet, what should be done?

1. Keep the baby skin to skin as much as possible, as this may encourage him to take the breast. Help the baby latch on as soon as he seems interested. It may be too late to get him to latch on if he's crying.

2. If the nipples and areolas are swollen (not always evident), reverse pressure may soften the area around the nipple. See the instructions on how to do this in the chapter "The First Few Days."

3. If the baby does not latch on and feed within the first few hours after birth, don't panic (too often doctors and nurses do panic). Begin hand-expressing colostrum. Anything you can express should be given to the baby by spoon (easier than using a cup or finger feeding). If there is concern about the baby's hydration, the colostrum can be mixed with 5% glucose or plain water and given with a cup or by finger feeding.

4. Express your milk regularly but only after attempting to get the baby to latch on.

5. Finger feeding is primarily used to prepare the baby to take the breast. If the baby is latching on and needs supplementing, it's better to give the supplement with the lactation aid at the breast.

6. Once the baby is sucking well, calm and awake (finger feeding is a good way to wake up a sleepy baby), attempt to latch him on. If the baby doesn't seem to prefer one side over the other, pick the

side you think will work best. Usually the left breast is a little easier for a right-handed mother, and the right breast for a left-handed mother.

7. Hold the baby in a cross-cradle position, the side of your forearm pushing in the baby's bottom, your hand palm-up and open like a pillow under his face (not on his shoulder or neck). If you hold the baby like this, he will come to the breast with your nipple pointing to his upper lip. Run your nipple along his upper lip from one corner to the other lightly, just a tickle. A hungry baby will usually open wide. Bring the baby onto the breast, *straight* on, so that his chin touches the breast first and is buried in it but his nose does not touch it. As a result, the baby covers more of the areola with his lower lip than with his upper lip. This is an asymmetric latch. It can be achieved with a football hold or a regular cradle hold or by lying down, but I think most mothers, at least at first, find it easier to use the cross-cradle hold to achieve this latch.

8. If the baby resists, let him move away from the breast and start again.

9. It often works to line up a lactation aid, with the tube full of the fluid to be given to the baby. The extra flow will encourage the baby to latch on. He will get a little fluid from the breast and a little from the tube and may be happy to remain there. Most of the babies we see are used to the rapid and continuous flow from the bottle, and if the flow is not maintained at the breast they may pull off. An opportunity to give the baby a full feeding at the breast will have been lost.

10. If the latch is not working, don't keep trying until everyone is exhausted and frustrated. It may be worth trying the other breast. But if neither side works this time, it's okay. You can feed the baby any milk you were able to express, mixed with water or sugar water if you need to. Once the baby is three or four days old, if you aren't able to express or pump enough milk and if donated milk is not available, you may need to use formula. But if you started expressing soon after birth, you'll probably have enough for your baby's needs. The most important thing during this time when the baby isn't latching is building up an abundant milk supply. It may be helpful to start taking fenugreek, blessed thistle or goat's rue, or malunggay.

11. We have given domperidone to mothers whose babies are not latching on, even if they are able to express all the milk the baby needs. The more milk, the faster the flow, and the more likely the baby will latch on. It's like having a lactation aid in place without the hassle.

12. We have seen some mothers resort to just finger feeding, not even trying the baby at the breast some days. This is not a good idea. Finger feeding can be very slow and once the baby's needs increase after three or four days, feeding this way can take up much of the day. We recommend finger feeding just to prepare the baby to take the breast, something that takes only a minute or two at most. If the baby does not latch on, finish the feeding with an open cup or spoon.

13. I am aware that many mothers will not cup feed or spoon feed the baby and will use a bottle. I am convinced that cup feeding works well and is better than a bottle (see the video clip "Cup Feeding" at www.breastfeedinginc.ca), but if a mother is going to use bottles, I'd encourage her to finger feed for a minute or two before trying the baby at the breast.

14. In our experience, if the mother develops an abundant milk supply, the baby will almost always latch on between four and eight weeks of age—often, with good help, even earlier. We have seen babies at our clinic latch on at three or

four months and continue happily breastfeeding even if they didn't latch at all before.

15. Even if the mother does not have a full milk supply, most babies will latch on if she does not give up. Many mothers find their milk supply increases substantially when the baby latches on and feeds directly at the breast.

16. Watch the video clip "Baby-Led Mother-Guided Started Upright Left Breast, Latches" at www. breastfeedinginc.ca. It shows how a baby can latch on by himself. A baby is quite capable of finding the breast and latching on by himself if he is allowed the time. Sometimes he literally falls sideways toward the breast. See also "Baby 28 hrs old, Baby-Led Mother-Guided Latching."

What if the baby just won't take the breast?

This can be an incredibly frustrating and disappointing situation for a new mother. What are her options?

If the mother has an abundant milk supply, as evidenced by being able to pump or hand-express substantial amounts of milk (although *not* being able to pump substantial amounts does not mean the mother does not have enough), and the baby is at least three weeks old, it *might* be reasonable to try a nipple shield, though I grit my teeth as I say that because I don't believe it. I'd want to be sure the mother has had help from someone skilled at latching babies on first. Even after a nipple shield has been started, the mother should keep trying the baby at the breast. Using a shield is probably better than pumping milk and giving it to the baby in a bottle for months at a time. But it can be hazardous to use a shield if the mother's milk supply is only adequate, as her milk production is likely to decrease. Pumping after feedings may help reduce this risk, but this involves yet more work for the mother. We have not recommended a nipple shield in our clinic for many years.

As mentioned earlier, some mothers have managed to get the baby to latch on after three or four months of bottle-feeding. If the baby has not latched by the time he starts solids, the mother may be able to reduce the number of bottles at that point or stop them altogether, and this will encourage the baby to take the breast. Keeping the baby skin to skin whenever possible is very important, and you can offer the breast at times when the baby is content and not especially hungry. Keeping the baby close at night can help, too, provided you follow the guidelines for safe co-sleeping. Many older babies latch on for the first time during the night when they are half-asleep.

By the way, if this is your first baby, don't worry that this will happen with your next baby, too. It rarely does.

The nursing strike

A nursing strike is when a baby who has previously been breastfeeding reasonably well abruptly stops taking the breast. I suggest that there are two different types of strike.

With the first type, there is some kind of precipitating event that causes the strike. For example, when Teresa's son Daniel was 10 months old, he bit her one day when she was breastfeeding (she was not paying close attention because she was supervising her two older children). She yelped and startled the baby, who pulled away, crying, and then refused to nurse again. Every time she offered the breast, he would cry and turn his head away—even though he was hungry. She did get him back to the breast after a couple of days, and he continued breastfeeding until he was three and a half. Other babies have gone on nursing strikes if they had a cold because they couldn't breathe and breastfeed at the same time.

Even a baby who is gaining weight well may stop nursing if the milk flow decreases. This generally happens when a once-abundant milk supply becomes insufficient. Just as a baby who has become accustomed to the rapid flow of milk from a bottle may reject the breast, a baby who is used to very fast flow from the breast may reject it if the flow slows down—*even if* the milk supply is still very good. Pulling off the breast after a short period of time may be the first sign of an impending nursing strike; the baby may soon reject the breast altogether. Babies can tell when there is little milk in the breast, even without suckling. I have noticed how a nursing strike and a decreased milk supply can result in a similar clinical picture.

In both situations:

1. The mother has or had a very good milk supply and the baby gained weight at a rapid rate, often faster than average.
2. In *most* cases, the baby was on the breast without getting any bottles, at least until he started refusing the breast.
3. The baby would often refuse the breast if wide awake but take it if he was sleepy.
4. The baby would take the breast during the night, especially if he and his mother were co-sleeping.
5. Typically, decreased milk supply occurs after the first few weeks, or even two or three months. This decrease can happen for various reasons; see the chapter "Late-Onset Decreased Milk Supply."
6. Increasing the milk supply, usually with domperidone, helped, even if the baby was still gaining weight well.

One explanation proposed for nursing strikes was that the baby was uncomfortable with the rapid flow of milk from the breast, so he resisted breastfeeding when the mother was sitting up but breastfed better when she lay down with him. This seemed plausible but didn't agree with my observations: by eight months, for example, the baby is usually taking solids, so the milk supply (and flow) should be decreasing. We have learned over the years that a lot of the discomfort that babies show at the breast is not due to too rapid a flow but rather to *too slow a flow*. Mothers are often surprised to hear this because the baby has been growing rapidly, but observation of the baby at the breast shows he is not drinking well (see the video clip at www.breastfeedinginc.ca). See also the chapter "Late-Onset Decreased Milk Supply."

Whether this is a nursing strike or a decrease in milk supply, the treatment is the same:

Avoid the bottle, even if it is breastmilk in it. Using a bottle will make the baby more likely to continue refusing the breast. It can be discouraging if the baby refuses the breast and then drinks eagerly from the bottle; his eagerness is due to the rapid and steady flow. It doesn't mean there is anything wrong with the milk. Pumping to maintain supply is a good idea and the baby can be fed with a cup or spoon. If the baby is eating solid foods, breastmilk can be mixed with the baby's solids.

If the baby is not nursing, pump or express your milk to maintain (or increase) your production. You want to have plenty of milk available when the baby does latch on. Keep your baby close, skin to skin if possible. A baby carrier that allows you to be skin to skin in a position where he can latch on if he wants is ideal. At naptime and night time, as much as possible, sleep or rest next to your baby, and give him access to your breasts. Be sure, of course, that you are bed-sharing safely.

Because it is likely that your milk supply has decreased, it helps to review the various reasons for it and eliminate what you can. See the chapter "Late-Onset Decreased Milk Supply." Don't try to force the baby to take the breast. For the older baby, you can add expressed breastmilk to his solids. He can take more solids than usual because he will want to make up for the decrease in milk. Avoid using pacifiers, and if he tries to suck his thumb or fingers, gently offer the breast.

14 Breastfeeding While on Medication

Myth: A mother who needs to take medication must wean her baby because the medication will make him sick.

Fact: In the *vast majority* of cases, the mother can and should continue breastfeeding. The medication will either have no effect on the baby or the effect will be minimal compared to the possible side effects of artificial feeding.

One of the most common kind of emails I receive concerns whether or not a mother can take such and such medication while breastfeeding. Somehow women and health professionals have gotten the idea that if the mother is taking any sort of medicine or is exposed to any sort of toxin or chemical, she must interrupt breastfeeding until the drug is eliminated from her body. They are so paranoid that I have received emails from mothers asking whether they can continue breastfeeding:

- while drinking green tea, Gatorade, protein shakes or amino acids
- while putting Vaporub on their feet
- while taking vitamins, probiotics or food supplements such as lecithin
- while going to a tanning salon, getting a tattoo, getting a perm, or using a tooth whitener.

Of course, the companies that make products don't help, as they often have labels advising against breastfeeding while using the product, or suggesting breastfeeding mothers consult a doctor first. The companies are simply protecting themselves, not the mother or the baby. But mothers end up afraid of using anything (seriously, vitamins? Green tea?).

The marketing of artificial baby milk (formula) has convinced parents and health professionals that breastmilk and formula are essentially the same. According to this mistaken belief, if even miniscule amounts of a drug appear in the breastmilk, it becomes inferior to formula, so it's safer to switch.

Some physicians will instruct mothers to interrupt breastfeeding because they fear being sued. Package inserts and info sheets from pharmacists often advise against using drugs while pregnant or breastfeeding. But taking a drug while breastfeeding is not at all like taking a drug during pregnancy, especially early pregnancy. The amount of drug that gets to the baby is *much* less during breastfeeding than during pregnancy. Furthermore, the fetus stage is a much more sensitive period.

In some cases a physician will refuse to treat a mother for a serious or even life-threatening condition unless she stops breastfeeding. Since, in the majority of cases, breastfeeding while taking a drug is of minimal or no risk to the baby, the physician's refusal to treat the mother unless she weans the baby is wrong and unethical, and it endangers both mother and baby.

Another point: Few people, other than breastfeeding mothers, appreciate how difficult it is to deprive a baby or a toddler of the breast. Babies breastfeed for more than milk and toddlers even more so. An older baby may be inconsolable for hours if he is refused the breast, especially at night.

Is formula almost the same as breastmilk?

Interrupting breastfeeding requires feeding the baby something else. Formula? How close is formula to breastmilk, really, putting aside the misinformation of the formula companies? Even in the second decade of the 21st century, formula is not even close to breastmilk. It is *superficially* the same in certain ways. It looks whitish, like breastmilk (although not like colostrum). The so-called improvements still leave formula a long way from breastmilk. Sometimes, in fact, the "improvements" have backfired and babies have gotten sick. In the 1970s, a formula with low salt content was introduced. This seemed like a good idea: decreasing the amount of sodium might prevent high blood pressure later in life (of course, breast-milk already has low, *but normal*, sodium content). However, in decreasing the sodium in the formula, the manufacturer also reduced the amount of chloride (salt is made from one molecule each of sodium and chloride). This resulted in a number of babies in the US developing "failure to thrive," developmental delays, metabolic abnormalities, kidney problems and other permanent problems. That was not the last time formula was manufactured incorrectly: in November 2003, the *Jerusalem Post* reported that three babies had died because the formula they drank did not contain enough vitamin B1. Of course, even if we could duplicate the components of breastmilk, we would not have the relationship that develops by feeding at the breast.

Why won't we be able to make formulas just like breastmilk?

First, there is no such thing as standard breastmilk. Breastmilk is different from woman to woman, just as blood and any other physiological fluid differ from person to person. Milk changes from one feeding to the next, from day to day, with changes in the mother's diet, to name just a few factors. Breastmilk is also different if the baby is born prematurely than if the baby is born at term; the milk is adapted to his particular needs (see the chapter "The Preterm and Near-term Baby").

Breastmilk will vary with the mother's diet. For example, if you are a vegetarian, you'll have different fatty acids (the components that make up fat) in your milk than if you eat a lot of fish or meat.

Breastmilk varies throughout the day, and it's unpredictable. One study showed that fat levels were on average higher in the morning and lowest in late afternoon. Another study showed the opposite: that fat concentrations in the milk were higher in the evening and lower in the morning. The differences in the studies' outcomes proves the point: breastmilk cannot be copied.

How can anyone make a reliable copy of breastmilk, given all these variations? Everyone knows that colostrum is different from the milk the mother produces one week after birth. But it is also different at three weeks than at three months, and different at three months than at three years.

Milk changes throughout the feeding. As the baby takes more milk, the amount of fat gradually increases. Other components change too. The less time between feedings on the same breast, the higher the concentration of fat in the milk. Sometimes it helps colicky babies if they feed on just one breast at a feeding or twice on the same side. But we shouldn't make a rule about feeding from only one side because milk supply may decrease to the point that this doesn't work anymore. Accurately measuring what is in breastmilk can be very difficult, because it changes so much and is so different from woman to woman. One study in Guatemala showed that to have a satisfactory estimate of how much iron was in the milk, they had to test it each day for 11 days, otherwise the result was not reliable. Many older studies were based on pooled mothers' milk, which does not reflect what each individual mother actually produces.

Let us return to the question of breastmilk changing with time. Here is a typical question from a lactation consultant: A woman who is going to be adopting a newborn baby also has her own 11-month-old child. She would like to breastfeed the newborn, but the lactation consultant is concerned that her milk might not be appropriate for the newborn. Now wait. The consultant is wondering whether the difference between the milk of a mother feeding an 11-month-old and that of a mother feeding a one-day-old is so great that formula would be more appropriate. Does this person also ask how old the calf is whose mother provided the milk for the formula? The underlying assumption here is that formula is just like breastmilk. Well, the breastmilk of a mother of an 11-month-old is still much, much closer to what the newborn baby needs than formula.

There is more, of course. The amino acids that make up proteins are different in breastmilk than in formula. Some amino acids found in breastmilk protein are not present in formula; others are present in much smaller or larger amounts. For example, phenylalanine is present in much lower concentrations in breastmilk than it is in most formulas. This means that babies born with phenylketonuria can usually breastfeed, at least partially (see the chapter "Sick Babies, Special Babies").

Furthermore, the amount of protein a baby gets from breastmilk is much less than the amount he gets from formula. *More is not necessarily better.* Although not all the protein from formula is absorbed, a lot less protein from breastmilk is absorbed. Breastmilk contains about 1 g of protein per 100 ml. If a baby drinks a litre of breastmilk in a day (a goodly amount), he will ingest about 10 g of protein. But 60% or more of the protein measured is lactoferrin, which is not absorbed by the baby. Another 5% or so is made up of antibodies (sIgA), which is also not absorbed by the baby. So the baby absorbs only about 3.5 g of protein per day, and grows very well. Because neither lactoferrin nor antibodies are present in formula, the artificially fed baby is getting too much protein, which is not necessarily a good thing. High intake of protein in infancy is associated with obesity and type 2 diabetes later in life.

Here's another example of the difference between breastfeeding and formula feeding. Peter Hartmann and his students in Perth, Australia, have shown that the amount of breastmilk an exclusively breastfed, well-gaining baby takes does not increase much, if at all, from one month to six months, even though the six-month-old usually weighs more than twice as much as the one-month-old. The amount of milk a formula-fed baby gets will steadily increase. How can this be? Is the metabolism of the baby different when he is breastfeeding than when he is getting formula? Possibly. Is the fat content of the milk actually higher than we generally believe? Also possible. A study from Israel published in *Pediatrics* in August 2005 showed that mothers breastfeeding a baby over a year had 10 or more grams of fat per 100 ml of breastmilk, far higher than the usually quoted 4 g per 100 ml in formula. Furthermore, at six months the fat content was also considerably higher than 4 g per 100 ml. The study compared the milk of mothers breastfeeding from one to three years with mothers breastfeeding only two to six months, and even the milk of the mothers breastfeeding the younger babies was higher in fat than the previous estimate (7 g per 100 ml of milk on average, but as much as 12 g per 100 ml) and almost double the amount in formula.

What else is missing in formula?

- Immune factors. Aside from nucleotides, that were minor factors added only in the late 1990s mainly as a marketing strategy, there is nothing in formula to protect the baby against infection. And you can't just throw in some antibodies and say, "Okay, now formula has immune factors also." Antibodies are not the only immune factors in breastmilk; there are dozens. The antibodies in breastmilk interact with other immune factors in the milk to protect the baby. Without the other immune factors, the antibodies will not work as they should. Plus, the antibodies the baby gets through breastfeeding are geared to his environment—the environment he shares with his mother.
- Breastmilk probably contains stem cells, which can change into any other type of cell in the body. We don't yet understand their function in breastmilk, but it is probably important. Indeed, if we can harvest stem cells from breastmilk, then the whole debate about using fetal tissue for stem cells will disappear.
- Prostaglandins are present in breastmilk and have useful functions.
- Growth factors are present in breastmilk. They stimulate the growth and maturation of the baby's brain, gut and immune system.

There are dozens of other factors in breastmilk that are absent from formula. Space does not allow us to go into these.

Do all these differences between formula and breastmilk matter?

See the chapter "Why Breastfeeding Is Important": the research shows that the very different composition of formula means babies fed formula have a higher risk of many illnesses, developmental problems, etc. It is absurd to expect studies to be perfect and "prove" breastfeeding is better. That's backward thinking. It's never been shown that artificial feeding is at least as good as breastfeeding, which, given the differences between breastmilk and formula, is what needs to be shown. And, as I've mentioned before, breastfeeding is much more than breastmilk. Often mothers are told that if they don't produce enough milk, they should just formula feed, as if some breastmilk is worse than none. Breastfeeding is valuable even if supplements are needed. This is why, if the mother must supplement the baby, it should be done at the breast with a lactation aid, not by bottle, spoon, finger feeding or syringe feeding.

Principles of drug use for breastfeeding mothers

1. Do not use drugs if they are not necessary. Patients often push doctors to prescribe something for any problem; they like to leave the office with a prescription in their hand. Doctors often prescribe medication when it's not necessary in order to placate a patient, avoid giving long explanations why medication is not necessary, out of ignorance or because marketing has convinced him/ her that something is a wonder drug. Too often, medications are prescribed when other treatments, such as changes in lifestyle, may be effective without the possible side effects of drugs. Antibiotics are often prescribed for colds or fevers caused by viruses, when they have no effect. Often, even bacterial infections will get better without antibiotics. Mastitis is an example. If the mother is not prescribed a drug for a problem that can be adequately treated without drug therapy, the question of whether she can continue breastfeeding won't come up.

2. Use drugs that are also prescribed for babies.

3. Use drugs that are less toxic. Most infections can be treated with relatively benign antibiotics such as penicillin or derivatives of penicillin. Why use a relatively toxic drug such as clindamycin when cloxacillin would be just as good?

4. Use established drugs that have been tested on breastfeeding mothers. Even a new drug from a family of medications that has been proven safe to take while breastfeeding may cause an unusual reaction in the baby. Physicians order new drugs because they are influenced by marketing (although they believe they remain unbiased towards it). New drugs are not necessarily better than tried-and-true ones.

5. All drugs have a half-life (T½, the time it takes for half the drug to be eliminated from the body), and in this case, the shorter the better. A short half-life means that the drug stays in the milk for less time and is eliminated by the baby's body more quickly.

6. A short course of treatment may be acceptable when a longer course is not. Methotrexate, for example, is used to treat certain cancers as well as some chronic inflammatory diseases such as psoriasis, rheumatoid arthritis and Crohn's disease. When used for these diseases, the drug is prescribed for months or years. Methotrexate is also used to treat an ectopic (tubal) pregnancy without surgery with just a single dose. This changes everything. Methotrexate comes out in the milk in only very small amounts, but it goes to the baby's ovaries or testes and stays there. It would be a concern for even small amounts of methotrexate to accumulate in the baby's reproductive organs for months and years. On the other hand, if the mother receives a single dose, I would consider that breastfeeding should continue without interruption.

7. Finding an alternative to a problematic drug is often possible. Again, methotrexate used chronically is a problem. But azathioprine, a drug very similar to methotrexate, is used to treat inflammatory diseases but does not accumulate in the testes or ovaries. A physician who is supportive of breastfeeding will look for alternatives to a problematic drug rather than simply tell the mother she has to interrupt breastfeeding.

8. Is the drug considered safe during pregnancy? If so, it should *usually* be safe for the baby while breastfeeding. But not always, because during pregnancy the mother breaks down the drug for the baby. Some drugs have much longer half-lives in newborn babies than in their mothers; however, the reverse is also true. Given the small amounts of most drugs in the milk, a drug which is considered safe during pregnancy is usually safe during breastfeeding. A woman taking a drug is exposing her baby's developing nervous system much more during pregnancy than during breastfeeding. During pregnancy the baby's blood levels are comparable to the mother's (very few drugs do not pass through the placenta).

So, can I continue breastfeeding when taking medication? Get to the point, please.

Here's the point. Given the risks of *not* breastfeeding, the real question is this: which is safer for the baby, breastfeeding with a tiny amount of drug (and it is almost always tiny) or formula? The answer is: *only rarely* is formula the safer alternative.

As well, interrupting breastfeeding for 7 or 10 days may mean that the baby will never again take the breast. We have seen case after case of mothers whose babies were breastfeeding well, and interrupted breastfeeding because they were told that it was dangerous with this or that medication. When the mother stopped the drug and tried to resume breastfeeding, the baby refused to latch on again, having got used to the bottle. Not to mention the hassles for the mother in pumping around the clock to keep her milk production up (and probably being told to throw the milk away).

Why does so little drug get into the milk?

Any drug a person takes is diluted throughout the whole body, though not uniformly. Some drugs do not get into the brain easily. Some drugs are stored in the fat. However, the only way drugs can get into the breastmilk is for them to be in the bloodstream, and the concentration of the drug is usually *extremely* low. As an example, paroxetine (Paxil), used to treat depression, goes mostly to the brain, so that only about 1% of all the drug taken is actually in the bloodstream. Amounts in the blood are usually measured in micrograms (millionths of a gram) per millilitre of blood or even nanograms (billionths of a gram) per millilitre of blood. These are very small amounts, and that means that only very tiny amounts can get into the milk.

Alcohol is one of the most commonly used drugs in the world. Many people tell mothers they have to interrupt breastfeeding if they drink alcohol: two hours for every ounce of alcohol taken is a typical recommendation. Let's look at this a little more closely. Whisky is 40% alcohol, beer 3% to 10%, wine 10% to 13%. Even de-alcoholized beer contains approximately 0.6% alcohol. Depending on the jurisdiction, you are considered too drunk to drive with more than 0.05% to 0.1% alcohol in your blood. Alcohol behaves differently from other drugs. The concentration of alcohol in blood and breastmilk is about the same. So, if the mother has 0.06% alcohol in her blood, she will have 0.06% alcohol in her milk—one-tenth

that of de-alcoholized beer! This is not a concentration of alcohol that is going to make the baby sick or cause brain damage (as some have suggested). This over-cautiousness with regard to alcohol reflects the emergence of neo-puritanical attitudes. Of course, if the mother is drunk much of the time and unable to take proper care of her baby, this is another story, but the milk alcohol level is not the concern.

Some drugs are used topically, on the skin, in the vagina, on the lining of the tubes of the lungs (as with inhalers for asthma) or in the nose or eyes. Because absorption into the bloodstream from these sites is usually much reduced and the total doses much smaller than if the drugs are taken by mouth or injection, it is even rarer to have to interrupt breastfeeding.

What, in addition to the concentration in the mother's blood, determines how much drug gets into the milk?

The proportion of drug that is bound to proteins in the blood is very important, since only the drug unattached to protein is available to enter into the milk. Some drugs are almost completely attached to protein. Ibuprofen (a nonsteroidal anti-inflammatory drug) is over 99% bound to protein. Thus, less than 1% of the tiny amount in the mother's blood is excreted into the milk. Though mothers may take close to 400 mg every six hours, the milk will contain less than 1 mg per litre. If we treated a baby with ibuprofen (for pain, for example), we would generally give 10 mg per kilogram of his weight, so that a 5 kg (11 lb) baby would get 50 mg as a *single* dose. The baby taking a litre of breastmilk would get only a milligram or two.

Paroxetine is 95% protein bound, which means that of the already small amount in the blood (most paroxetine is in the brain and other parts of the body), 95% will not be available for transfer into the milk.

Another important factor is the size of a molecule of the drug. Not all drug molecules are small enough to enter the milk. Drugs too large to get into the milk include heparin (for preventing or treating blood clots), insulin (for treating diabetes), interferon (for treating multiple sclerosis, hepatitis C and other chronic diseases), glatiramer (Copaxone, also for treating multiple sclerosis), the monoclonal antibodies (Enbrel, Remicade and others, used to treat rheumatoid arthritis, Crohn's disease, ulcerative colitis, multiple sclerosis and other inflammatory diseases) and pituitary hormones (used to treat infertility). Most of these drugs are also digested by stomach acid, so that even if they did get into the milk they would be destroyed before being absorbed into the baby's blood.

Many mothers have been told they must stop breastfeeding for drugs such as gentamicin (a relatively toxic antibiotic). But gentamicin is given by injection because it does not get absorbed into the body if taken by mouth. If the mother is breastfeeding, the tiny amount of gentamicin the baby gets won't be absorbed. It will just come out in the baby's bowel movements. Gentamicin is frequently given to tiny premature babies in neonatal intensive care units without much worry. It is possible that the gentamicin will kill some bacteria in the baby's gut, changing the proportions of the bacteria that live there. It's not likely, because the amounts are so small. But even if that were true, formula also changes the proportion and types of bacteria in a significant and profound way. In fact, breastmilk encourages the growth of probiotics in the baby's gut.

People also worry that the baby might become allergic to the antibiotic. This is possible for any antibiotic, but it rarely occurs in infants. However, the baby might become allergic to cow's milk or soy milk protein if he is taken off the breast and given formula. Allergy to cow's milk or soy protein is a lot more inconvenient and life-restricting than allergy to gentamicin. Why risk these allergies to avoid a possible but unlikely allergy to a medication?

The following are just a few of the commonly used drugs that are not well absorbed from the gut and thus cannot get into the baby's body and or cause any problems. They just end up in the baby's diaper.

These are the drugs I am asked about most often.

Vancomycin. This drug is being used more and more because it is usually effective against methicillin-resistant *Staphylococcus aureus* (MRSA) and is used in the treatment of pseudomembranous enterocolitis caused by *Clostrium difficile*, both of which have caused severe illnesses in recent years. When treating *Clostrium difficile*, the drug is given by mouth and cannot enter the milk because it does not get into the mother's bloodstream. Vancomycin is minimally excreted into the milk, but it is not absorbed from the gut. Several other antibiotics, including tobramycin and amikacin, are also very poorly absorbed from the gut.

Lidocain. This is used both for local anaesthesia as well as for cardiac arrhythmias. It is given intravenously. Although a very small amount gets into the milk, the oral absorption is very poor.

Zafirlukast. This is used for the prevention of asthmatic attacks. It is poorly absorbed from the gut and even less well absorbed when taken with food.

Follicle-stimulating hormone and luteinizing hormone. I am asked frequently about the suitability of continuing breastfeeding while receiving these and other pituitary hormones given to stimulate fertility. Even if they entered the milk, which is extremely doubtful, they would not be absorbed from the gut. However, they may decrease the milk supply. On the other hand, if the mother gets pregnant, her milk supply will diminish anyway.

Some drugs that are poorly absorbed from the gut are given in larger doses so that enough gets into the body. That's not a concern, though, because only a small amount will get into the mother's bloodstream and a smaller amount into the milk, and an even smaller amount will be absorbed by the baby. An interesting example is omeprazole, a proton pump inhibitor, and other drugs of the same family, which are used to decrease acid secretion in the stomach. The pills are coated to protect them from stomach acid, but this coating has disappeared by the time the drug reaches the mother's milk, so any amount that enters the baby's stomach would be destroyed.

Some "problem" drugs (anti-infection drugs such as antibiotics)

Almost all antibiotics are compatible with continued breastfeeding. Although side effects may happen even with small amounts, they should be weighed against the very significant side effects of formula.

Tetracycline. Tetracycline is sometimes used to treat acne, Rocky Mountain spotted fever, Q fever, chlamydia infections and psittacosis. There is no question that tetracycline is contraindicated during pregnancy or for children under the age of 8 (some say 12) because it will attach itself to calcium and cause weakening and browning of the teeth and bones. Because of this, many health workers believe that it is a problem for mothers to breastfeed while taking tetracycline. But it is not.

Tetracycline in breastmilk binds to the calcium and is not absorbed; it comes out in the baby's bowel movements. Newer forms of tetracycline, such as doxycycline, are less well-bound to calcium, but then are less likely to cause problems with the bones and

teeth, given how little gets into the milk. Doxycycline is considered the drug of choice for Lyme disease.

Metronidazole is used frequently to treat infections, especially in the gut (*Clostridium difficile* for example), pelvic and vaginal infections (*Trichomonas*) in women, and *Giardia lamblia* in children and adults. *Giardia lamblia* frequently causes epidemics of diarrhea in daycare centres.

Metronidazole caused mutations in bacteria and cancer in rodents, so many recommended not using it if breastfeeding. However, the rodents received metronidazole for their entire lives, and the drug has never been shown to cause cancer in humans. But some doctors still recommend interrupting breastfeeding for 24 hours after a 2 g dose of metronidazole. If we are so worried about cancer, which has never been shown to be a risk in humans who took metronidazole, why do we give the drug to the mother? If the mother can handle it, the baby should continue breastfeeding without interruption.

Ciprofloxacin and other fluoroquinolones (norfloxacin, ofloxacin and others). This family of drugs is used to treat a wide variety of infections. Based on studies showing damage to the cartilage of the joints in baby beagles that were given ciprofloxacin, it was recommended that ciprofloxacin not be used in breastfeeding mothers. However, the beagles did not get ciprofloxacin through the mother's milk but rather were given it directly. There is no evidence in human children that ciprofloxacin causes damage to the joints and in fact there is evidence that it doesn't cause joint damage, even in children with cystic fibrosis who have received it many times over many years, often with the first treatments in the first months of life. If the mother must take one of this family of medications, she should continue breastfeeding.

Nitrofurantoin and sulfa drugs. These drugs are used frequently to treat urinary tract infections. In theory they can displace bilirubin from protein in the blood and increase the risk of toxicity from bilirubin, but in practice this seems unlikely. There are other drugs available for treatment of urinary tract infections that do not present this problem.

Other "problem" drugs

Antidepressants. These drugs are among the most commonly prescribed to women of childbearing age. Some suggest that if the mother needs to be treated she should not be breastfeeding, since we don't know what effect there will be on the baby's developing brain. Even though the baby receives only tiny amounts through the milk this is true. However, we do have good evidence that not breastfeeding negatively affects the baby's developing brain. Study after study shows the baby who is breastfed has better brain development compared to the baby fed artificially, and the more exclusively and longer the baby is breastfed, the greater the difference. Here is the conclusion of an article reporting a study that looked at almost 14,000 children, followed from birth until six-and-a-half years old, published in 2008: "These results, based on the largest randomized trial ever conducted in the area of human lactation, provide strong evidence that prolonged and exclusive breastfeeding improves children's cognitive development."

Studies continue to be published on babies' cognitive development and future mental health. One study published in *Biological Psychological* in 2004 compared the brains of one-month-old babies (using EEGs). They found that the babies (whether breastfed or bottle fed) of mothers who were not depressed were developing normally. The brains of bottle-fed babies whose mothers were depressed showed some abnormal development. However, the brains of breastfed babies whose mothers were depressed developed normally.

Too many physicians don't appreciate the value of breastfeeding to the health of the mother, baby or toddler. Some psychiatrists or family doctors go beyond advising women to stop breastfeeding. They tell them that they will not treat their depression unless they wean. Considering the lack of evidence of harm from these medications, and the evidence that harm can occur if the child is not breastfed, I think this is a despicable approach to patient care, particularly because any new mother—but especially the depressed mother—is very vulnerable. As with most drugs, very little of the antidepressants gets into the milk. I have mentioned paroxetine (Paxil); sertraline (Zoloft) does not get into the milk in significant amounts either. These are older drugs, the ones about which we have the most information, but many doctors are convinced by drug reps to prescribe newer medications with less research.

There are a couple of drugs that do concern me, however. One is fluoxetine (Prozac) and the other is bupropion (Wellbutrin).

- **Fluoxetine**. Many mothers have breastfed their babies without problem while taking fluoxetine; however, it has a long half-life, much longer than that of most other antidepressants, and when it breaks down, one of the breakdown products stays in the body and also has a very long half-life. So I would not consider it the drug of choice for the breastfeeding mother, or rather for her baby. There are many others to choose from.
- **Bupropion**. Bupropion is used to help stop smoking and is also an antidepressant. A few women have contacted me because they believed bupropion caused their milk production to decrease. No research has been done to support this, but with so many other antidepressants to choose from, why take the chance?

Lithium. Lithium is used for the high or manic phase of bipolar disorder, previously called manic depression. It is not effective against depression. This drug has always been considered contraindicated during breastfeeding. However, a change of attitude is slowly taking place.

It has been found that lithium comes out in the milk in variable amounts. If a mother excretes only small amounts, it may be safe for her baby if she takes the drug and breastfeeds. The baby should be watched for untoward side effects and the amount of lithium in his blood should be measured from time to time, but the mother can and should breastfeed or continue breastfeeding.

If, however, the amount of lithium in the baby's blood causes concern, there are alternatives. They don't always work as well, but they often work well enough. Both valproic acid and carbamazepine are compatible with breastfeeding, even in the large doses often used in bipolar disorder.

Drugs for psychosis. The first drugs used to treat psychosis were phenothiazines. There was always a concern with these drugs because they are quite sedating and the commonly used chlorpromazine has a relatively long half-life (about one day). Although little gets into the milk, sedating drugs are a worry, because they may increase the risk of sudden infant death in susceptible babies. This family of drugs also increases prolactin secretion and can increase milk supply. I used it frequently in Africa to help mothers stop formula or to relactate. As this was done in hospital, we had an opportunity to observe the babies and did not see problems with sedation.

More recently, we have quetiapine (Seroquel) and olazepine (Zyprexa, Symbyax) for breastfeeding mothers, drugs that are much less worrisome than the phenothiazines. Very little gets into the milk and babies seemed to suffer no negative side effects in the studies that have been done. Risperidone (Risperdal, Invega) and trazodone (Dysyrel, Trazorel) also seem safe to use for breastfeeding mothers. However, other drugs in the same family, such as nefazodone (Serzone, Dutonin), are more of a concern and should be avoided. Just because several drugs in the same family are considered compatible with breastfeeding does not mean that *all* drugs in the same family are compatible.

Corticosteroids (prednisone, prednisolone, hydrocortisone and others). Corticosteroids (not to be confused with the drugs used by some athletes to enhance performance) are drugs used for their anti-inflammatory effects. Often the most distressing symptoms of many ailments or diseases are those caused by inflammation. Corticosteroids are prescribed frequently (as pills, injections, inhalers, enemas or creams), so I get many questions from breastfeeding mothers about these medications. Corticosteroids are normally found in the mother's milk and, in most studies, mothers taking corticosteroids will not have a measurable increase in the amount of corticosteroids in the milk.

Though corticosteroids can be very helpful, bringing relief to patients suffering from various diseases such as asthma, multiple sclerosis, ulcerative colitis and many others, they can also have significant side effects, including weight gain, high blood sugar, loss of calcium from the bones and activation of dormant illnesses such as tuberculosis, especially when given orally for long periods of time. For this reason, mothers are often told, incorrectly, that they must interrupt breastfeeding while taking these drugs.

If a mother gets a corticosteroid injected into her knee, for example, there is absolutely no reason to interrupt breastfeeding for even a second. The drug stays in the joint and does not get into the mother's bloodstream and therefore cannot get into the milk.

If a mother must take an inhaled steroid to treat her asthma, she should not worry about the steroid getting into the milk. With inhalers, the drug is delivered where it is needed (the lining of the airways in the lungs), so smaller doses can be used than if the steroid were given by mouth. Furthermore, the amount of the drug that actually gets absorbed into the mother's bloodstream is less than half the total amount of the drug she inhales. And of that, the amount that gets into the milk is hardly measurable.

The same can be said of creams and ointments used to treat skin problems. Treating "locally" decreases the amount of corticosteroid needed to treat a problem. Also, it is not that easy for drugs to get through intact skin, unless there is a lot of inflammation.

However, even oral corticosteroids or corticosteroids given by injection into the vein or muscle— even high doses given to treat a relapse of multiple sclerosis—do not increase the amount of corticosteroid in the milk significantly.

Drugs used to treat inflammatory diseases by interfering with tumour necrosis factor alpha. These include infliximab (Remicade), etanercept (Enbrel) and others. These drugs are being prescribed more and more and are used to treat Crohn's disease, ulcerative colitis, rheumatoid arthritis and many other diseases that are classified as autoimmune or whose main symptoms may be due to inflammation. These drugs stop the inflammatory process by interfering with a factor called tumour necrosis factor alpha. Mothers are almost universally told that they cannot breastfeed while getting these medications. This is simply not true; the mother can and should continue breastfeeding.

Why? These drugs are huge molecules. They are proteins and at the same time antibodies and their molecular weights are measured in the tens of thousands or hundreds of thousands of Daltons. Any drug with a molecular weight of more than 600 to 1000 Daltons cannot get into the milk. And because they are proteins, if by some fluke they did get into the milk, they would be digested in the baby's stomach and intestines. This should be the end of the story, yet here's what the drug company writes in its package insert with regard to infliximab (Remicade): Nursing Women: **It is not known whether infliximab is excreted in human milk or absorbed systematically after ingestion. Because human immunoglobulins are excreted in milk, women must not breastfeed for at least six months after Remicade treatment.** (Bold print in the original.)

Let's look into these statements. "It is not known whether infliximab is excreted in human milk or absorbed systematically after ingestion." Not true: a few studies (small ones) showed no excretion into the mother's milk. There is no reason why the baby would absorb the drug. On top of that, the fact that breastmilk contains antibodies (the human immunoglobulins mentioned above) does not mean that any old antibody is excreted into the milk. The antibodies (sIgA) that are present in breastmilk and protect the baby have a special chain attached to them that allows them to enter the milk-producing cells and then enter the milk. Infliximab and other similar drugs do not have that chain. The antibodies (sIgA) present in breastmilk also have another chain that protects them from being digested in the baby's stomach.

". . .women must not breastfeed for at least six months after Remicade treatment." For six months? The information in the insert says that women treated with Remicade have undetectable levels of the drug in their blood by *eight weeks* after the last treatment. Why would they have to stop breast-feeding for six months after the last treatment? Out of interest, do the math. How would a mother be in a position to breastfeed within six months of receiving Remicade if it's contraindicated during pregnancy?

Unfortunately, too often doctors don't look for other resources beyond these inserts, which are clearly meant primarily to limit the company's liability.

Drugs used to treat high blood pressure (anti-hypertensives). Again, as with most medications, the amount that gets into the milk with these drugs is very small. There are numerous drugs used to treat high blood pressure, and most are compatible with breastfeeding.

The separation of drugs into families is useful, not only for drugs for high blood pressure, but also for many other drugs, such as antibiotics. Drugs in the same family often have the same effects and side effects as other members of the same family (though this is not universally true). In the case of anti-hypertensive medication, if a member from one family is not effective, the doctor could try a drug from a different family. Or if the drug doesn't bring down the blood pressure enough, the physician might add a member of another drug family to help control the blood pressure better.

Beta-blockers. Propranolol is the original beta-blocker and it is still quite effective for the treatment of high blood pressure. It is also used for the prevention of migraine headaches and for symptoms of an overactive thyroid gland (hyperthyroidism). Being older, it is not as often used as some of the new beta-blockers, which is unfortunate because from the breastfeeding point of view it is one of the best; the amount that gets into the milk is extremely small and extremely unlikely to have any effect on the baby. Other beta-blockers that can be used with

confidence during breastfeeding include labetalol (which seems to be the obstetrician's drug of choice in the Toronto area) and metoprolol.

Atenolol, on the other hand, does get into the milk in larger quantities and there is at least one case report of a baby getting into trouble while the mother was taking it. Many mothers have taken atenolol and breastfed without problems, but this case does point out that, in rare cases, drugs may affect the baby, even if very little gets into the milk. Since we have so many alternatives, even in the same family as atenolol, it makes sense to use a different drug.

Calcium channel blockers. In general, members of this family are strongly bound to plasma proteins (this is good, since only the unbound drug can get into the milk) and have low oral bioavailability (which is also good because that means little of what gets into the milk is absorbed by the baby). Levels in the mother's blood are usually very low. Nifedipine, one of the more commonly used calcium channel blockers, fits this pattern and is compatible with continued breastfeeding. We use it to treat vasospasm of the nipples (see the chapter "Sore Nipples"). Verapamil is another drug that gets into the milk in only tiny amounts. Verapamil is sometimes used for babies with heart problems.

Angiotensin-converting enzyme (ACE) inhibitors. Again, in general, this family of drugs is characterized by strong binding to plasma proteins and low bioavailability. Benazepril is a commonly used ACE inhibitor. It is estimated that the baby would get less than 0.1% of the total maternal dose, which means virtually nothing. Captopril has long been used for children, even infants, with cardiac problems. Because of the drug's low excretion into the milk, the baby would get only an estimated 0.002% of the mother's dose, an amount that is essentially zero.

Magnesium sulphate. This drug, used for treating high blood pressure around the time of delivery, has sometimes been said to be incompatible with breastfeeding. But magnesium is normally found in the blood, the amount that gets into the milk is very small and absorption from the baby's gut is very low. There should be no concern at all about magnesium sulphate during breastfeeding.

Diuretics. Diuretics are drugs that decrease blood pressure by increasing the amount of fluid that is lost in the urine. They are also used to treat heart failure and other causes of fluid retention. Some have suggested these drugs may decrease the milk supply because mothers need plenty of fluid in order to make milk, but we don't know this for sure. Mothers don't need to drink lots of fluids, just enough not to feel thirsty. Given that there are so many alternatives to diuretics, it would probably be better to avoid them.

Other medications used for hypertension. Some drugs are in a category of their own. Hydralazine is one such drug. It has been used for treating high blood pressure for many years, even in infants. The baby gets very little in the milk. Methyldopa enters the milk only in tiny amounts and may have the beneficial side effect of increasing the mother's milk supply.

Codeine. In 2005, there was a case in Canada of a baby who died at 13 days old. An investigation showed that the baby died from morphine intoxication. The mother had been taking codeine with acetaminophen for episiotomy pain and continued to take the drug until the baby's death. Codeine is metabolized to morphine in the mother's milk but normally only very small amounts of morphine are passed into the milk. However, this mother had a rare genetic variation that caused her to metabolize unusually high levels of morphine in her milk.

Because this event got so much press at the time, many mothers became concerned about taking codeine post-partum or thought they would need to wean in order to take pain medications.

I don't think we should say that codeine should never be prescribed. However, if a physician wishes to treat a mother's pain with codeine, it should be taken for only a short period of time in the days after birth. Because of the small (but normal) amount of milk a baby gets in the first few days, the amount of morphine (metabolized from codeine) he'll get will be small. Once the milk comes in after three or four days, it is usually possible to change the mother's medication to a nonsteroidal anti-inflammatory. If the mother needs codeine for longer than five or six days, she needs to be checked for possible infection or some other cause of continued pain. I do think that it was unusual that the mother of the baby who died needed the codeine for so long. It has been suggested that if a baby gets excessively sleepy on standard maternal doses of codeine, the codeine is metabolizing to morphine very quickly. Also, several studies comparing the pain relief of codeine to nonsteroidal anti-inflammatory drugs showed no difference between the two.

Medical investigations that do not involve radioactive compounds (X-rays, CT scans, MRI scans)

These scans do involve radiation, but not radioactive compounds that stay in the body. I frequently get emails about this. The American College of Radiologists published a bulletin in 2001 stating that interrupting breastfeeding after CT scans, MRIs and other radiological investigations using iodine-containing contrast media was *not necessary*; however, too often mothers are *still* being told that they must interrupt breastfeeding for 24 to 48 hours after such investigations. Here is what the bulletin recommends with regard to MRI scans:

"Review of the literature shows *no* evidence to suggest that oral ingestion by an infant of the tiny amount of gadolinium contrast agent excreted into breast milk would cause toxic effects. We believe, therefore, that the available data suggest that it is safe for the mother and infant to continue breastfeeding after receiving such an agent." (My emphasis) Then, inexplicably:

"If the mother remains concerned about any potential ill effects, she should be given the opportunity to make an informed decision as to whether to continue breastfeeding or temporarily abstain from breastfeeding after receiving a gadolinium contrast agent. If the mother so desires, she may abstain from breastfeeding for 24 hours with active expression and discarding of breast milk from both breasts during that period."

The phrase "abstain from breastfeeding" makes it sound as though the mother is the only one involved (apparently the baby is expected not to even notice, and there is no mention of what he will eat while the mother is "abstaining").

Since it is clear that iodine-containing contrast media pose no risk, the mother doesn't need to be concerned about interrupting breastfeeding. And there are definite risks to temporarily stopping breastfeeding; first, the baby may need to be given formula, and second, the baby may not come back to the breast.

It boggles the mind that mothers are sometimes told they must interrupt breastfeeding even after a simple chest X-ray. X-rays pass right through the body. They don't stay in the chest or in the breast. Nothing to worry about in terms of breastfeeding.

As for tests with iodine-containing contrast, the reason they are not a problem is that the iodine is attached to a carrier, rendering the whole compound too big to get into the milk. Iodine *without the carrier* is concentrated in the milk, but it is rare for women to need iodine-containing medicines.

Every radiologist I have spoken to has acknowledged that it is not necessary to interrupt breastfeeding after investigations using iodine-containing contrast. Nevertheless, the prohibition on breastfeeding for 24 to 48 hours continues because the manufacturer of the contrast media says so.

As for MRIs, the contrast medium is gadopentetate (gadolinium). Gadopentetate has a half-life of less than an hour. Thus 97% to 98% of it will be eliminated from the mother's body in less than five hours. So why are mothers told to stop breastfeeding for 24 to 48 hours after an MRI, even in the ARC bulletin? If it were necessary (it's not), six hours would certainly be enough. The total amount of gadopentetate that gets into the milk has been calculated at 0.04% of the maternal dose. Of that tiny amount, only 0.8% gets absorbed by the baby. Let us not forget that we do MRI scans in small babies (even premature babies) using contrast media.

What about investigations using radioactive compounds?

Investigations using radioactive compounds present a different dilemma. Although we do not want to expose young babies or toddlers (or anyone for that matter) to radioactivity, radioactive investigations are indeed done on children when needed (and sometimes when not needed). The most commonly used radioactive material in scans is technetium. It has a half-life of about six hours, which means that 97% to 98% of it will be eliminated from the body in about 30 hours. So should the mother stop breastfeeding for 30 hours? Some are told to stop for 48 to 72 hours, which is likely to lead to breastfeeding problems. However, I believe that even 30 hours is excessive. If the mother waited 12 hours (two half-lives) after the investigation, 75% of the technetium would have been eliminated from her body and thus, much less would get into the milk.

Is this acceptable? It's a complicated question, but I would say yes. Feeding the baby expressed milk by cup, finger feeding or even a bottle for 12 hours is much less of an issue than feeding him this way for 24 to 30 hours.

I also urge physicians to consider whether the investigation might be done with an MRI or CT scan rather than a radioactive scan. For example, if a mother is thought to have had a blood clot in the lung, a radioactive scan is usually done to see if the clot will cause chest pain and difficulty breathing. But a CT scan is more accurate, and as a bonus, takes very little time to do compared to the radioactive scan. So why do the radioactive scan and interrupt breastfeeding for X hours?

Radioactive iodine

Of all the radioactive scans, I am asked most frequently about a scan to distinguish between two different problems affecting the thyroid gland: postpartum thyroiditis and Graves' disease. The thyroid gland is scanned with radioactive iodine. There is no question that we don't want a baby to get radioactive iodine since it is *not attached to a carrier* and is actually concentrated in the mother's milk. Is there a way to avoid interrupting breastfeeding?

It is said that 2% to 15% of new mothers develop postpartum thyroiditis. This usually causes an overactive thyroid; then the thyroid returns to normal or becomes underactive. The overactive phase tends to show up around three to six months after birth. The symptoms are irritability, insomnia, tremor, weight loss despite adequate intake of calories, fatigue, heart palpitations, muscle weakness and more, though not everyone with hyperthyroidism has all these symptoms. The symptoms tend to diminish and disappear after a couple of months, possibly followed by the symptoms associated with an underactive thyroid: fatigue, constipation, more

than usual sensitivity to cold and depression (worth knowing, given the frequent diagnosis of depression in women who have recently given birth).

When hyperthyroidism is due to Graves' disease it is not a temporary problem and can be quite serious.

Physicians like the mother to have a scan of the thyroid with radioactive iodine in order to distinguish between Graves' disease and postpartum thyroiditis, but the usual test, done with the isotope I^{131}, requires the mother to interrupt breastfeeding for several weeks, since the half-life of the isotope in the body is eight days. This means it would take at least a month for 97% to 98% of the isotope to be removed from the body, essentially ending breastfeeding, since very few babies would return to the breast after a month. However, the scan can also be done with isotope I^{123}, which has a much shorter half-life. The mother would have to interrupt breastfeeding for only 12 to 24 hours, depending on the dose.

But does the scan have to be done in the first place? Are there options to distinguish between postpartum thyroiditis and Graves' disease? One way to determine the cause is to wait and see what happens. Within about four to eight weeks, the overactive phase of postpartum thyroiditis gets better even without treatment, whereas Graves' disease is very *unlikely* to get better spontaneously. So if it is postpartum thyroiditis, blood levels of thyroid hormones will be decreasing by six to eight weeks after diagnosis. The mother can be treated, usually with propranolol, to keep the symptoms under control while her blood levels are monitored. If the blood tests continue to show evidence of hyperthyroidism after six to eight weeks, then Graves' disease becomes much more likely. The mother can then be treated with a drug to suppress the thyroid's activity. Methimazole or propylthiouracyl (PTU), used to treat Graves' disease, are both compatible with continued breastfeeding.

Sometimes mothers are told the best treatment is the destruction of the thyroid with radioactive iodine, I^{131}. There are other options that should be offered. One possibility is to continue the medication. Along with propranolol, either methimazole or PTU can be used indefinitely.

If the mother does not tolerate the medication, then surgery is an option. The mother can breastfeed immediately before going into surgery and as soon as she is awake and up to it afterwards. Anaesthetics and painkillers do not require a mother to interrupt breastfeeding. Perhaps the situation is such that radioactive iodine is indeed the best choice and the baby will have to stop breastfeeding. But options should be explored.

Pollutants and toxins in breastmilk and infant formulas

Every so often the question of pollutants or toxins in breastmilk comes up in the media. These stories frighten many pregnant women out of breastfeeding and many women who are already breastfeeding into stopping. Why all these studies that look at toxins in breastmilk? It's not because breastmilk is so polluted it must be urgently studied; it's simply because breastmilk is easily available to study.

When a mother decides to feed her baby artificial milk instead of breastfeeding, she is not avoiding the problem of her baby getting toxins.

There are toxins in *all our food,* and that includes formula. The press reports on contaminants in breastmilk rarely mention that formulas contain heavy metals in quantities much higher than those in breastmilk. Lead, manganese, cadmium—all metals that can damage the central nervous system—are found in disturbing quantities in formulas. In a study published in *BMC Pediatrics* in 2010, the researchers seemed shocked that the formula companies have not heeded warnings about the high

concentrations of aluminum in formulas. Note the first sentence, which shows that these researchers are not crazed breastfeeding radicals:

"Infant formulas are integral to the nutritional requirements of preterm and term infants. While it has been known for decades that infant formulas are contaminated with significant amounts of aluminum there is little evidence that manufacturers consider this to be a health issue. Aluminum is non-essential and is linked to human disease. There is evidence of both immediate and delayed toxicity in infants, and especially preterm infants, exposed to aluminum and it is our contention that there is still too much aluminum in infant formulas."

Really? Infant formulas are *integral* to the nutritional requirements of preterm and term infants? With regard to term babies and *most* preterm babies, that's simply not true. Aluminum is particularly harmful to premature babies.

Why are we worried about toxins in our food, in particular breastmilk?

1. **Toxins increase the risk of cognitive deficits.** However, studies show that breastfed babies do *better* on cognitive tests than formula-fed babies, and the longer the baby is breastfed, the greater the difference. The long-chained polyunsaturated fatty acids in breastmilk (DHA and ARA) probably have an effect, an effect that has never been shown when these same fatty acids have been added to formula. The heavy metals in formula may also play a part. Another important factor in the higher cognitive functioning of breastfed babies may be the close physical relationship, often skin to skin, between the mother and the baby.

2. **Toxins interfere with immune function.** Yet breastfed babies have fewer infections of all

kinds *and a* more mature immune system than formula-fed babies.

3. **Toxins increase the risk of cancer.** And yet, breastfed babies have a lower risk of several childhood cancers and may even be protected against certain cancers when they are adults. There is some evidence that breastfed girls are less likely to develop breast cancer, for example. Why might this be? Well, first of all, the breastfed baby has a more mature immune system. We all have cancer cells in our body from time to time, but usually our immune system kills them. Furthermore, breastmilk contains alpha-lactalbumin, which is transformed in the baby's gut by a biochemical reaction into HAMLET (Human lactalbumin made lethal to tumour cells). This protein-lipid complex essentially makes tumour cells "commit suicide" (apoptosis).

It's interesting that none of the articles or television programs I've seen about toxins in breastmilk mentions toxins in formula. There *are* toxins in formula. After all, the cows do eat the grass in the countryside where the fields are sprayed with pesticides, and eat grains that are treated with pesticides of all kinds as well.

What is best to do?

A mother who breastfeeds is doing the best for her baby, for herself, for her family (and for the world, for that matter). Breastfeeding is very environmentally friendly. Formula feeding pollutes the environment. The fact that there are pollutants in breastmilk can be likened to the situation of the canary in the coal mine. We should be worried about what we are doing to our planet, *but this should not lead us to encourage mothers to feed their babies artificially.* Killing the canary doesn't decrease the level of poisonous gases in the coal mine.

Child spacing, use of hormones and breastfeeding

The question of child spacing is an important one for all families. Generally, breastfeeding mothers do not want their babies too close together because pregnancy will decrease the milk supply, often quite considerably, and this may mean the older child will be supplemented or weaned. I do, however, sometimes hear from mothers who want to have another baby quickly because of their age or because it took a long time to conceive for the first pregnancy. More about this later.

The Lactation Amenorrhea Method (LAM) of child spacing

Though many physicians are not aware of this, breastfeeding can decrease the chances of pregnancy considerably. Research shows the lactation amenorrhea method is 98%+ effective in preventing pregnancy if the following conditions apply:

- The baby is breastfeeding exclusively. He may receive vitamins, for example, but no other milk. Even expressing milk and giving it by bottle can diminish the effectiveness of this method. So will holding off feedings by using a pacifier or not feeding according to the baby's cues.
- The mother has not had a normal menstrual period. (Bleeding up to eight weeks after birth is not considered a true period.)
- The baby is less than six months old. This age is recommended because most babies start solids around six months and the addition of solids decreases the effectiveness of LAM.
- The baby is not getting pacifiers or bottles—all sucking is done at the breast. If the baby sucks on his fingers, it may be that he wants the breast but feedings are delayed. Breastfeeding is not really on demand.

- Mothers and babies have as much skin-to-skin contact as possible. Swaddling babies, or having them sleep separately from the mother, may also interfere with LAM. It is important for LAM to breastfeed on demand, not to space out feedings and not to train the baby to sleep through the night.

Mothers who don't follow these steps will want to take precautions if they wish to space out pregnancies. However, any hormonal method can decrease the milk supply, and even dry it up.

Here is an an example: The mother had been breastfeeding without any problems, but had a Mirena IUD inserted when her baby was four months. Within five days, her milk supply dropped dramatically. She told me she would be having the IUD removed in two weeks. When I asked her why she was waiting, she said that her doctor was not convinced that the Mirena was affecting her milk supply and insisted on waiting, hoping she would change her mind. Yes, there could be other reasons for milk supply to decrease, but the timing of the sudden decrease after 15 weeks of problem-free breastfeeding is very typical of what we hear from mothers over and over. Too many doctors believe the manufacturer of the Mirena but don't believe the mothers.

At one time, there were concerns about breastfeeding mothers taking birth control pills because the hormones would get into the milk. In fact, breastmilk contains the same hormones (different versions) that are used in birth control pills, and research showed the amounts do not change significantly when the mother takes the pill. So physicians started prescribing the pill to breastfeeding mothers. Unfortunately, we soon began hearing from mothers who had a significant decrease in milk production within 7 to 10 days of starting on the pill.

Waiting until the milk production is well established (say, after six to eight weeks) doesn't make any difference. Even after five months of successful exclusive breastfeeding, mothers have had a significant decrease in milk production after starting the pill, even the progesterone-only pill. The fact that there is no estrogen in the pill does not mean the mother cannot have a decrease in milk production. It may be that the decrease is less common with a progesterone-only pill, but we don't know this for sure.

Why does this happen? The birth control pill simulates pregnancy, and milk supply decreases significantly during pregnancy.

It is true that not all mothers experience this decrease in milk supply. Perhaps the mother with an abundant milk supply has a reduction but it is not obvious if the baby doesn't fuss.

We also see a difference with different babies. Some mothers who started taking the pill six weeks after birth had no problems with babies one and two but had a big drop in milk supply with baby number three. Mothers do not always produce the same amount of milk for every baby and this may be an explanation. On the other hand, the problem may be more evident when the mother has a lot of milk, because the baby, expecting rapid flow, gets fussy when it slows down even a little. Or it may be more evident when the milk production is low already, as perhaps the breast is more sensitive to the hormones in this situation.

So what to do about birth control? Physicians should discuss options with the parents and mention the possibility that the milk supply might decrease with the use of hormonal methods. Not every couple is ready to resume sexual relations in the first few weeks or months after the birth. The fatigue and change of lifestyle associated with having a young baby is not always conducive to a vigorous sexual relationship. Temporary celibacy is not a horror from which all new parents recoil. In addition, intimacy between two people does not require "going all the way," as we used to say. A satisfying, intimate physical relationship can continue without actual ejaculation into the vagina.

When couples do want to have sex, there are many good birth control options that don't put breastfeeding at risk. Barrier methods (condom, diaphragm) are an extra reassurance for those who worry about the reliability of breastfeeding as a good method of child spacing. The IUD without progesterone is a good method as well.

IUDs bring up yet another unexpected barrier to breastfeeding. The IUD containing progesterone is quite expensive, about $500 in our area. The copper-T IUD is much less expensive, about $135. Drug plans will pay for the expensive one because it contains a drug, but not for the less expensive one because it doesn't. So mothers opt for the expensive one if they have a drug plan. Okay, there are other issues with the copper-T such as breakthrough bleeding, but many mothers have used it quite happily and didn't have a decrease in milk supply, and the progesterone in an IUD does not prevent bleeding in all women.

If the pill is the only option acceptable to the couple, the progesterone-only pill *may* be worth trying, although there does seem to be a risk of decreased milk production with this pill as well. I believe it would be best to avoid any hormonal method of birth control until the baby is at least six months so that he can compensate for any decrease in milk production by eating more food. He may still fuss at the breast, though, because the flow will have slowed.

Medroxyprogesterone (Depo-Provera) is an injectable progesterone given as a single dose every three months. There is no need to place an IUD or fit a mother for a diaphragm; from the couple's point of view, the mother doesn't have to remember to take a pill every day or make sure a diaphragm is well placed and add the spermicide properly; there's no worry about a broken condom. But medroxyprogesterone is a hormone and, once given, it cannot be taken away.

Here's the problem: research suggests that it is the drop in progesterone levels when the placenta is delivered that sensitizes the milk-producing cells of the breast to the action of prolactin, the hormone that stimulates the production of milk. If there is no drop in progesterone levels, there is no milk production, which explains why even a small piece of placenta remaining in the uterus may prevent the milk from coming in. So the mother who is given an injection of medroxyprogesterone before her milk even comes in may not be able to produce enough milk—and the effects of the injection last for three months. New mothers should resist the temptation to accept the medroxyprogesterone injection immediately after birth. In fact, even the manufacturer suggests that breastfeeding mothers not be given the injection before six weeks after birth. Even if the mother does not plan to breastfeed, this method is best avoided; mothers often change their minds about breastfeeding. Even at six weeks after birth I would urge mothers not to take the injection. If considering it, better to try the progesterone-only pill for one cycle first. If there is a problem, stop the pill. If milk production is unaffected, the risk from the injection *may be* lower.

You have started on the pill or a progesterone-releasing IUD and your milk supply is down? First, stop taking the pill or have the IUD removed. You don't need to wait until the end of the cycle of pills. At this point I usually prescribe domperidone, a drug that increases milk production (see the chapter "Increasing Breastmilk Intake by the Baby"). I do this because stopping the pill (or removing the IUD) does not always bring back the milk supply rapidly, even if the mother starts expressing her milk.

Please let your doctor know what happened. You want to make sure he or she tells the next mother about this possible side effect. Your doctor is also obliged to report the medication's side effect to Health Canada. The doctor does not need proof that the hormones caused a drop in the milk supply; if there is a possibility that the hormones caused a drop, it should be reported. In fact, you don't have to be a doctor to report a possible drug side effect to Health Canada.

Drugs of recreation and abuse

Alcohol. I have already discussed why a drink or two of alcohol should not be a reason to tell mothers to "pump and dump" their milk. Indeed, as long as the mother is not so impaired she cannot take care of her baby, she should continue breastfeeding. I believe "pump and dump" is a horrible expression because it treats breastmilk as some sort of disgusting fluid.

The formula that the baby would receive while the mother is throwing away her precious milk undoubtedly puts him at greater risk than the tiny amount of alcohol in the milk after one or two drinks.

A woman who is constantly under the influence is a different case, but her baby is probably at greater risk of neglect or accidental injury than of the alcohol that might pass into the milk.

A study several years ago suggested that if a breastfeeding mother has more than two drinks daily, her baby's motor development at one year is not as good as that of babies whose mothers drank less or not at all. One fault of this study is that the researchers depended on the mother's word that she did not drink during the *pregnancy*. The effects of alcohol during pregnancy were already well known at the time of the study. What heavy drinker will tell a researcher that she drank heavily during her pregnancy? Many won't. We already knew that alcohol

during pregnancy can affect the fetus's development and this may have been the real factor here.

It is also said that alcohol may decrease the mother's milk ejection reflex and decrease the milk supply. I have seen no proof of this. A glass of wine with dinner or a couple of beers while you hang out with friends is not going to be a problem for your baby.

Tobacco. There is no doubt that babies exposed to cigarette smoke are at greater risk of respiratory illnesses, sometimes severe, and are more likely to die of sudden infant death syndrome (SIDS, or crib death). However, babies are generally healthier if their mothers smoke and breastfeed than if they smoke and not breastfeed. Given that the baby is already at some risk from exposure to nicotine and carcinogenic compounds in the tobacco smoke, why add the risks of not breastfeeding?

The presence of any smoker, not just the mother, living in the same area as the baby increases his risk of SIDS, even if that person smokes outside. Breastfeeding decreases the risk of SIDS.

If the mother can stop smoking, all the better. If she can't, she should cut down. If the parents cannot stop, they should smoke outdoors, away from the baby. The mother should continue breastfeeding even if she cannot stop or cut down. Breastfeeding is still better for her and for her baby.

Marijuana. I am not advocating the use of marijuana, but some mothers will use it, whatever its legal status or advisability. Is this a reason to deprive a baby of breastfeeding and use formula instead?

If a mother is using marijuana occasionally, and is capable of taking good care of the baby, there is no reason to advise formula. There is no evidence that the small amounts present in the milk will harm the baby.

Chronic heavy marijuana use is a different story. THC, the active ingredient in marijuana, is concentrated in the milk (but still present in tiny amounts) and chronic exposure could result in the drug accumulating in the baby's tissues. The long-term effects of this accumulation are unknown. The mother should breastfeed, and if she lights up, she should make sure it is only occasionally.

Narcotics. Occasional use of narcotics is not a contraindication to breastfeeding. After all, women breastfeed while they are taking narcotics for medical reasons. The problem is that too often recreational use becomes frequent use and then daily use. A baby needs his mother, and regular heavy users are not usually in good enough shape to take care of their babies. A new life depends on the mother. Of course, she can rid herself of the responsibility, have someone else take care of the baby and formula-feed him. But she is giving up something that some women have told me is better than drugs. Yup—breastfeeding.

To reiterate: using meperidine (Demerol) or morphine for pain relief after surgery, for example, is not a reason to interrupt breastfeeding, again because the amount that gets into the milk is tiny and unlikely to affect the baby. This is understood by most, though unfortunately not all health professionals. A mother who occasionally abuses narcotics does not pass on more in her milk than she would if the drug were taken for medical reasons. Of course, one needs to realize that street drugs may contain dangerous contaminants.

What about the mother who was a chronic user during pregnancy? Should she be required to take an oath never to use narcotics before she's allowed to breastfeed? Most women will simply opt not to breast-feed, given that choice, and will believe that formula is better for their babies because of their drug use.

Health professionals should not let this oppor-tunity slip by. Giving birth and breastfeeding can be life-affirming and life-changing events. Here is a

chance to break with the past. Many drug abusers have low self-esteem. If we tell a new mother she can breastfeed only if she stops drugs first, we are telling her that she is no good, that she and her milk are contaminated, and we are setting her up for another failure. A better message is that we trust her with this baby and that we think she can make a go of it.

I realize the above scenario does not always fit. Some drug users are too far gone. They will not be able to take care of their babies. But let's not write off everyone.

When babies are born to mothers who were reg-ular users during the pregnancy, the babies may pass through several days to several weeks of withdrawal symptoms. These withdrawal symptoms are often treated with narcotics, such as morphine, intrave-nously. At the same time, mothers are often told they cannot give their milk to the babies because it might contain narcotics. This is absurd. The tiny amount of extra narcotic present in the milk will do no harm to the baby who is already getting narcotics to treat his withdrawal. However, if we say to the mother that we cannot use her milk, we are sending a very strong message: it's not the drug, it's you. And we are not giving the mother the opportunity to become involved with her baby in a way that is potentially far more fundamental and meaningful than merely touching the baby in the incubator. This is an oppor-tune time to mention that Kangaroo Mother Care could probably do much to help calm the baby and decrease his need for medication.

The mother and baby will have to be monitored carefully by their physicians and if drug abuse con-tinues, breastfeeding and even her ability to take care of her baby will have to be re-evaluated. However, the mother just might make it work!

Methadone. The mother on methadone is usually trying to get off her dependency on street drugs. She should be encouraged to breastfeed. Discouraging breastfeeding only decreases the mother's feelings of self-worth, which may impair her abilities as a mother.

At one point the American Academy of Pediatrics recommended allowing breastfeeding only if the mother was taking 20 mg or less of methadone a day. Where this 20 mg came from is not clear, but the AAP has changed its stance and does not limit quantities of methadone. Women have taken 180 mg a day without significant effects on the baby.

Cocaine. Cocaine taken by the mother will appear in the breastmilk, and since it is a very strong stimulant and completely absorbed from the gut, a mother who uses cocaine should not breastfeed her baby for at least four or five hours after taking the drug. Occasional use coupled with such a wait does not pose a danger to the baby through the milk. But the baby needs a mother who can take care of him without the effects of a drug that can cause paranoid delusions.

If the mother is using cocaine daily, breastfeeding is too dangerous for the baby.

If the baby has received cocaine through the milk, his urine will test positive for breakdown products of cocaine for several days to a week or even longer. The mother should know this if she is being monitored by child protection services.

LSD. We do not know much about LSD and its transfer into milk. Undoubtedly some gets in, and it is a powerful hallucinogen even in tiny amounts. Mothers should not take LSD while breastfeeding. If they do, it is advisable that they wait 12 hours before breastfeeding the baby again.

Mothers receiving vaccines while breastfeeding

It bewilders and concerns me that mothers are often told they can't have an immunization (vaccination) while breastfeeding. This includes vaccinations we give to babies such as diphtheria, polio and tetanus, for example. Why would it be okay for a baby to receive the immunization directly into his thigh by injection, but be a problem for the mother to get the very same immunization? If anything, the baby might even boost his own immunity by being exposed to the antigen in the milk, *if the antigen got into it.*

An antigen is usually a protein or part of a protein that provokes an immune response. The antigen of the tetanus immunization is called tetanus toxoid, a weakened version of the toxin that causes tetanus. It is a very large molecule and unlikely to get into the milk. The same is true of diphtheria toxoid. And even if these antigens could get into milk they would be destroyed in the baby's stomach, which is one reason they are given as injections. This is also true for immunizations given with parts of the bacterial cell wall (a polysaccharide), such as pneumococcus, meningococcus or haemophilus influenza. Again, the molecule is too big to get into the milk and even if it did, there would be no risk of infection since these vaccines use only a small, non-infectious part of the bacterium.

As for an immunization made from an inactivated virus such as hepatitis A, it probably would get into the milk, as many viruses can, but one wonders why there would be a concern. After all, the virus is inactivated! The vaccine for hepatitis B is made up from a protein from the capsule of the virus, much like the vaccines for pneumococcus and haemophilus influenza. Indeed, most jurisdictions strongly recommend the vaccine for hepatitis B at birth for all babies whose mothers carry the virus. In some jurisdictions, *universal* immunization of newborns with hepatitis B is recommended. So how can continued breastfeeding be a problem?

The polio vaccine given in North America by injection is also an inactivated virus, as is the rabies vaccine. There is no risk to the baby from either one.

On the other hand, could live but weakened viruses such as rubella (German measles), influenza (there is also an inactivated virus vaccine available), measles or mumps cause the baby harm? In theory, it is possible. However, it is extremely unlikely if the baby has a normal immune system. The rare cases reported are babies whose immune systems are compromised in some way. A recent reported case of a baby who became sick with yellow fever after the mother received the vaccine (a weakened live virus vaccine) should not make us panic—it is a highly unusual case, and that's why it was reported. If the mother needs the vaccine, then she should get it. Breastfeeding mothers and their babies are usually travelling together or at least they should be, and the breastfed baby has *normal* immunity while the formula-fed baby does not. Taking an artificially fed baby to areas where yellow fever is endemic, usually places where clean water and medical care may not be easily available, is the height of folly. The WHO recommends continued breastfeeding when the mother is immunized against yellow fever.

Babies may actually benefit from vaccinations given to their mothers. In one reported case several years ago, a breastfeeding mother was mistakenly given rubella vaccine immediately after the birth of her baby. The baby did not get sick and was found to have immunity to rubella when he was tested. Influenza immunization is also strongly encouraged in the autumn for *everyone*, with only a few exceptions.

Local and general anaesthesia

Local anaesthesia is medication given to numb the area when surgery or dental procedures are done; for example, lidocaine used to freeze a tooth for a filling. There is no reason mothers would need to interrupt breastfeeding after an injection of lidocaine. Although some of the drug may be absorbed into the mother's blood, this amount, especially if given with epinephrine (adrenalin), would be very small indeed, and the amount that would get into the milk would also be negligible. Given that lidocaine is very poorly absorbed when ingested orally (as the baby would be getting it), the risk would be extremely small.

Lidocaine is also given to treat some arrhythmias of the heart. In this case it is given intravenously, but again the amounts that get into the milk are very tiny and are poorly absorbed by the baby. No need to interrupt breastfeeding even for a minute.

Most drugs used for general anaesthesia (halothane, for example) are gases and are almost completely eliminated from the body quickly through the lungs. Amounts getting into the milk are extremely small. Furthermore, it is unlikely that any would be absorbed when the baby drinks the milk.

Other drugs are given in addition to gas, (for example, atropine), in order to dry up secretions temporarily. Atropine does not get into the milk in significant amounts.

Bottom line? After anaesthesia, local or general, the mother can breastfeed as soon as she is awake and feeling up to it.

Breastfeeding in times of disaster

We tend to imagine that natural and man-made disasters won't happen to us. Yet none of us is immune. What are some of the concerns?

Radiation. After the earthquake and tsunami in 2011 in Japan, many people, including nursing mothers, were exposed to radiation released from the nuclear plant that was damaged.

Supposedly intelligent people went on television to tell mothers that they should not breastfeed because of the possibility of passing radioactive substances, particularly radioactive iodine, to the baby. At first glance, this seems to make sense. After all, we don't want the baby, who undoubtedly received radioactivity along with his mother, to get even more.

But what are the practical issues? First of all, think of what happened in northeastern Japan. Whole towns, including shops, were destroyed. Getting milk from a cow or goat might seem reasonable, but weren't they also irradiated? And were the cattle not also killed? Where would the mothers get clean water even if they did have formula available? From the rivers—which were also irradiated? And was the river water, full as it was with dead people and animals, free of bacterial contamination? Ah, but the mothers could boil the water, right? With what fuel? A little thinking could have helped these intelligent people to understand the absurdity of their recommendations.

They also recommended that the mothers take potassium iodide (KI) to displace radioactive iodine from their thyroids. Assuming KI was available, shouldn't the babies take it as well? Large amounts of iodide saturate thyroid receptors and prevent uptake of most radioactive I^{131}, although it does not protect from other radioactive isotopes. The protective effect of KI lasts approximately 24 hours, so it must be dosed daily until there is no further risk of radiation.

Formula donations. Every time there is a devastating earthquake, flood or famine in some unfortunate part of the world, formula companies, being "good corporate citizens," donate formula for the "benefit" of mothers and babies. Actually, this is also to their benefit. After all, mothers will be grateful to the company. And in places where formula feeding is still a rarity, the gift will establish formula feeding as a good thing, planting a seed for the future. Yet so often during disasters it is impossible to get clean water or fuel to sterilize bottles, and the risk of infection can be very high. In these situations, breastfeeding is the best protection for the child. In many situations it can be lifesaving. The policewoman in China who breastfed babies whose mothers had died shows that breastfeeding is best in these times.

15 | Breastfeeding and Maternal Illness

Myth #1: When a mother has an infection she should not breastfeed.

Fact: Breastfeeding *protects* babies against infection. When a mother has an infection this is precisely the time *not* to interrupt breastfeeding because it will help the baby fight off the infection. The baby may pick up the virus, but breastfeeding will usually prevent him from getting as sick as he might have otherwise, and will help him recover more quickly if he does. This is exactly what immunization does: it infects the baby with the virus or bacterium so that he can develop antibodies against it that prevent him from getting sick.

Myth #2: When a mother has a non-infectious illness, it is better for her not to breastfeed.

Fact: If the mother is seriously ill she may not be able to breastfeed. However, in the vast majority of situations, the mother should get appropriate treatment and if she needs rest, take the baby to bed with her. Family and friends (or a home care nurse) take care of the mother, the mother breastfeeds the baby, and the others handle the rest of the baby care. Illness sometimes seems to decrease the milk supply, especially if a mother has a fever; keeping the baby at the breast and skin to skin as much as possible reduces this risk.

A mother may worry that if she has an infection her baby will catch it from her, so she thinks she should stay away from the baby and not breastfeed. But by the time the mother has symptoms, she and the baby have already been sharing the germs for several days.

So it doesn't make sense to stop breastfeeding to prevent the baby from getting the virus through the milk. The virus is likely to get into the milk in only very small amounts and the chance of the baby getting sick depends on the dose of virus he receives. Breastmilk protects the baby from getting seriously ill (usually) while, at the same time, he is exposed to the virus. It is, in effect, an immunization. This answers the question: should an exclusively breastfed baby be cocooned at home for the first few months, as many doctors and family suggest? I would say no. Without deliberately exposing the baby to sick people, taking him out in the world is a good way to help build his immunity, especially if he is breastfed exclusively.

As for bacteria, they are normally not found in blood; if the mother has bacteria in her blood, she is likely ill enough to be in hospital, probably too ill to breastfeed, at least without help.

So how is breastfeeding like an immunization? When we immunize a child, we give him a weakened virus—for example, the measles virus. This weakened virus elicits an immune response so that if, in the future, the baby is exposed to measles, his immune system will be able to fight off the virus more effectively, and he may not get sick at all.

The virus or bacterium the child might get from his mother is not weakened, but the baby already has an immune response in place from breastfeeding.

The baby doesn't have to start fighting off the infection from scratch. He may have no symptoms, or only mild ones, and rarely becomes seriously ill. But because his body, with the help of breastmilk, fought off the infection, the baby is now immune to that virus or bacterium.

How does breastfeeding protect the baby?

Health professionals often talk about how breast milk contains antibodies and other immune factors and why breastfeeding is important. But too many act as if these immune factors are there only so that questions can be asked on medical or nursing school exams. How else can we explain that so many doctors will tell mothers to interrupt breastfeeding when they have a cold or diarrhea or a cough? Let's look at the power of breastfeeding in more detail to see why continued breastfeeding is usually the best plan when mothers are sick.

Antibodies

These are certainly the best known of the many immune factors in breastmilk. Indeed, some people seem to think they are the only immune factors, whereas antibodies are actually only a part of a whole system that protects the baby from illness. The immune factors interact with one another, reinforcing one another's effects.

There are several antibody types. IgG is the most common; it fights off a virus or bacterium our body has encountered before. IgA is the antibody that protects our mucous membranes. IgM is a large antibody that is the "first responder" when we are exposed to an infection we haven't encountered yet. IgE is associated with allergy.

All these antibodies are found in breastmilk, but the most common antibody in the milk *by far* is sIgA. This antibody is made up of two IgA molecules. In addition to two IgA molecules put together, this antibody has a secretory chain that other antibodies don't that allows it to be excreted into the milk. Thus, other antibodies in the mother's bloodstream do not usually get into her milk in any significant amounts. Also, sIgA contains what is called a J chain. This J chain protects sIgA from being digested by stomach acid and other enzymes.

Sometimes a mother with an autoimmune disease (such as lupus erythematosis) caused by antibodies in her own body attacking her own tissues is told that she should not breastfeed because the antibodies will enter the milk and attack the baby's tissues. This is nonsense, and it's easy to see why. The antibodies in the blood of a mother with lupus do not have the special secretory chain that allows them to get into the milk. If the antibody did get into the milk, it doesn't have the J chain, so it would be digested in the baby's gut. If, by some miracle, the antibody survived digestion, it would not be absorbed by the baby. This is also true of antibodies that cause other autoimmune diseases such as autoimmune thyroid disease, idiopathic thrombocytopenic purpura, rheumatoid arthritis, etc.

Many of the immune factors in breastmilk, including sIgA, mucins, lysozyme and others, are involved in what is called mucosal immunity. Mucosae are the linings of the gut, respiratory tract and vagina. By forming a layer of almost impenetrable defences along the mucous membranes, breastmilk helps prevent bad germs from gaining entry into the baby's body. Some people who do not understand how immune factors work have written articles saying that breastmilk cannot prevent most infectious diseases, with the exception of gastroenteritis (infectious diarrhea and vomiting), because the antibodies are not in the blood. The immune factors don't need to enter the baby's bloodstream. Which makes better sense? Fight off infectious agents once they are in the baby's body or prevent their entry? Clearly it is better to prevent entry into the baby's body in the first place.

The enteromammary system or circulation

I find the protective abilities of breastmilk quite fascinating, but this particular aspect is especially impressive. Let us say that a mother is exposed to a bacterium, such as methicillin-resistant *Staphylococcus aureus* (MRSA) or *Clostridium difficile*. Some health care providers would tell her to stop breastfeeding, just in case.

But here's why that advice is incorrect. There are special cells called M cells in the lining of the small intestine. Most intestinal cells try to repel bacteria, but the M cells actually absorb them. Under these cells, in the intestinal walls, are special white cells. The M cells pass the bacteria over to the white cells, which send information to other white cells. These white cells start producing antibodies, and within 24 to 48 hours they are in the mother's breastmilk, protecting the baby. In the meantime, the baby is being protected by other immune factors always in the milk.

Other immune factors in breastmilk

Breastmilk immunity is very complex. Cells, cytokines (chemicals that transmit messages) and lactoferrin, lysozyme and complement, and many other immune factors interact to help protect the baby. Breastmilk also contains factors that decrease the inflammation that usually occurs when the body is fighting off an infectious process.

Inflammation helps fight infection, but it is also responsible for many of its unpleasant symptoms and the damage it causes. An infected finger will be swollen, red, painful and hot. The heat and swelling help to fight off the infection, but that inflammation can also cause damage to the tissues. Breastmilk

helps the baby fight off the billions of bacteria, fungi and other microbes found in the intestine *without* inflammation. Not only does the prevention of inflammation decrease the risk of damage, it also saves energy.

White cells

White cells are found in breastmilk in large numbers, particularly in colostrum, and for several months they are present in much higher numbers than are present in blood. The majority are leukocytes, which fight off infection, but all types of white cells, including lymphocytes, are present in the milk. The various white cells do not seem to be capable of all the same functions as the white cells in blood, but lymphocytes produce cytokines, which send information to the baby's developing immune system to help it mature more rapidly. Some lymphocytes in breastmilk have been found in the baby's blood, which means they were absorbed from the baby's intestine.

Lysozyme

Lysozyme is a protein that helps protect against infection by destroying bacteria's cell wall. It is very effective. Lysozyme increases in concentration in the milk as the months go by and is highest after the baby is a year old. This makes sense, because toddlers need *more* protection. They are frequently picking things up off the floor and putting them in their mouths. And they tend to be in contact with other toddlers who are sick. This is why it's particularly important to continue breastfeeding if your baby or toddler is in daycare.

B12-binding protein

This protein may interfere with bacterial use of B_{12}, a vitamin essential for bacterial growth. If the bacteria can't grow and multiply, they can't cause illness.

Bifidus factor

This factor encourages the growth of non-harmful bacteria in the baby's intestines that inhibit the growth of more dangerous bacteria that can cause disease.

Oligosaccharides

These polymers protect babies in an interesting way. They have endings that resemble receptors on the lining of the gut. Disease-causing bacteria that enter the stomach will attach themselves to the oligosaccharides instead of the gut. The bacteria then end up in the baby's diaper rather than invading his body. Formula manufacturers are now adding oligosaccharides to their milk, but these prebiotics have always been present in breastmilk.

Interferon

Interferon is a protein that helps protect against viral diseases. It is produced in the body in significant amounts when a person has a viral illness and inhibits viruses from multiplying.

Lactoferrin

Lactoferrin is able to kill several types of bacteria. Together with lysozyme, it acts on the cell wall of bacteria, destroying it. Lactoferrin also has antiviral and antifungal properties and acts against *Candida albicans*. Like the oligosaccharides, lactoferrin decreases the ability of certain bacteria, including the enteropathogenic *E. coli* (which causes "hamburger disease") to attach themselves to the cells of the intestinal mucosa. At one time, it was thought that lactoferrin slowed or stopped the growth of bacteria by making iron unavailable to them, but this is no longer thought to be correct. Lactoferrin does, however, encourage the growth of good bacteria, such as bifidobacteria, in the baby's gut.

Fat

The fat in breastmilk is an immune factor. Free fatty acids liberated from the breakdown of breastmilk fat are capable of killing enveloped viruses such as chicken pox and herpes. They are also capable of killing some bacteria and some parasites such as amoebas, and the scourge of daycares, *Giardia lamblia*.

Cytokines

Cytokines are proteins that have a wide range of immune effects. They stimulate immune responses in white cells, but their main function may be to help the baby's immune system mature.

These are just a few of the many immune factors in breastmilk. You can see how these work together to keep your baby healthy. For example, formula companies have been adding a group of substances called nucleotides to their formulas, claiming that they protect the baby the way breastmilk does. Studies have not shown important effects of nucleotides on the baby's immune system. Nucleotides may have a role in immunity when the baby is under stress, such as after surgery, but this is unproven.

It seems the main reason to add nucleotides is marketing, convincing both parents and health professionals that the immune factors of breastmilk have now been added to formula. In this way, the companies perpetuate the notion that formula is similar to breastmilk. It isn't.

I want to mention one more interesting compound that is found in breastmilk: alpha-lactalbumin. While not, strictly speaking, an immune factor, it does induce cancer cells to commit suicide. The presence of this compound in breastmilk may account for the decreased incidence of certain cancers in breastfed babies and children.

In summary, breastmilk contains a variety of

immune substances that give the baby excellent, though not guaranteed, protection against infection. If the mother develops an infectious illness, it is almost always in the baby's best interests for her to keep breastfeeding.

Illness

Babies who are breastfed, especially those exclusively breastfed, are not likely to get sick even when the mother has fever, cough, rash, vomiting, diarrhea or any number of symptoms. If the baby does get sick, he is likely to have a much milder illness than if he weren't breastfed. If he is partially breastfed, he may still not be as sick as if he were not breastfed at all.

In the presence of many illnesses, some health professionals will counsel mothers to interrupt breastfeeding "just to be safe," but it's *not* safe to stop breastfeeding when a baby has been exposed to an infection. "Just to be safe," the mother should continue breastfeeding so that the baby can get the immune factors we've described.

Some specific situations are discussed here. It is not possible to discuss every illness that may strike a breastfeeding mother. I'll cover those for which mothers are most often advised to wean.

Infectious Diseases: some general notes

- The ending "itis" denotes infection or inflammation or both. Although many infections have the "itis" ending (otitis, infection of the ear; sinusitis, infection of the sinuses), the ending does not necessarily mean infection; it may mean inflammation only.
- It is generally true that by the time a person knows she's sick, she is less infectious than during the incubation period.
- Most viral infections have a "viremic" phase, when the virus circulates in the blood after gaining access to the body. This is the only time, practically speaking, that a virus can pass into the mother's milk and infect the baby directly. The viremic phase, which lasts only a few hours, occurs before the mother knows she is sick.
- Viral and bacterial infections can be transmitted through direct contact with sores (chicken pox, herpes), secretions (colds), and even very small amounts of bowel movements (hepatitis A, intestinal infections caused by several sorts of bacteria and viruses), or by inhaling sneezed or coughed secretions (colds caused by a large variety of bacteria and viruses). Illnesses can also be transmitted through contaminated food (food poisoning, hepatitis A) or by contact with infected blood (blood transfusions in the past, or needle sharing). Except for the viremic phase, bottle-feeding mothers are just as likely to pass on an infection in these ways as breastfeeding mothers. And the viremic phase occurs before the mother suspects she is sick.

Hepatitis

Hepatitis is an infection of the liver. The symptoms of hepatitis include fatigue, nausea, jaundice and abdominal pain. There are several viruses that can cause hepatitis, including hepatitis A, B, C, etc., all the way to hepatitis G. Other viruses can also cause hepatitis, including infectious mononucleosis (Epstein-Barr virus), cytomegalovirus, and even some viruses that cause the common cold. Reactions to drugs or toxins can also cause hepatitis; in this case, it is not infectious. The symptoms of infectious hepatitis may be so mild that the affected person doesn't even know he has it, or the illness can be very severe, even fatal.

Hepatitis A. Typical hepatitis A, the most common infectious hepatitis, is passed on by contact with the infected person's bowel movements, small amounts of which are found on hands through poor hand washing. But the virus is in the bowel movements before the person knows he's sick, and usually no longer present by the time symptoms develop.

Unlike hepatitis B and C, hepatitis A does not result in chronic infection or cause the person to become a carrier. The acute illness is usually relatively mild in children. Symptoms in adults may last a long time, weeks and even (rarely) months, and in general are more severe than in children. Because loss of appetite and fatigue are typical symptoms, this is a real problem for the mother who has a new baby.

However, by the time the mother notices a yellow discolouration of her skin, if she hasn't already passed the infection to the baby, she almost certainly will not. The viremic phase, when the virus is in the blood, has long passed and even the excretion in the bowel movements has virtually if not completely stopped. Interrupting breastfeeding at this point merely puts the baby at higher risk of getting sicker, without the protection of the immunity of breastmilk.

But what if the mother has had contact with someone who turns out to have hepatitis? I bring this up because I have been asked this question. Should she interrupt breastfeeding to prevent the virus from getting to the baby through the milk during the viremic stage? I think this is a terrible idea. First of all, just because the mother comes into contact with someone with hepatitis, she will not necessarily be infected. As well, the incubation period (the time between the infection and the appearance of symptoms) can last anywhere from two to six or more weeks. Taking the baby off the breast and giving him a bottle for two weeks or longer means that the baby will likely not breastfeed again because he will refuse the breast. If the mother does get the infection, the baby may get infected even if he is bottle-fed, but he's now lost the important protection

that breastmilk provides and is likely to be much sicker. The risks of artificial feeding, outlined elsewhere in this book, are far greater than the risks of the baby getting hepatitis A.

If the parents are truly concerned, both the mother and the baby could be immunized against hepatitis A or given hepatitis A immunoglobulin, which is often recommended if exposure and infection are *likely*.

If the mother develops hepatitis, the baby can still get the injection of immunoglobulin while the mother continues to breastfeed.

Most adults want to stay in bed when they have hepatitis. The mother can take the baby into bed with her and just breastfeed as the baby requires, with as much help as possible from family, friends or other caregivers.

Hepatitis B. This virus is very similar to hepatitis A, and its severity is also quite variable: some have no symptoms, some are mildly ill and some very ill. Hepatitis B is often transmitted through sexual contact, sharing needles or getting a tattoo with improperly sterilized equipment.

Unlike with hepatitis A, about 10% to 15% of all people infected with hepatitis B become chronic carriers, meaning their bodily fluids are infectious even once the acute phase of the disease is over and they no longer have symptoms. Many chronic carriers of hepatitis B have never had symptoms of hepatitis.

Hepatitis B may be passed from the mother to the baby during childbirth, so pregnant women are usually tested for this disease. If the baby is given immunization and immunoglobulin against hepatitis B within 12 hours of the birth, infection can be prevented. It should be pointed out that even before immunization and hepatitis B immunoglobulin were available, the rate of infection after birth for babies who were breastfed was no higher than for those who were not.

Hepatitis C. Like hepatitis B, hepatitis C can be transmitted through sharing needles or improperly sterilized tattoo equipment. Sexual transmission may be possible but seems rare in vaginal intercourse. The disease can be passed to the baby during childbirth, whether he is born vaginally or by Caesarean section, but the incidence is not high. The baby can be infected during the pregnancy.

Infection with hepatitis C is similar to hepatitis A and B, though often the infection is milder or not noticeable. However, a chronic carrier state results in a significant percentage of those infected. This may cause continued inflammation of the liver and eventual cirrhosis.

Breastfeeding does not seem to increase the risk of the baby being infected. However, the evidence is based mostly on small studies and since the baby can be infected during pregnancy or birth, it is hard to analyze the data. In any case, the studies do support encouraging the mother to breastfeed, preferably exclusively so that the baby gets the best protection from the milk's immune factors and to maximize the effect of mucosal immunity.

There are concerns that if the mother's nipples are bleeding, the risk of the baby getting hepatitis C might increase. If the mother has any nipple soreness, she should get immediate help so that it does not progress to bleeding. Hepatitis C is often treated with interferon, and mothers may be told that they can't breastfeed while taking this medication. Not true; interferon is a molecule that is too big to get into the milk.

Given the risks of not breastfeeding, mothers with hepatitis C should continue to breastfeed.

Human Immunodeficiency Virus (HIV) or AIDS
HIV is thought to be a relatively new virus in the human population and acquired immunodeficiency syndrome (AIDS) has been recognized as a disease only since the early 1980s. HIV can certainly be called an epidemic. In spite of treatments, many people, especially in resource-poor areas, are dying of the disease. There is much we still need to learn about HIV and AIDS, but we know it is serious and usually fatal if not treated aggressively.

The virus can be passed from mother to child. It has been said that about one-third of the cases of transmission occur during the pregnancy, another third during the birth and another third during breastfeeding. But there is a problem in saying that the baby gets infected during breastfeeding.

The early studies on transmission of HIV from the mother to the baby through breastfeeding compared exclusively formula-fed babies to partially breastfed babies. These studies found that the virus was transmitted at higher rates in the partially breastfed babies. Newer studies comparing exclusively breastfed babies to exclusively formula-fed babies showed no difference in transmission of HIV.

In theory, exclusive breastfeeding, providing mucosal immunity, helps to prevent the virus from passing through the gut into the blood. Probably even more important, it is known that exclusive breastfeeding results in gut closure much earlier than partial breastfeeding or formula feeding. When the baby's gut is "leaky," proteins can more easily get through the mucous lining and into the baby's body. The foreign proteins in formula may actually injure the baby's mucosal lining, allowing invasion of the virus. The presence of the virus in the milk doesn't mean that the baby will get the infection. It needs to get into the baby's body, and breastmilk has ways of preventing that.

In August 2011, the British HIV Association (BHIVA) and the Children's HIV Association (CHIVA) put out a statement saying they did not recommend HIV-positive mothers breastfeed under any circumstances, but added: "In the very rare instances where a mother in the UK who is on effective HAART [an antiretroviral medication protocol] with a repeatedly undetectable viral load chooses to breastfeed, BHIVA/CHIVA concur with the advice from EAGA (Expert Advisory Groups on AIDS) and do not regard this as grounds for automatic referral to child protection teams. Maternal HAART should be carefully monitored and continued until one week after all breastfeeding has ceased. Breastfeeding, except during the weaning period, should be exclusive and all breastfeeding, including the weaning period, should have been completed by the end of six months." The EAGA stated that if a well-informed mother on effective antiviral therapy chose to breastfeed, she should be given the best help possible to breastfeed exclusively and should know that even with effective treatment and exclusive breastfeeding, the risk to the baby was no greater than if he was not breastfed.

This is debatable, if the mother and baby are on effective treatment. Remember that there are mothers even in affluent countries who live in very poor conditions: in many First Nations' reserves, the water must be boiled because of contamination; in the Inuit village where I worked, there was no sewage treatment. In many communities, babies who are not breastfed are given inexpensive homemade formulas (made up from evaporated milk) that we would consider inadequate by current standards. The infant morbidity and mortality on First Nations' reserves is much higher than in the rest of Canada and many of the conditions that kill babies could be prevented by breastfeeding, especially exclusive breastfeeding. The same could be said of intravenous drug users who are at high risk of getting HIV and whose babies are at high risk of death.

Herpes simplex

There are two herpes simplex viruses, which from the point of view of breastfeeding can be treated as one. Many of us have been infected with these viruses without actually knowing it. Type 1 virus causes mouth sores in children and cold sores in adults, and can cause sores similar to chicken pox at any age. Often, though, people who have evidence of infection (antibodies against the virus in their blood) never have any symptoms.

Both viruses can cause severe illness at any age, but are more dangerous for a baby younger than a month. However, the most severe disease occurs in the baby when he gets infected during the pregnancy, particularly during the first trimester; this may cause severe birth defects or even fetal death.

How is herpes virus transmitted? This virus is transmitted by contact with open sores. During pregnancy, the virus passes to the baby through the placenta when it is in the mother's blood.

How can herpes be prevented or reduced? As long as the baby is not in contact with an open sore, there is no reason to avoid breastfeeding. If there is a sore on the nipple, breastfeeding should be avoided on that side. Sores elsewhere on the mother's body can be covered (with a dressing) to protect the baby.

Once the baby is about a month old, there is much less risk of severe illness (although it is possible at any age). Some babies or young children get ulcers in their mouths (herpetic stomatitis) from herpes virus. These can be quite painful, and in some cases the child will refuse to eat or even drink, resulting in dehydration. Breastfeeding babies may be willing to breastfeed and avoid dehydration. However, the mother *may* get inoculated with the virus on the nipple and areola, causing painful sores. If at all possible, however, breastfeeding should continue.

Herpes viruses are enveloped. Breastmilk contains, among other immune factors, fatty acids that kill enveloped viruses.

Chicken Pox

Chicken pox is caused by the herpes zoster virus. Usually it is a mild disease in children but can be serious in adults, particularly pregnant women. Even in children, it can in rare cases cause inflammation of the brain (meningo-encephalitis). The virus is transmitted by direct contact with open sores or coughed or sneezed secretions. Sores are infectious until they have crusted over, usually five to seven days after their appearance.

The incubation period (the time between infection and appearance of symptoms) is 10 to 21 days. This means that before the mother knows she has chicken pox, the baby has already been exposed. If the mother develops chicken pox, she should continue breastfeeding. She has free fatty acids and other immune factors in the milk to help prevent the baby from getting serious chicken pox.

What happens if the mother develops chicken pox around the time of delivery? This is a special case. If the mother develops chicken pox within four or five days before delivery or about two days after, she has not yet developed antibodies to protect the baby through the placenta or in the milk. Very young babies (less than a month) can become very ill with chicken pox.

If the mother develops chicken pox four or five days or more before birth, she actually got infected 10 to 21 days before she started getting sick. Thus, the baby was probably exposed to the virus, since it can cross the placenta. The baby can be infected at birth as well, since the virus is highly infectious. Once the sores develop, the virus has disappeared from the mother's blood and doesn't enter the milk.

If a woman gets chicken pox more than about five days before her baby is born, the baby will get antibodies through the placenta, but if he is born sooner he won't; in this case, about 20% of the babies

will develop severe chicken pox. It is best not to induce labour, to give the baby more time in utero. Infected babies should be given zoster immune globulin (antibodies against the virus) immediately at birth and acyclovir or a similar drug to prevent the baby from getting very sick. The baby and mother should *not* be separated. The baby should be breastfed to get the immune factors present in the milk that will help protect his mucous membranes from invasion by the virus.

Herpes zoster (shingles)

Shingles is caused by the same herpes virus as chicken pox. The affected person had chicken pox in the past; the virus became dormant, then, years later, reawakened and caused shingles to appear. The rash looks like chicken pox but the blisters are not itchy but are usually painful, sometimes agonizingly so. As with chicken pox, the sores are infectious to touch, but a person with shingles is not infectious through coughing or sneezing.

So, if the mother gets shingles, should she stop breastfeeding? Absolutely not. She is immune. She had chicken pox in the past and the baby got antibodies from her during pregnancy. These antibodies remain in the baby's blood for about six months; plus, he will receive immunity through breastfeeding. If the mother is treated with acyclovir or a similar drug and painkillers, she does not have to interrupt breastfeeding. See the chapter "Breastfeeding While on Medication."

Influenza

Influenza is commonly called "flu," a respiratory infection not related to what people call "stomach flu," which is a gut infection leading to nausea, vomiting and diarrhea.

There are three types of influenza viruses: A, B and C. Influenza A, the most common, is the usual cause of the yearly epidemics of influenza. H1N1, which caused much concern in 2009 and 2010, is an influenza A virus. Typically, every time there is a new strain of influenza, mothers are told to stop breastfeeding even though continued breastfeeding provides protection for the baby. Another group of viruses called parainfluenza viruses cause a similar but usually milder illness than influenza viruses.

Influenza can cause severe illness and every year people whose immunity is compromised die from the disease. The elderly are particularly at risk, as is anyone with chronic lung disease. Premature babies sometimes have chronic lung disease and are thus at risk. As with any virus, the range of influenza symptoms can be extremely variable, from no symptoms to illness requiring intensive care. Luckily, most infections are not severe.

As with most viruses, influenza is most infectious just around the time the mother gets sick, from a day or two *before* she has symptoms to a few days after. The best protection for the baby is to continue breastfeeding. The baby will become immune, almost as if he had been vaccinated. If they are breastfeeding, most babies, even if they do get sick, will get only a mild illness. To repeat, any medication the mother needs can be taken while breastfeeding. However, many cold medications contain antihistamines, which can reduce the milk supply. See the chapter "Breastfeeding While on Medication." Pseudoephedrine, found in many cold medicines, *may* also decrease milk supply, so oral cold medicines should be avoided. A stuffy nose, for example, can be treated with nose drops (xylometazoline, for example).

Cytomegalovirus (CMV)

This is yet another member of the herpes virus family, which means that the fatty acids in the milk have the ability to attack it. Generally, infection with CMV in children or adults passes unnoticed or causes only very mild symptoms (fatigue, fever, feeling unwell). Occasionally CMV causes a syndrome similar to infectious mononucleosis.

If a pregnant woman contracts CMV during the first trimester, the fetus can develop serious problems, including poor growth, neurological issues or even liver disease. Some fetuses will have mild symptoms or no symptoms. Babies and adults who are infected with CMV may excrete virus in their urine off and on for years and thus can transmit CMV.

In the previous edition of this book, I mentioned that some very premature babies who got infected with CMV, presumably from the mother's milk, got quite sick. I recommended freezing the milk, which kills off most of the CMV, before thawing it and feeding it to the baby. More recent research suggests that this is unnecessary and that the premature babies, even the very small ones, can get their mother's milk without freezing and thawing the milk beforehand.

What about the baby who is born with CMV infection? If the mother contracted CMV during the pregnancy, especially in the first trimester, and the baby was born with liver or neurological problems, he should breastfeed. If he is not able to breastfeed immediately, he should get his mother's milk. The baby already has the infection and breastfeeding may help to diminish some of its effects. I think worries about adding more virus to the baby's system are unnecessary; the mother may transfer virus to the baby even if she is not breastfeeding, whereas if breastfed, the baby gets the immune factors.

Of course, sometimes babies are born so sick that they cannot suckle well. Nevertheless, breastmilk given by nasogastric tube is still better for them than formula. As mentioned in the previous edition, if there is truly a concern, the breastmilk can be frozen to kill the CMV, but this is not necessary. Freezing destroys some of the important components of breastmilk; however, frozen breastmilk is still better than formula, which never had any of these important factors to start with.

What happens if CMV is acquired after birth?

A mother infected with CMV after the baby's birth usually has mild symptoms or may not know she's sick. The baby may get the infection from the mother simply by being close to her; the virus may appear in her milk. The infection in the baby is usually also very mild or he may have no symptoms at all.

Infectious mononucleosis

Mothers are frequently told to stop breastfeeding when they have this illness, presumably because it is *usually* caused by a herpes virus. This herpes virus, called Epstein-Barr, causes a variety of symptoms. Again, one can be infected with this virus and have no symptoms at all, have a mild cold-like illness, or have an increasingly severe sickness that includes fever, severe sore throat, fatigue, enlarged and tender lymph nodes, enlarged spleen and evidence of hepatitis. The illness can last several weeks. Most people are exposed to and infected with the virus as children. Symptoms in children are usually mild and short-lived.

There is absolutely no reason a mother should have to stop breastfeeding because she has infectious mononucleosis. Breastfeeding protects against illness and this disease is, in any case, almost always quite mild in young children. It is much better to get the infection as a child than as an adult.

Human papillomavirus (HPV)

There are many species of human papillomavirus. Some cause common warts, others are associated with genital warts and still others are associated with cancer of the cervix.

The only real issue relating to breastfeeding is when a baby is born with papillomas (warts) in the trachea and on the vocal cords. This is rare, but I've had several questions about breastfeeding when the baby has this condition. The infection comes from genital warts caused by papillomavirus 6 or 11. When the mother also has warts on the nipple, she is frequently warned not to breastfeed for fear of worsening the baby's condition, which causes difficulty breathing and stridor (a "musical noise" when the baby breathes in). But the papillomas on the vocal cords are not caused by the papillomaviruses that create warts on skin. The baby may not be able to breastfeed because he has difficulty breathing. That may require surgical treatment to remove the warts, but until this has been done, the baby should still get the mother's milk, by nasogastric tube if he cannot feed directly from the breast.

German measles

German measles (rubella) is also caused by a virus. If a woman develops the illness during the first trimester of pregnancy, the baby can be very seriously affected. The baby could be born small, blind or deaf, have severe neurologic abnormalities or liver disease, among other problems. If a mother develops rubella while breastfeeding, but is not pregnant, there is absolutely no need for concern. She should keep breastfeeding. At worst, the baby will develop a very mild form of German measles, which is a mild illness in children.

West Nile virus (WNV)

When a new virus, such as West Nile, shows up, panic ensues and infected mothers are often warned not to breastfeed, even though there is no evidence of harm to the baby. Breastfeeding is usually considered guilty until proved innocent. Eventually, research shows that breastfeeding is safe.

In 2002, a breastfeeding mother was diagnosed with West Nile virus. Material from the virus was discovered in the mother's milk and the baby had antibodies to the virus in his blood. However, researchers were frustrated trying to grow the virus from the mother's milk because something was inhibiting the virus's growth. The Center for Disease Control (CDC) reported the presence of the virus in the mother's milk and suggested the baby might be at risk. Larry Gartner, a US neonatologist who often speaks on breastfeeding issues, pointed out: "The West Nile virus (WNV) report from the CDC is of great importance, but we need to look at the facts. This is only one child. The child was entirely well and asymptomatic. The child is now apparently immune and presumably protected from future risk of infection. The mother continued to breastfeed the child throughout her illness. There is no evidence yet that any breastfeeding child has been ill from WNV infection. Finally, if the mother develops symptoms of WNV while breastfeeding, the greatest risk to the infant may come from interrupting breastfeeding. Transmission of the virus almost certainly occurred during the period prior to the mother developing fever and headache, when the viremia was at its peak. Shortly thereafter, through her breastmilk she provided the infant with some immune protection as well as nonspecific antiviral agents. If the infant had not continued to receive breastmilk from the mother, the child might well have become clinically ill. Thus, the advice we need to give is to continue breastfeeding even if the mother is symptomatic with what may be WNV infection—or any other infection—as long as the mother is clinically able to do so." (*Academy of Breastfeeding Medicine News and Views*, volume 8(4), 2002, p. 36)

Bacterial infections

Bacteria rarely get into breast milk or are found in milk in insignificant amounts. If the mother has bacteria in her blood, she is almost certainly very ill.

There is a normal flora of bacteria growing on our skin, in our throats, and in our lower intestines. These are usually benign or "good" bacteria, which help prevent disease by stopping "bad" bacteria from proliferating. Some people carry disease-causing bacteria as part of their flora but, being carriers, live in equilibrium with the bacteria. *Staphylococcus aureus*, for example, is often found in the nose or throat of many hospital workers.

Mothers and babies tend to share the same bacteria (and fungi, of course). The mother is resistant to her bacteria and she passes this resistance to her baby through her milk.

What if the mother becomes sick, say, with strep throat? Should the baby be separated from her? Should she interrupt breastfeeding? Of course not. Group A haemolytic *Streptococcus*, the cause of strep throat, is commonly carried in the throat without actually causing infection. In winter, about 20% of all schoolchildren have this streptococcus in their throats yet are not sick. If the mother continues breastfeeding, chances are the baby will not get sick, or may get only mildly ill. If the baby is taken off the breast and given formula, he could easily become seriously ill since an important part of his immune response has been taken away.

The vast majority of bacterial diseases require no separation of the mother and baby and no restriction of breastfeeding.

Mothers are frequently advised to interrupt breastfeeding if they have the following bacterial infections:.

Tuberculosis (TB)

Tuberculosis is a bacterial infection caused by *Mycobacterium tuberculosis*. It is generally thought of as an infection of the lungs, but it actually can affect *any* part of the body. TB was once thought to be almost eradicated, but it is making a strong comeback and is resistant to many drugs used in the past. If the mother has tuberculosis, she can infect the baby in three ways. One is if she coughs up sputum (phlegm), which is laden with *Mycobacterium tuberculosis*. In affluent countries, it is rare that tuberculosis has advanced to the stage where the mother is coughing up bacteria.

Another way the mother could infect the baby is to have the tuberculosis bacterium in her milk. Bacteria can get into the milk in two ways. The first is when bacteria are in her blood. Bloodstream spread of tuberculosis happens only in adults whose immune function is compromised because of illness. HIV is one example. (Being "immune compromised" is not what most people think: it doesn't simply mean "I'm tired" or "I haven't been eating well.") The second is from a tuberculosis infection of the breast. Although tuberculosis can affect any part of the body, it is extremely rare for a tuberculoma (something like a tuberculosis abscess) to form in the breast and communicate with a milk duct.

In other words, the chances of passing the bacteria from mother to baby and infecting him are very low indeed. If the mother is coughing up sputum that is positive for tuberculosis, she can breastfeed wearing a surgical mask. Once the mother is treated and her sputum no longer contains bacteria, there is no reason to wear a mask.

If there is concern the baby will get infected, he should be given an immunization against tuberculosis and treated with anti-tuberculosis medication.

The use of anti-tuberculosis medication by the mother is also not a contraindication to breastfeeding. See the chapter "Breastfeeding While on Medication."

Syphilis

Like tuberculosis, syphilis is making a comeback. It is a sexually transmitted disease caused by the bacterium *Treponema pallidum*. The illness has three different stages according to its clinical manifestations, which can be so varied that syphilis has been called the great masquerader.

The primary stage is an open sore, usually on the genitals. It is highly infectious and if the mother has an open sore when the baby is born, he can be infected by contact. The secondary stage is a rash that often covers much of the body, including, typically, the palms and the soles of the feet. The rash is also infectious through contact. If there are sores on the nipples, transmission to the baby is likely.

Syphilis is usually easily treated in its early stages with penicillin or other antibiotics. Ideally, the mother should be treated during pregnancy. If both mother and baby are adequately treated after the birth, there is no reason to stop breastfeeding.

Lyme disease

The bacterium that causes Lyme disease in North America is called *Borrelia burgdorferi*. A similar bacterium causes infection in Europe. The bacterium is transmitted to humans through the bite of a deer tick. Because these ticks are very small it is hard to see them. The tick must feed on the skin for at least 24 hours for infection to be transmitted.

Lyme disease in Canada was at first restricted to southern Ontario, particularly the area of Point Pelee, but with changes in global temperatures it has now been reported in the southern areas of all provinces and it moves farther north every year.

What are the signs, symptoms and progression of Lyme disease? Lyme disease usually starts with a very particular rash called *Erythema migrans*. After a few days the rash takes on the appearance of an expanding target or bull's eye. The centre is a red circle surrounded by a paler area, which in turn is surrounded by another area of redness. The appearance of *Erythema migrans* is virtually diagnostic of Lyme disease. It is seen in the vast majority of people infected and thus allows for early confirmatory diagnostic tests and treatment, preventing delayed symptoms and problems.

After a few days to a few weeks, the bacterium spreads into the blood and can cause various neurological problems. If not treated adequately, chronic problems such as arthritis can occur.

Can a mother with Lyme disease continue breastfeeding?

Since the bacteria spread through the bloodstream after the initial infection, can they appear in the milk and infect the baby? The bacterium causing Lyme disease has been found in breastmilk in a couple of cases, but I have not heard or read of any baby that was infected through breastmilk. It seems very unlikely. These bacteria need direct access to the bloodstream, and that access needs to last at least 24 hours. Babies almost always have very rapid transit through the gut and the bacteria would probably be excreted before 24 hours. Even if the baby has bowel movements only every few days, breastfeeding forms a protective layer of immune factors over the entire gastrointestinal system, preventing bacteria, viruses and other microbes from invading his body. Of course no system is perfect, but again, the possibility of the bacteria of Lyme disease invading from the gut seems extremely remote.

Many mothers taking doxycycline for Lyme disease are told to stop breastfeeding. In fact, this is not necessary. About 20% of the doxycycline is bound to calcium (from the milk) and thus does not get absorbed by the baby. Amoxicillin is also used to treat Lyme disease and is compatible with continued breastfeeding, without question.

The bottom line? The mother should be treated as soon as the typical rash appears to prevent long-term problems, and she should continue breastfeeding.

Food poisoning

Food poisoning is a common problem around the world. It is an infection of the gut that causes vomiting and/or diarrhea and sometimes fever. It is usually caused by bacteria or toxins in food due to improper handling or cooking. Many different organisms cause food poisoning, including *Staphylococcus aureus, Salmonella* (several kinds), *Listeria monocytogenes, Escherichia coli* (*E. coli,* "hamburger disease"), *Clostridium perfingens, Clostridium botulinum* and others. All can be serious. In 2008, several deaths occurred in Canada due to *Listeria monocytogenes*. In 2011, *Listeria monocytogenes* caused illness in the United States, apparently transmitted through cantaloupes. Some organisms cause direct infection of the gut. Others, such as *Staphylococcus aureus*, produce a toxin that causes illness.

Most cases of food poisoning last only a day or two, at least the worst of it. As with any infection, mothers with food poisoning can and should continue breastfeeding. This is not to underestimate the importance of careful hand washing, especially after going to the toilet, but the baby's best protection is continued breastfeeding. Medications used to treat food poisoning do not require a mother to interrupt breastfeeding.

Non-infectious maternal illness

It is, of course, impossible to discuss every illness a mother might possibly develop while breastfeeding. However, it is a rare situation that requires a mother to stop breastfeeding, even temporarily. We discussed thyroid problems in the chapter "Breastfeeding While on Medication"; here are a few non-infectious diseases we are often asked about.

Rheumatoid arthritis

There is a general feeling among physicians that rheumatoid arthritis is worsened by breastfeeding. There is no evidence for this. Some chronic illnesses such as rheumatoid arthritis and multiple sclerosis improve during pregnancy and get worse after the baby is born, so it may not be breastfeeding that causes a relapse.

Another concern is medications used to treat pain and inflammation. See the chapter "Breastfeeding While on Medication." There are several drugs that mothers can take while continuing breastfeeding. Acetaminophen and nonsteroidal anti-inflammatory drugs (NSAIDs) are safe. The monoclonal antibodies such as etanercept (Enbrel), adalimumab (Humira) and infliximab (Remicade) are extremely unlikely to get into the milk because of their very large size, so they are safe to take during breastfeeding no matter what the manufacturers say.

With regard to some of the other drugs, there are differing opinions. One authority states that gold injections are not compatible with breastfeeding while another says they are. One says that hydroxychloroquine (Paquenil) is compatible with continued breastfeeding; the other says it's not. I believe both gold and hydroxychloroquine are definitely compatible with breastfeeding. If there is concern, drug levels in the milk can be measured.

A mother who has joint pain and muscle weakness may not be able to handle her baby easily, but pillows or splints to support her wrists, if needed, can help. A mother with arthritis can feed her baby while both are lying down, face to face, which will take most of the baby's weight off her arms and may decrease pain in her hips, sacroiliac joints and leg joints. Carrying the baby in a carrier or a sling rather than in her arms may also help. A smaller sling to support the breast may be helpful if the mother has pain holding it.

Multiple sclerosis

There are several treatments for multiple sclerosis and relapses. Steroids are often given in large doses, but usually for only short periods of time and often as intravenous infusions. There is a perception that a drug given by intravenous infusion is somehow more of a problem than a drug given by mouth. Not true. See the discussion on the use of corticosteroids in the chapter "Breastfeeding While on Medication."

Interferon is often used to treat multiple sclerosis. Mothers are told that they can't breastfeed while on interferon, but it is a large molecule, too large to get into the milk. The mother should continue breastfeeding.

Glatiramer (Copaxone) is also used to treat multiple sclerosis, but it is also too large to get into the milk. The mother should continue breastfeeding.

As in the case of rheumatoid arthritis, mothers with multiple sclerosis may have muscle weakness or spasticity that interferes with holding the baby and helping him to latch on. With ingenuity, the right approach for the mother's particular situation can be determined.

Inflammatory bowel disease (Crohn's disease, ulcerative colitis)

With the increased use of monoclonal antibodies to treat mothers with Crohn's disease and ulcerative colitis, I have received many questions about breastfeeding while on these medications. Etanercept (Enbrel), adalimumab (Humira) and infliximab (Remicade) are *not* contraindicated during breastfeeding. The corticosteroids that are often used to treat inflammatory bowel disease are also safe. How the mother gets the corticosteroids does not make a difference, though many are told that getting them rectally is a problem. Not true.

One issue that comes up is the use of domperidone to increase milk production in mothers with inflammatory bowel disease. It is true that domperidone can cause abdominal cramps and diarrhea, but for the vast majority of mothers with inflammatory bowel disease that we have treated with domperidone, these symptoms are no more severe or prolonged than those of untreated women.

Postpartum depression

Postpartum depression is a common problem that can range from mild to serious with a significant risk of harm to both the mother and the baby. There are many theories about possible causes. I believe that the way we manage labour and birth and separate mothers and babies after birth are important factors in the development of depression.

There are various treatments for depression, such as psychotherapy or exercise (one study found that daily outdoor exercise was more effective than medication), but in severe cases the mainstay of therapy is medication. Several antidepressants are now available; they are unlikely to get into the milk in significant amounts. See the chapter "Breastfeeding While on Medication."

Some physicians treat postpartum depression with hormones, believing that it is due to low estrogen levels. There is no evidence for this. Estrogen therapy may result in drying up of the milk.

A new approach is to separate mothers from their babies at night for five days immediately after birth so that the mothers get uninterrupted sleep. This study is going on right now at Mount Sinai Hospital in Toronto. Unfortunately, this approach seriously undermines breastfeeding, and I believe that the ethics of such a study are questionable to say the least. The hormones of attachment released when the baby has uninterrupted, skin-to-skin contact with his mother would probably be far more effective in preventing depression, and breastfeeding would be protected. Mount Sinai's program involves feeding newborns with formula overnight. Babies get artificial feeding with known risks, and most likely breastfeeding fails.

Surgery and anaesthesia

This question has already been addressed in the chapter "Breastfeeding While on Medication," but since it comes up frequently, a short recap seems worthwhile.

Most drugs used for general anaesthesia are short-acting and are not absorbed from the intestine. Thus, even if a small amount gets into the milk, it is not absorbed by the baby. Drugs that can be absorbed from the gut will be present in the milk in only tiny amounts and for only a very short time. Once the mother is no longer receiving medication, whatever is left in her body is very rapidly eliminated. The risk of the small amount of any of these anaesthetics or tranquilizing drugs being a problem for the baby is virtually zero. The mother can breastfeed as soon as she is awake and up to it.

Drugs used for local anaesthesia for dental surgery or fillings are even less of a problem; they may appear in the milk, but they are not absorbed from the baby's digestive system, so the baby will just get rid of them in the bowel movements. There is no need for concern.

To summarize, it is not possible to cover all the illnesses that a breastfeeding mother might develop, but through an understanding of the importance of breastfeeding for both the baby and the mother and an awareness of the risks of artificial feeding, a way to continue breastfeeding can be found in most situations.

16 Sick Babies, Special Babies

Myth: When a baby is sick, it is usually better that he not be breastfed or given breastmilk.

Fact: Not only is this untrue, but in the vast majority of cases, it is significantly better for the health of the baby that he be breastfed. Sick babies don't need breastfeeding or breastmilk *less*; they need them *more*.

Breastfeeding and breastmilk are not only for healthy, full-term babies. Most of the prohibitions on breastfeeding the sick baby arise from not understanding that breastmilk is different from formula and breastfeeding is different from bottle-feeding. Unfortunately, too many health professionals have been trained to believe that breastfeeding is better (or equal) only for healthy, full-term babies and that a sick baby needs formula—possibly one of the "special formulas" for "special situations."

There are very rare instances when a baby's illness requires interruption of breastfeeding or that he stop receiving breastmilk. One is the presence of galactosemia, an inborn error of metabolism in which the baby is unable to metabolize galactose properly. (Galactose is one of the two sugars that make up lactose. The other is glucose.) An alternate pathway of metabolism is taken that results in the formation of a toxic compound, galactitol. There is no way to remove the galactose from the milk, so a baby who has the full syndrome of galactosemia cannot breastfeed. However, some babies have only partial galactosemia (Duarte variant), in which they have some enzyme to metabolize galactose (as much as 10% to 25% of normal levels). These levels of enzyme mean the baby can metabolize galactose adequately and does not suffer the effects seen in classic galactosemia. He can and should breastfeed, just as any child. Babies with lower levels of enzyme can be partially breastfed.

Other inborn errors of metabolism may also make breastfeeding more hazardous than artificial feeding. Tyrosinemia is, *perhaps*, one of them, but it is so rare that this has not been studied. Another rare condition is called maple syrup urine disease. We don't know about breastfeeding with this condition either.

Often breastfeeding is prohibited because the physicians and dietitians who are treating the baby need to control the intake of certain elements in the diet very strictly and believe this cannot be done when he is breastfeeding. Galactosemia occurs in about one in 40,000 to 60,000 live births; tyrosinemia and maple syrup urine disease are about one-third less common than galactosemia. There are several other rare metabolic diseases for which we don't know the impact of breastfeeding.

It is not possible in this book to discuss all the illnesses that might befall a baby, but here are the points to consider: Breastfeeding has a significant positive effect on the short-term and long-term health of both the mother and child; it is very different from any artificial feeding that has been devised. Breastmilk is a living, dynamic fluid whose various components interact to help the child fight off infection and help the development of the immune system, intestinal tract, lungs and brain. Breastfeeding also helps the mother and child develop a close relationship.

Breastfeeding comforts the sick child and the fact that the child breastfeeds comforts the mother. Through breastfeeding, the child helps reassure the mother that he is not so sick. It gives her a way to console her baby. A calm, comforted baby has more resources to fight off illness. Research has shown that breastfeeding has an analgesic effect and reduces pain better than many pain-relieving drugs. It may also help the baby go to sleep easily and calmly. Doctors often forget these important aspects of breastfeeding. On the other hand, a child who is so sick he won't breastfeed requires urgent evaluation by a physician.

When mothers are told they must wean their children because they are ill, they should remember health professionals don't always understand or appreciate the intense emotions mothers may feel. When the nursling is a toddler, the mother too often hears, "He's breastfed long enough" or worse, "You are causing him to be over-dependent." When told they must wean, mothers should do further research on their own, possibly with the help of a breastfeeding-friendly health professional, to determine if the recommendation (and it is a recommendation, usually, not a commandment) is valid. It almost never is.

What if the child gets really sick?

Yes, unfortunately this can happen even if he is exclusively breastfeeding, but it is very unusual. If he is also getting other milk (formula or cow's milk, goat's milk, etc.) or is eating solids, it is more likely that the illness will be more severe. But even if the child is admitted to the hospital and put on intravenous fluids, it does not mean that breastfeeding should be stopped or discouraged. Breastfeeding keeps up the baby's nutrient intake and helps his gut recover more

quickly. It also comforts the child who feels unwell and must undergo numerous painful procedures (having blood taken, for example). And the fact that the baby is breastfeeding also comforts the mother.

What is normal?

To understand what is *not* normal, it is important to understand what is. Many health professionals have never learned about the normal breastfed baby who is doing well—how to know he is actually drinking from the breast, what the normal bowel movement pattern is, what the weight gain should be like and so on. Too many have no idea how the exclusively breastfed baby is different from the exclusively artificially fed baby. So below is information on what to expect from the healthy baby who is breastfeeding well.

Bowel movements

During the first few days after birth, babies pass meconium, a very dark green, almost black, sticky substance that accumulated in the intestines while the baby was in the uterus.

After the first two or three days, a baby who is breastfeeding *well* exclusively will start to have bowel movements that are getting lighter, becoming lighter green or a golden brown or even yellow. Giving formula in the first few days will change the appearance of the bowel movements and it becomes harder to assess how things are going. However, one can still judge how well the baby is breastfeeding by observing him at the breast (see the video clips at www.breastfeedinginc.ca). Once the baby is three or four days old, he should, if he is exclusively breastfeeding well, have yellow or yellowish-brown (mustard-coloured) bowel movements, several a day.

On the other hand, a baby who still has meconium-type bowel movements on day four or five is not getting enough milk from the breast. That baby needs to be seen urgently to prevent dehydration and save the breastfeeding. If it is determined that the baby needs supplementation, it should be done *at the breast* with a lactation aid. However, by fixing the latch and making sure the baby gets milk well (following our Protocol to Increase Breastmilk Intake, found in the chapter "Increasing Breastmilk Intake by the Baby"), it is often possible to save the situation without giving supplements.

Usually during the first few weeks, exclusively breastfed babies will have many bowel movements every day. Ten a day is not rare and if the baby is content, drinking well at the breast and gaining weight, there is no issue. Furthermore, the amounts of each bowel movement and the colour can be quite variable. One day a baby could have 3 bowel movements, the next day 10 and 5 the day after. What matters is whether the baby is content and drinking well at the breast, not the colour of the bowel movements. Of course, the very dark green, almost black, bowel movements that are meconium are not normal after three or four days of life.

After the first three to six weeks, some babies may have very infrequent bowel movements. It is not uncommon for some exclusively breastfed babies at this age to have one bowel movement every three or four days. Ten days or two weeks without a bowel movement is not rare. Since the previous edition of this book, the record I am aware of is 32 days without a bowel movement in a healthy, exclusively breastfed baby, beating out the previous record of 31 days. To repeat, the issue is whether the baby is content, gaining well and drinking well at the breast, not the frequency of the bowel movements.

Some mothers say the baby is fussy after he hasn't had a bowel movement for a few days. If that is the case, putting the baby to the breast when he's straining will recruit the gastrocolic reflex and help him to have a bowel movement. What is *not* a good idea is giving the baby prune juice or some sort of laxative. The baby is *not* constipated. When he finally goes, the stool will still be soft.

However, if the mother is convinced that the baby is truly unhappy, a pediatric glycerin suppository may help. The parent cuts about 3 cm (an inch) of suppository and inserts it into the baby's bottom, holds his bottom cheeks together for a minute or so to make sure the suppository doesn't come out, and then lets go. (Stand away from the line of fire.)

I have never seen or heard of an *exclusively* breastfed baby who was truly constipated, meaning having *hard* bowel movements. Infrequent bowel movements do not mean constipation. If an exclusively breastfed baby has hard bowel movements, he should be seen by a doctor.

Spitting up; choking at the breast

Spitting up is common in all babies, not just breastfed ones. If the baby is content, gaining weight well and drinking well from the breast, spitting up is not a bad thing. In fact, as stated earlier, it's probably a good thing, since breastmilk protects against infection by painting the baby's mucous membranes (the linings of the gut and respiratory tract) with immune compounds (mucosal immunity). A baby who spits up has double protection: once on the way down to the stomach and again when he spits up. I frequently use this example of how breastfeeding is so different from formula-feeding and bottle-feeding: Spitting up formula, if all else is going well, is probably not bad. Spitting up breastmilk, if all else is going well, is probably good.

Spitting up can sometimes be lessened by having the baby finish the first side before offering the second, a good idea anyway. It is often helpful for the mother to use breast compressions to keep the baby drinking longer on the first side. If she does this, the baby will have the advantage of continuing to receive more calories and fat (since there is more fat in the later milk) while not drinking a larger volume of milk, which would increase his spitting up. A baby whose mother has an abundance of milk can spit up a lot, have frequent, watery green bowel movements and sometimes be unhappy. See the chapter "Colic (The 'C' Word)." That's not gastroenteritis. It may simply be that the mother has a lot of milk but got poor breastfeeding information (such as being told to feed the baby 10 minutes on each side, for example).

The same can be said about choking at the breast. When the flow of milk is rapid, babies often inhale a few drops of breastmilk that go down the wrong way. Though this appears dramatic, after pulling off the breast and coughing a bit, the baby is fine again. And that milk lined the trachea (breathing tube) with immune factors, helping protect the baby against infection. We all choke sometimes on our food, but usually the choking and coughing stop the food from going down too far.

The frequency of choking at the breast can be diminished by getting the best latch possible. This allows the baby to control the milk flow better.

Sometimes when babies choke frequently at the breast, doctors suggest a feeding study. But a feeding study does not duplicate breastfeeding in the slightest. The baby is given something to drink, something that is not breastmilk, in a bottle, which is not at all like a breast. If some of the drink goes down into the trachea, the baby is said to be aspirating and is often taken off the breast and given, at best, thickened breastmilk. This is unnecessary in the vast majority of cases and undermines breastfeeding completely.

Spitting up also often prompts physicians to test the baby to see if he has reflux. After fasting and breastfeeding, the baby is given an ultrasound. On pushing the ultrasound probe onto the baby's stomach, it is decided that he indeed has reflux and is put on thickened breastmilk or formula or, at best, anti-reflux medication. All these steps—from the test to taking baby off the breast—are unnecessary and harmful.

Acute illness (temporary illness)
Gastroenteritis (diarrhea and/or vomiting due to a virus or bacterium)

An infection of the digestive system in an exclusively breastfed baby is very unusual and when it does occur it is rarely severe. Once a child is eating other foods, especially if he is in contact with many other children, as happens in daycare centres, gastroenteritis does become more common.

It is not easy to decide if an exclusively breastfed baby has diarrhea. Breastfed babies' bowel movements are often quite watery, seem to contain little or no solid material and can be quite frequent. They are often green. This doesn't mean there is an infection or a problem; it simply means milk passed through the gut quickly. This may occur in many situations, including so-called lactose intolerance. If the baby has watery and/or green bowel movements and is content and drinking well at the breast and gaining weight well, he is just fine and nothing should be done. In fact it is *undesirable* to treat green bowel movements.

As well, true vomiting is different from spitting up (regurgitation). True vomiting is forceful and sometimes painful, but not always easy to distinguish from spitting up. One needs to look at the whole baby. If he is content and drinking well, but also brings up milk after each feeding, he is probably just spitting up.

For many years, physicians said that babies with gastroenteritis should be taken off milk or formula, because babies with a gut infection temporarily lose the enzyme lactase, which breaks down lactose, resulting in continued diarrhea. As usual, this advice was based on the formula-fed, bottle-fed baby. And in the 1980s, doctors realized that keeping babies and toddlers on clear fluids—starvation, really—was the real reason diarrhea continued. Lactase (the enzyme that breaks down lactose) will recover if the baby is not starved. Most physicians now know this and don't advise temporary weaning, even if the baby is formula-fed. Unfortunately, there are still some holdouts who not only tell parents to stop milk or formula but tell mothers to stop breastfeeding.

The best treatment for the breastfeeding baby with acute gastroenteritis is continued breastfeeding, even if he is vomiting and doesn't seem to tolerate it. Breastmilk contains a host of immune factors, not only antibodies, that help protect the baby from the worst effects of a gut infection. Furthermore, he will recover more quickly if breastfeeding is continued. Babies and toddlers often tolerate breastmilk better than other liquids because it leaves the stomach relatively quickly and thus they may vomit less. Furthermore, the nutrients in breastmilk are better and more rapidly absorbed than those in other foods (including formula), so the baby is not starving. As mentioned above, one of the causes of prolonged diarrhea is that we starved babies to "cure" them. When food was reintroduced to their diets, physicians frequently suggested rice, apple and banana, which are all low in fat; it turns out that returning fat to the diet was what was actually needed. Continued breastfeeding will prevent "starvation diarrhea." Furthermore, the child is comforted by breastfeeding and the mother is comforted by the fact that the baby breastfeeds.

The main worry with an intestinal infection (gastroenteritis) is that it can lead to dehydration; babies are much more susceptible than older children and adults. Gastroenteritis almost always gets better with time, without any specific treatment, so the key is to maintain the baby's hydration. As long as he keeps down more than he loses, he will usually be fine. A child who is urinating six or seven times a day, even if the urine is concentrated, is probably managing to stay ahead. It is true that when babies wear diapers, it is not easy to know how often they urinate and if the baby is having frequent diarrhea, it's not easy to tell what constitutes watery bowel movements and what constitutes urine in the diaper.

Parents are sometimes advised to check the baby's fontanelles for sunkenness to see if he is dehydrated. This unnecessarily causes many parents to panic. If a baby is sitting up there is a good chance he will have a sunken fontanelle. See the photo below. This perfectly hydrated baby who is not vomiting and does not have diarrhea has what appears to be a sunken fontanelle. It's not; it's normal.

One of the principles of feeding children with gastroenteritis is to give small amounts of fluid frequently. Large amounts are more likely to be

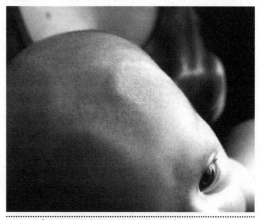

Many information sheets about breastfeeding suggest that parents check their baby's fontanelle as an indicator of dehydration, but even most doctors don't know how to tell if a fontanelle is sunken. A baby will often appear to have a sunken fontanelle if sitting up. Gaining weight and drinking well from the breast, this baby is perfectly normal and is definitely not dehydrated.

CREDIT: **JACK NEWMAN**

vomited. Furthermore, due to what is called the gastrocolic reflex, a full stomach tends to stimulate a bowel movement, increasing fluid losses because the intestine does not have as much time to absorb fluid from the gut. We all have this reflex, but babies have a much more sensitive one than older children or adults. However, what do small, frequent feedings mean when a baby or child is breastfeeding?

Babies rarely spit up or vomit while they are suckling at the breast, probably because waves of muscle contraction in the esophagus and stomach move the milk down in the opposite direction of vomiting. Vomiting while suckling is more likely to occur if the baby has gastroenteritis, but still less likely than when he comes off the breast. So it is a good thing to let the baby drink from the breast; then, when he is no longer drinking, stay on the breast and "nibble." The baby will not be getting much milk, but the continued sucking may prevent vomiting. Most young babies who are nibbling at the breast will fall asleep. Sick older babies may also fall asleep. That's good, because sleep helps fight off infection. The baby may continue to nibble while sleeping, preventing him from vomiting. The best treatment for a vomiting breastfed baby is keeping him on the breast as much as possible so that he is getting small amounts of milk continually.

What about electrolyte solutions? In resource-poor areas such as the Transkei in southern Africa, where I worked as a pediatrician for 18 months, gastroenteritis is very common and often fatal. In Toronto, where I trained, we rehydrated dehydrated babies with intravenous fluids. But intravenous fluids are expensive and not practical in resource-poor areas, partly because laboratory tests to guide intravenous therapy are not easily available and also because babies frequently arrive in a very poor state, and finding a vein to start an intravenous is

extremely difficult. We soon learned that oral rehydration was not only practical, it was often better.

Intravenous replacement of fluid and salt losses can be tricky, especially if the child has abnormally high sodium in the blood, and pediatricians in training spend much time learning how to rehydrate children intravenously.

As mentioned above, blood tests are a guide to treatment, but they do not tell us what is going on inside the baby's cells or in the brain. Too rapid rehydration of a baby with a very high sodium level (hypernatremic dehydration) can be dangerous. Oral rehydration was found to be effective much of the time and, for the majority of children, safer and cheaper. Even if they vomited, they were usually able to keep down enough fluid to overcome dehydration.

On the other hand, commercial products in North America are expensive. I did an informal survey of various pharmacies in Toronto in September 2011 and found the cost of a litre of oral solution averaged about $12. This is outrageous, considering that all it is is salt and water and one of the major reasons for developing these solutions was to decrease the cost of rehydration. A child who is dehydrated might require a litre or more of oral solution a day. What is perhaps not well known is that the major oral solution sold in Canada is made by a formula company. Gastroenteritis is much more common in artificially fed babies.

Because the severity of gastroenteritis in exclusively breastfed babies tends to be mild and self-limited, the vast majority of breastfed babies with gastroenteritis need only continue breastfeeding without oral rehydrating solutions. Only in the unusual situation where breastfeeding does not keep up with the child's needs should oral rehydration solution be considered. For example, if the mother's milk supply has decreased because she is weaning the child from the breast or the child is breastfeeding less because he is eating more food, breastfeeding *may* not, at first, be able to keep up with his need. However, even in this situation, more frequent breastfeeding will quickly bring up the milk supply and the extra fluid may no longer be necessary after a day or so. If breastfeeding alone is unable to keep up with the child's needs because the losses are so great, he needs to see a doctor urgently, not just be given oral rehydrating solution. It is rare indeed that breastfeeding cannot keep up.

Older children will often not drink these oral solutions because they taste bad. When I worked at the Hospital for Sick Children emergency department, I often used the willingness of the baby to take oral rehydrating solution as a measure of dehydration. If the baby would actually drink the stuff, he was probably dehydrated. (This sign of dehydration is not found in standard pediatric textbooks.) Manufacturers of oral rehydrating solutions have added flavour to the liquids, but unless they add sugar as well, the taste is not better. Adding sugar, on the other hand, can actually increase fluid loss from the gut. The Canadian Paediatric Society, very wrongly, I believe, suggests starting oral electrolyte solution at the *very first sign of a gut infection*. But what is the first sign in the breastfed baby? Breastfed babies can *normally* have many bowel movements every day. One day a breastfed baby could have 5 bowel movements, all fairly liquid, and another day 10 bowel movements, also very liquid. Does that mean he has a gut infection? Not necessarily.

Furthermore, young babies can have increased numbers of bowel movements with *any* infection. It makes little sense to start giving a baby oral rehydration fluid when he has an ear infection, for example. Breastfed babies can have yellow bowel movements one day, orange the next and green the day after.

Many breastfed babies spit up a lot. If they spit up and the bowel movements turn green as well,

does that mean a gut infection? Not necessarily. We have to look less at the bowel movements and more at the baby. A happy, content, baby drinking well at the breast and gaining weight well who has 12 green bowel movements a day and lots of spitting up is fine and should not be given oral rehydrating solution. The fact that some pediatricians call those green bowel movements "starvation stools" shows how little they know about breastfeeding.

Breastfeeding and breastfeeding alone is all the majority of babies with gastroenteritis need. If a baby who is eating some solids stops eating solids when he is ill, he can start eating again as soon as he shows interest. Breastfeeding comforts the baby who is sick, and the fact that the baby will breastfeed comforts the mother.

What about lactose intolerance? Transient lactose intolerance can sometimes be a cause of continued diarrhea after a bout of gastroenteritis, but it is not a reason to stop breastfeeding. Though it used to be said that the virus causing diarrhea injured the walls of the intestines, this may not be the only, or even the most important, factor. It is likely that the "starvation" we imposed on babies and older children with these infections was at least a part of the problem of lactose intolerance. "Starvation" prevented the lactase (the enzyme that breaks down lactose) from recovering.

The best way to prevent lactose intolerance during a bout of gastroenteritis, therefore, is to maintain the baby's nutrition, and the best way to do this is continued breastfeeding. Eventually the gut will recover, as will the lactase. With the growth factors present in the milk, such as prostaglandins and epidermal growth factor (to mention only two), the gut and the lactase are likely to recover more quickly. Breastmilk also hastens the recovery of the villi, which are frequently damaged during severe gastroenteritis. (Villi are tiny fingers of the gut wall that project into the space of the intestine and are the surfaces from which nutrients are absorbed.)

In other situations, lactose intolerance may be diagnosed without gastroenteritis. A lactation consultant I know describes a scenario she sees too often: a three- or four-month-old is pulling away from the breast, crying, and/or has stopped gaining weight well, and the pediatrician refers him to hospital where, instead of watching the baby at the breast (finding that the mother's supply has decreased), a lactose tolerance test is performed. The baby is overloaded with lactose for the purpose of the test and diagnosed with lactose intolerance, so the mother is told to stop breastfeeding and put the baby on lactose-free formula. To learn the real reason the babies mentioned above are pulling at the breast, see the chapter "Late-Onset Decreased Milk Supply."

Other causes of vomiting and diarrhea

Many babies have sensitive stomachs. Something as mild as a cold or as serious as meningitis or anything in between may cause a baby vomiting or diarrhea. If the baby does not look right or react normally, parents should not assume that vomiting and diarrhea is gastroenteritis. A child who just doesn't seem right should be examined by his physician urgently. Whatever the problem, a mild illness or a serious one, there is rarely ever a reason to stop breastfeeding. Even if the baby is too sick to drink, breastmilk can be given by syringe or with a tube into the stomach. One exception is if the baby has a blocked gut, but in this case, nothing should be put into his stomach.

What about prolonged diarrhea? Vomiting during an acute gut infection usually lasts a day or two and then slows down and stops. Diarrhea usually lasts longer, up to a week or two, occasionally longer. But what if the diarrhea goes on for weeks?

The most common cause of prolonged diarrhea (we used to call this toddler diarrhea), as suggested earlier in this chapter, is a too-slow return to a normal diet, especially a normal amount of fat. Obviously, if the baby is under six months, his normal diet is breastmilk and breastfeeding should continue throughout the course of the infection. If he has frequent or even watery bowel movements on breastfeeding alone, this is normal, *if* he is content, drinking well, gaining weight well and generally in good humour.

However, the older child may continue having watery bowel movements if his diet includes a lot of sweet drinks (even diluted) and not much food containing fat. Apple juice is a big offender. Once the worst of the vomiting and diarrhea is over and the child wants to eat, he should be encouraged to do so, even if the diarrhea temporarily gets worse. The toddler should start eating normal food (including dairy products, if those are part of his usual diet) as soon as he is willing, and his diarrhea will almost always settle quickly enough.

"Allergic" colitis

This is a not uncommon problem in babies, judging by my emails. Often within weeks or months of birth, the baby starts to have blood in his bowel movements. When the parents notice the blood, they rush to the doctor, who suggests a battery of tests, often resulting in the baby being taken off the breast and put on a "hypoallergenic formula." Even if the baby is not taken off the breast, the first step suggested by many physicians is for the mother to stop dairy products in case cow's milk protein in her milk is causing this allergic reaction. See the chapter "Colic (The 'C' Word)." This *does* seem to work occasionally, but if it doesn't, the mother's diet is often restricted more and more until she is eating nothing but white rice and drinking nothing but water. This is neither good nor necessary.

The mothers of babies with "allergic" colitis usually have an abundance of milk and the babies often grow very quickly. They are *usually* calm, happy babies. They are drinking well at the breast. Almost always, the blood is present only as streaks or little mucousy globules no bigger than a drop of water. In such a situation, I would encourage the mother to see her doctor to rule out other causes of blood in the bowel movements such as:

1. An anal fissure. This is a small tear in the anus of the baby that may be caused by an explosive bowel movement, not a rare event in babies who are exclusively breastfed. An anal fissure will cause streaks of red blood in the bowel movements, but not blood mixed with mucus. If the baby has an anal fissure, there is obviously no need to take him off the breast or to pass a scope into his large intestine to make sure the blood is not coming from there. The fissure should heal without treatment. Some doctors will stretch the opening with a gloved finger and this may help.

2. Swallowed blood from a mother's nipple or breast. Even if the mother does not have visible bleeding from her nipple, blood from the nipples or breast ("rusty pipe" syndrome: see the chapters "Sore Nipples" and "Sore Breasts") can appear in the baby's bowel movements. The baby will usually have had blood in milk he spits up, too, showing that the blood is not coming from inflammation of the intestine.

3. Meckel's diverticulum. This is a pouch that protrudes from the intestine like a finger, not far from the area where the small and large intestine join. It is said that about 2% of the population have a Meckel's diverticulum. The bleeding comes from ulcers due to cells in the diverticulum that produce gastric acid; only a small number of those affected have these cells, so this is an unusual problem. Meckel's diverticulum should be considered in a baby who has more than a few streaks or globules of blood in the bowel movement. The diagnosis is made with a radioactive scan after the baby is given technetium.

4. While gastroesophageal reflux disease (GERD) is way over-diagnosed, in those few cases where the baby's esophagus is irritated, blood may get into the baby's bowel movements.

There is a large number of very uncommon problems that can also cause blood in the bowel movements. Unless there is something unusual about the way the baby's symptoms present, these problems do not need to be investigated.

Why does the blood appear? Some babies may be reacting to something the mother is eating or drinking that is passing into her milk. But many such babies have irritation of the intestinal wall because they are getting a lot of milk very rapidly and the transit time through their gut is very fast. These babies often have very irritated bottoms from watery, acid bowel movements. The vast majority of babies eventually improve with time, especially once they are on solids, which slow the transit time through the gut. This is not a reason to start solids early, however. The approach to treatment, if deemed necessary, should be to slow intestinal transit time by making sure the baby gets adequate fat in his milk. See the chapter "Colic (The 'C' Word)" on how this can be done.

What to do? In the usual case of "allergic" colitis, where the baby is generally content (no baby is ever always content), drinking well, gaining well, and the amounts of blood are small, I would recommend the mother do nothing at all. She should just continue to breastfeed as usual and forget about the blood. The blood eventually disappears when the baby starts to take solid foods because intestinal transit time decreases once solids are added to the diet. On the other hand, if the baby is colicky, his fussiness and crying are often due to something else, not necessarily inflammation of the gut. Often the treatment for "oversupply," colic and pulling at the breast is block feeding: the mother is advised to feed the baby on the same breast for a certain period of time; for example, on the right breast for 12 hours and then the left breast for the same period of time. But this rigid approach may result in a decrease in milk supply and the baby being fussy—not because his gut is bleeding, but because he is not getting enough milk. I have had mothers contact me with exactly this scenario. Here it is:

1.   The mother is told that the baby is colicky because he is not getting enough high-fat milk, so she is advised to feed on just one breast at each feeding, sometimes even two or more feedings before switching to the other side.
2.   As a result, milk supply decreases even if the baby continues to gain weight well. Especially in the evenings, but possibly at every feeding, the baby fusses when the flow of milk slows down.
3.   When I advise the mother to feed the baby on both sides again and/or to take domperidone to bring back her milk supply, the fussiness disappears, but the blood in the bowel movements does not.

And what about the baby who has blood in the bowel movements and is not gaining weight well? First of all, it is important to make sure the baby is getting as much milk as he can. It is also possible that the baby is fussy and not gaining for reasons other than blood in the stool. Work to improve the breastfeeding and investigate other causes.

Eosinophilic esophagitis

Eosinophilic esophagitis is thought to be an allergic reaction. This syndrome has been described only in the last few years. The diagnosis is made by putting a scope into the baby's esophagus (the tube from the mouth to the stomach) and taking a biopsy as the walls of the esophagus contain large numbers of eosinophils; white blood cells associated with allergic responses.

The condition sometimes responds to removing certain allergens from the patient's diet. If necessary, corticosteroid in liquid form taken by mouth should help. Presumably the contact of the corticosteroid with the esophagus decreases the allergic reaction.

This syndrome has become yet another excuse to tell mothers to interrupt breastfeeding and put the baby on hypoallergenic formula. Since there is a treatment that we can give the baby to improve the symptoms, stopping breastfeeding seems to me inappropriate.

Respiratory infections

Some older physicians still recommend taking babies and children off milk products when they have respiratory infections or acute asthma attacks. It was thought that dairy products would increase phlegm production. Some children do have allergic responses to dairy products, and possibly increased mucus production. However, breastmilk is *not* a dairy product, and what may be true for dairy products is not true for breastmilk.

If a child is having difficulty breathing, he may breastfeed poorly. Putting a little breastmilk or salt water in the baby's nose, then using a baby aspirator, will often help. If that doesn't work, a nasal decongestant for babies usually does. If

Is the baby's nose too stuffed up to breastfeed easily? The following may help:

- Use a rubber-bulb aspirator (available in drug stores) to gently suction some of the mucus out of the baby's nose.
- Put a drop of breastmilk or water—just a drop—in the baby's nostril(s) to make him sneeze and clear out his nose.
- Close the bathroom door and turn on a hot shower; the steam may loosen up secretions. This is a traditional treatment for croup (which causes the baby to cough like a barking seal).
- If necessary, use a medicated nasal spray (xylometazoline for children).

If a child with breathing difficulties needs to be in hospital, breastfeeding can and should continue. It is *less* stressful and *less* difficult for a child to breastfeed than to take a bottle. And it comforts him. Indeed, a baby or toddler who has never taken a bottle will be even less inclined to take one when he is sick and in a strange place. Ignore the nurse who says, "I can make any baby take a bottle." Forcing a breastfeeding child to take a bottle can cause distress and worsening of symptoms. If the child is in hospital he may have an intravenous infusion and that can keep him hydrated while he is close to his mother or father, skin to skin. I can think of no circumstance when it would be better for the child to take formula or regular milk than to breastfeed and get breastmilk. Even a tube into the stomach (if for some reason the child needed to get some nutrition), would be better since, uncomfortable as it is, the discomfort of trying to give the baby a bottle must be repeated every few hours.

there's no improvement, the baby should be seen by a physician, even if you need to go to emergency.

Fortunately, most colds, wheezing and even pneumonia are not so severe as to interfere with the child's breastfeeding.

Other infectious illnesses
Meningitis and encephalitis
Children with meningitis (an infection of the fluid that surrounds the brain and spinal cord) and encephalitis (an infection of the brain itself, usually due to a virus) can be very sick. Usually children with suspected meningitis or encephalitis are admitted to the hospital until the diagnosis is confirmed and the course of the illness is clarified. Some children with obvious viral meningitis who are only mildly ill can be sent home.

Sometimes with meningitis or encephalitis, too much hormone is released from the pituitary gland, which reduces the amount of urine produced. Giving lots of IV fluids in this situation may result in potentially dangerous dilution of the blood. In the past, it has been traditional to restrict the fluid intake of the child with meningitis or encephalitis to about two-thirds of the usual iamount.

This restriction on the amount of fluid causes problems because when a baby is breastfeeding, doctors don't know whether he is getting only two-thirds of his required intake. Generally, the baby is taken off the breast and given expressed milk in a bottle so that he gets only two-thirds of his daily requirement (minus, of course, the quantity of intravenous fluids). But this sick and often miserable child does not get the comfort of the breast. In addition, some of the immune factors in breastmilk are lost when milk is pumped and given by bottle. And what do we do with the baby who won't take a bottle or cup?

My approach would be different. The more serious the infection, the more likely it is that this problem of over-diluted blood will arise. But the sicker the child, the less likely he is to take the breast; by the same token, the less sick he is, the more likely he is to do so. So I would say that breastfeeding can and should continue during these illnesses even if it means the lethargic child only allows the breast into his mouth and sucks a little without getting much milk. In any case, blood is checked every day and if there is concern about the sodium levels (which drop with dilution of the blood), restriction of fluid can be done at the IV, not the breast. Furthermore, the chance of the sodium dropping too low decreases as the child improves and after the first few days, restriction of fluid is no longer necessary. Though many children's hospitals have moved away from prohibiting breastfeeding while these illnesses are present, not all have done so.

Should there be a real need to restrict fluid, the mother can express her milk before a feeding and, with a lactation aid, give the appropriate amount to the baby on her "emptied" breast. The breast will still supply small amounts of breastmilk, but in any case, two-thirds is an approximation. More or less can be given the next time, depending on the blood work results. And mother and baby are both comforted by breastfeeding.

This approach to meningitis and encephalitis is an example of the attitude to breastfeeding of pediatricians of my generation. Breastfeeding during my training was often seen as an obstacle to good medical care. The doctors needed to know how much milk the baby was getting and could not measure breastmilk intake. But breastfeeding mothers knew that their children would be unhappy if they couldn't breastfeed and objected to taking the baby off the breast. This led many pediatricians and nurses to believe that these mothers were choosing breastfeeding over the best medical care for the child. But there is more to good medical treatment than measuring precise amounts of fluids and there is considerable value in continuing breastfeeding to help the sick child. If physicians see the true value of breastfeeding, they will be able to find creative ways to base their care on it and to use it to their advantage.

Other infections

There should be no question of prohibiting breastfeeding in the presence of any other infection that a child might have. For example, breastfeeding is still better for the child with tonsillitis, an ear infection or a bone infection. The value of breastfeeding and breastmilk to the sick child is irreplaceable.

Other medical problems

There are very few medical or surgical problems that require a mother to stop breastfeeding or wait to begin breastfeeding. Some surgical problems of the gut require that the baby receive nothing by mouth until the problem is fixed, and this includes breastmilk. These babies are usually fed by intravenous fluids until they can start taking nutrition through the gut.

Cardiac problems

Some babies are born with cardiac abnormalities that can range from very mild, requiring no treatment, to life-threatening and requiring immediate surgery. Breastfeeding and breastmilk (not as good as feeding at the breast, but in some cases necessary temporarily) are valuable for the baby with a cardiac problem. Infection is a major problem for a baby who may spend weeks, even months, in the hospital, where super bacteria that are resistant to many antibiotics live happily. The immunity that the baby gets from breastfeeding may make the difference between resisting infection and becoming ill. For some children with cardiac problems, even a mild case of gastroenteritis or respiratory illness may result in significant setbacks in progress or a threat to their survival. Unfortunately, some pediatric cardiologists do not see the advantage of breastfeeding or even of breastmilk and may discourage these for invalid reasons such as the following:

"The baby needs to have his fluid intake and output calculated exactly." In certain situations, such as congestive heart failure, exact calculations and fluid restriction may be necessary. In many circumstances, pediatric cardiologists disagree about the need for exact measurements. But what if the cardiologist insists on strict fluid intake and output measures?

As mentioned earlier, the mother can express her milk before the baby goes to the breast and feed him on an "emptied breast" using a lactation aid to give him the required amount of fluid. The baby *may* get some milk from the breast, so perhaps decreasing the amount in the lactation aid slightly may reassure the cardiologists that the baby is not getting too much.

If necessary, babies can be weighed before and after the feeding to see how much they took in, a technique I do not particularly like, but if it helps keep the baby at the breast, it's okay. It is necessary to weigh the baby carefully both times, with the same diaper. I do not recommend this for routine use because the test weights do not tell us how much the baby is supposed to get when he is healthy, but if knowing the intake is that important the test may help.

Concerns about fluids can also be addressed by careful physical examination and daily weighing. If a baby cannot suckle at the breast, bottles are more work for him than feeding by cup or by a tube in the stomach. The baby should be cuddled and held skin to skin if he is not breastfeeding.

"It's more work for the baby to breastfeed than to bottle-feed." This is not true, and you can see why by watching the video "Inserting a Lactation Aid" on www.breastfeedinginc.ca and reading the text that accompanies it. Babies respond to milk flow, and premature, young and sick babies tend to fall asleep at the breast when the flow of milk is slow. In the chapter "The Preterm and Near-term Baby," I explained how health professionals believe this myth, but the data show that it is false. The baby's oxygenation and blood pressure are better when breastfeeding than when bottle-feeding, and the risk of apnea (arrested breathing) and bradycardia (too slow a heart rate) is lower. When the baby is on a respirator, skin-to-skin contact decreases stress, increases oxygenation and heart rate and decreases risk of low blood sugar. Overall, breastfeeding and skin-to-skin contact result in less stress and less anxiety in both the mother and the baby.

The argument that the baby must learn to bottle-feed before he can learn to breastfeed is probably the most common myth of all. It makes hospital staff and others push bottle-feeding to the detriment of breastfeeding. We give babies bottles and then when they don't latch on or don't breastfeed well, we say it's proof that bottle-feeding is easier and babies take more time to learn to breastfeed than to bottle feed. It's completely backwards and wrong.

"Babies with cardiac problems need extra calories without increasing fluid intake." Breastmilk makes babies grow better than formula. We don't understand exactly why, but I have mentioned earlier that exclusively breastfed babies do not increase the volume of milk they take in between one and five months of age, even though the five-month-old is usually twice as heavy as the one-month-old. How can we account for this? There are theories, but the point is that we can't just count calories, protein, fat, etc. and say that, based on what formula-fed babies get, breastmilk is not rich enough to help the cardiac baby grow adequately.

"Babies with heart transplants can't breastfeed because antibodies in the mother's milk will cause rejection of the heart." Heart transplants are not very commonly done in very young babies, but it is likely that, with time, they will become more common for problems such as hypoplastic heart syndrome. In this congenital (present at birth) heart malformation, the left side is hardly developed and unless urgent surgery is performed the baby will die. But the surgery is complex and usually requires three separate operations. It surprises me that doctors say the antibodies in the milk will cause rejection of the heart. Most of the antibodies that appear in breast-milk are sIgA, which are not absorbed into the baby's circulation but stay in the gut to protect him from germs. Neither are the tiny quantities of IgG and IgM absorbed from the gut.

There are other immune factors in the breast-milk, but it seems far-fetched that they would cause rejection of a transplanted heart, especially since most are not absorbed into the bloodstream, and the baby would be taking powerful immune suppressants.

Chylothorax

Some babies with cardiac problems develop chylothorax because the thoracic duct (which carries lymph back into the general circulation via the heart) has been nicked during surgery. With some types of surgery, this injury is almost inevitable. With a chylothorax, the baby's lung cavity fills with lymph, which can compromise his breathing. A tube is placed in the chest to allow the lymph to drain out while the baby is given formula with medium-chained fatty acids that do not (unlike the short- and long-chained ones in breast milk) enter into the lymph but rather directly into the bloodstream. In this way, the volume of lymph decreases.

But it is not necessary to give this special

Mothers' Stories

Trish

My son, Bobby, had just undergone open-heart surgery for the correction of a congenital heart defect. He had sustained a chylothorax, a complication that, according to his surgeon, 30% of pediatric open heart patients will encounter.

Bobby was allowed no food by mouth for two weeks, but the lymph did not subside. The next strategy was to implement Portagen, a specialized formula that consisted of 15% long-chained fatty acids, as opposed to breastmilk, which has 40%. For the next two days, Bobby was given Portagen via a tube placed in his nose, but instead of subsiding, the lymph increased. He was put back on intravenous feeding.

During that time I continued to pump and freeze my milk, praying for the day that Bobby would be able to receive it. Pump, freeze, wait. After weeks of drainage and no food by mouth, Bobby's condition was deteriorating rapidly. I contacted a network of La Leche League leaders and lactation consultants and we came up with a plan.

We needed a centrifuge but didn't have one. My husband, John, decided we could spin the milk in our own Maytag washing machine. He drilled holes in pine boards and put them in the washer so the bottles could sit at the right angle as they spun. We also worked with researchers at the university to find a way to aspirate the fat out of the milk, leaving the skim behind. I found an organic dairy farm that told me about the lab where they had their milk tested for fat content. The results showed that our "Maytag" sample had a lower fat content than the Portagen.

John then purchased a lab-quality centrifuge and set it up in our home. The tests showed that the centrifuged milk had .02% fat per 100 cc of milk. We finally had fat-free milk! We took turns making the skim milk at night, and every day we brought in a fresh batch for Bobby.

As Bobby began receiving my milk, the lymph started to subside. We slowly increased the amount of milk he was receiving and by the end of the week, Bobby was receiving one ounce (30 cc) per hour. When he could tolerate it, the milk was fortified with protein, carbohydrates and special fats he needed.

Bobby began to thrive. The infections subsided, his skin began to heal, the bruises faded away and his vital signs improved. After three months in intensive care, Bobby finally came home. Initially we continued on the skim milk, but after a month, he had trouble gaining weight. We decided it was time to try full milk again, which we introduced very slowly. A month later, Bobby was receiving full-fat breastmilk. We are now doing the whole process backwards and feeding the cream to Bobby at night to increase his calorie content. He is gaining weight beautifully and his strength is increasing.

There was not a doctor at that hospital who would deny that breastmilk saved Bobby's life, and several doctors bluntly told us just that.

---

formula. Medium-chained triglycerides can be added to breastmilk. See the story that follows.

The mother should have been advised to express her milk and then feed the baby the skimmed breastmilk by lactation aid while he sucked on a "dry breast."

Surgery on the baby's gastrointestinal tract

There are several congenital malformations of the intestinal tract that require stopping feeding until the problem is fixed. Most common, I believe, are esophageal atresia (where the esophagus or swallowing tube is a blind pouch with no opening to the stomach), tracheo-esophageal fistula (where there is a connection between the esophagus and the trachea), and gastroschisis (where the intestines have come out of a large hernia in the abdomen).

Below is the story of a mother who succeeded in breastfeeding her baby born with gastroschisis. Normal skin-to-skin contact is not possible with a baby who has gastroschisis since there is often a large amount of intestine outside the body. But the baby's back could be skin to skin with the mother!

Mothers' Stories

My son was diagnosed before birth with gastroschisis, a defect in which the bowel protrudes through the abdominal wall. He was rushed from the maternity hospital to the children's hospital on the other side of the city immediately after he was born.

In preparation for what I knew would be a hard task I took the advice of a lactation consultant before his birth, and began hand-expressing and freezing colostrum four days before he was delivered by elective C-section at 38 weeks.

Once he was born, I began expressing using a hospital pump and soon had an excellent supply of milk in the freezer. Because of his condition he was not allowed to take anything by mouth and was getting fluids and nutrients called TPN (total parenteral nutrition) by a central IV line. He underwent surgery the day after he was born and the large and small intestines that were outside his body were put back in. Following advice from Dr. Jack Newman, as soon as we were able to hold him my husband and I took turns to do as much skin-to-skin contact with him as possible; this was something we had to instigate ourselves; it was never suggested to us by hospital staff, and while all of the nurses seemed to know the term "Kangaroo Care," some were plainly unfamiliar with how it worked, often asking what we would like him wrapped in when they took him from the incubator. Because of his surgery, belly to belly was not possible at first, so I held him, side lying against my belly so the umbilical scar wasn't in contact with my skin.

It took some time before he got to the stage of being able to tolerate oral feeds, and when we reached that point, he was given one millilitre of colostrum per hour by a tube inserted into his stomach via his nose (NG tube). The quantity was very slowly increased over the course of a few weeks and he was weaned off TPN. I was determined to breastfeed exclusively and had done some research and reading about possible pitfalls so I thought I was quite well prepared. The hospital environment was far from ideal. While I was able to sleep in the same room with my son, I had no access to cooking facilities or a fridge, so all food had to be brought in from outside. I did have access to a room with a bed and kitchen facilities, but on the far side of the hospital from my son, so I used it to store my clothing and food.

My son was tolerating the NG infused breastmilk quite well, so we began to try and establish breast-feeding. The NG tube was still in so it was awkward to latch him on; initially his feeds lasted only minutes and he was then "topped up" by NG tube. Gradually the feeds got longer, and the NG tube was removed. Possibly due to overzealous pumping, I had an oversupply of milk, so feeding was pretty difficult. Nursing staff rotated each day so I had different people offering advice all the time (out of interest we counted up the number of nurses and there were 35 in all, and each one had some piece of well-meaning advice regarding breastfeeding, but none were really trained enough to help out with the difficulties I was experiencing). The hospital did not have a lactation consultant. I stayed in touch with my own LC by text message as I wasn't allowed to bring her to the hospital as an outside consultant.

My son was weighed every day—usually at 5:30 a.m. to suit nursing rosters! This daily weighing made me a nervous wreck, waiting to see if he was up or down. He started to have projectile vomiting, which was very distressing for him, causing him to arch his back and paddle his hands while screaming—I was distraught watching him. He was diagnosed with reflux and started on medications for that. He was constantly straining with gas and pain, and developed both umbilical and inguinal hernias. He got a perianal burn and the nurses took a stool sample for testing. The sample was tested for "reducing substances" (considered a sign of lactose intolerance), and came back +3. A consultant neonatologist determined that his weight gain was not adequate, diagnosed transient lactose intolerance and wanted to put him on a lactose-free formula. I was dead-set against this since I had looked into lactose intolerance and oversupply both online and in publications. The dietitian, nurses and neonatologist all said to put him on the formula to let the bowel rest. I knew this was not the right thing to do and kept arguing against it. My husband and family all tried to persuade me to switch to formula and because the neonatologist had diagnosed a problem, they said that I should trust him as he was an expert in caring for surgical and sick babies. I tried block feeding. I tried giving him lactase drops. His weight dropped a few days in a row and I caved in with a heavy heart and he was started on a lactose-free formula.

Five days later there was no improvement and in fact he seemed much worse; his skin was translucent and grey and he was still vomiting. His belly became distended. A senior nurse took a look at him and ordered a battery of tests. All of a sudden there were lots of doctors, lots of questions, X-rays, IV antibiotics. Thirty 15-ml syringes full of air and milk were removed from his belly via the NG tube. Four hours later we were taken aside by the surgical registrar, who explained that our baby had necrotizing enterocolitis (NEC), a life-threatening disease of the bowel. For some reason my husband asked if it was related to formula feeding. It was.

Subsequently we were told NEC was a very common complication of gastroschisis with an incidence rate of 20% and that it might have happened whether we had been feeding breastmilk or formula. We will never know for sure. With tears in his eyes my husband said how sorry he was for having doubted me. I repeatedly stated that if my son pulled through from NEC, we wanted him fed breastmilk. He was given TPN by central IV again, which required a general anaesthetic to put in. After 22 painful days the slow process of reintroducing oral feeds began all over again and soon we were ready to resume breastfeeding. Again I had the same oversupply problems, but my son didn't have the malabsorption symptoms and I found an experienced nurse who helped me with positioning him to improve matters. Slowly he started to gain weight and this time I insisted that he should be weighed only twice a week. Nine long weeks after he was born, we were discharged. He is now four months old, breastfeeding comforts him, and the fact that he breastfeeds comforts me.

The baby with trisomy 21 (Down syndrome)

A baby with trisomy 21 should be able to breastfeed. Many have difficulty in the beginning but once they get going, they usually do well.

Babies with trisomy 21 are hypotonic (they have low muscle tone or are "floppy") to a greater or lesser degree, which can cause difficulty in latching on. In addition they often have large tongues or small mouths. Finally, they tend not to be demanding and thus may not show obvious cues for feeding, and can get into a vicious cycle of not feeding well and not asking to be fed.

Some babies with trisomy 21 have cardiac defects ranging from the very mild to the severe. The approach to the baby with trisomy 21 and a cardiac problem is the same as with any baby with a cardiac abnormality, but the combination of the two conditions can be very challenging.

Some babies with trisomy 21 have intestinal problems, the most common being duodenal atresia, where the duodenum (the part of the gut below the stomach) is not open. A baby with a blockage anywhere in the gut cannot be nourished except by intravenous infusion until the defect has been corrected, usually by surgery. Until then, the mother should express and store her milk and feed it to the baby as soon as he can take tube feedings into the stomach. This is usually done after the surgery if the baby can't go directly to the breast.

Unfortunately, some pediatric surgeons are sold on the notion that predigested formula is better for babies who just had their esophagus or intestines operated on. This is irrational, as breastmilk is not only easy to digest but also includes enzymes that help digestion. Because breastmilk also contains anti-inflammatory properties, the healing of the gut is likely to be less traumatic and more rapid for the baby. Furthermore, the growth factors present in breastmilk help the gut develop and mature. Predigested formulas have no such properties.

Time and patience are necessary to breastfeed the baby with trisomy 21, but the effort should pay off. Alternative feeding methods should be used until the baby can learn to latch on to the breast (see the chapter "When the Baby Does Not Yet Take the Breast"). The mother and baby need experienced and skilled help. As with any baby who does not latch on right away, the most important thing is that the mother develop an abundant milk supply.

Most babies with trisomy 21 will, with good and skilled help, be able to latch on by the age of three or four weeks.

Cystic fibrosis

Cystic fibrosis is an inherited disease most commonly found in people of northern European origin. In order to inherit the illness, the baby has to receive one gene for the disease from each parent.

Children with cystic fibrosis have difficulty digesting their food because they lack, to varying degrees, the pancreatic enzymes that break down fat and protein and allow them to be absorbed. Thus, even if the child takes in a lot of food, he may not gain weight well.

In addition to these problems with digestion, the mucus in the lungs is abnormal and difficult to clear, leading to recurrent infections and damage to the lung. Children with cystic fibrosis can now live into adulthood and with the success of lung transplants can often expect to live a fairly normal life.

Some women with cystic fibrosis are now having their own children. At first there was a concern about the quality of their milk, but there is now sufficient evidence that the milk is fine and that the baby of a mother with cystic fibrosis will thrive on breastfeeding. The baby of a mother with

cystic fibrosis will be a carrier for the disease but won't have it unless he also inherits a gene from the father.

Very few babies with cystic fibrosis are breastfed, unfortunately. Yet these children benefit greatly from breastfeeding. The immune factors in breastmilk help to protect them from infections which can often be very difficult to treat. The enzymes in the breastmilk usually cannot make up for the lack of enzymes produced by the pancreas, but breastfeeding may reduce the need for supplemental enzymes.

There is now evidence that the baby with cystic fibrosis has better preservation of his lung function when breastfed. Considering that deterioration of lung function and lung infections are what cause the most difficult health issues, this is very important.

Why are so few babies with cystic fibrosis breastfed? Some health professionals believe that when a mother is faced with a devastating diagnosis for her baby, it is better not to add the "stress" and "pain" of breastfeeding. It is much easier to formula feed. At best, mothers are told to express their milk, put it into a bottle and add the enzymes to it. At worst, they are told to forget their milk and give formulas that are predigested. It is really a shame that health professionals think this way.

This approach does not take into account the special relationship that develops during breastfeeding, never mind the protection against infection, the digestive enzymes and the preservation of lung function associated with breastfeeding. The special relationship provides significant benefits to the child facing a lifelong disease which in many cases entails frequent hospitalizations and treatments. And the comfort to the mother should not be ignored, as it frequently is.

In order to determine the amount of enzymes to use to help the baby digest protein and fat, he is put on formula with a known amount of fat and bowel movements are collected for five days. Most normal babies lose less than 10% of the fat in their bowel movements. Most babies with cystic fibrosis lose a lot more. Breastfed babies bottle-fed formula for five days often won't return to the breast.

The amount of enzyme used is, in any case, a guess, and is adjusted depending on the growth of the baby. A trial and error approach to the amount of enzymes given helps to preserve the breastfeeding. I am hearing that many centres treating children with cystic fibrosis no longer do the five-day stool collection, and I hope the rest abandon the practice.

Most babies with cystic fibrosis will need enzyme replacement. For bottle-fed babies, this is simple enough and the enzymes are added to the formula.

How should a breastfeeding baby receive enzymes? The mother expresses a little milk, mixes it with the enzymes and gives it to the baby with a lactation aid at the breast toward the *beginning* of the feeding. The enzymes may irritate her skin, but given early on, milk will bathe the nipples and the baby will suck actively, so the enzymes will be washed off. Using a little of our all-purpose nipple ointment before feeding can help, too.

Some doctors say that because CF babies become dehydrated more easily they need to be bottle-fed to ensure that they are drinking enough. This is a classic example of how breastfeeding is sacrificed on the altar of ignorance: if doctors know how to tell when the baby is drinking at the breast, and share that information with the mother, then it is easy to know if the baby is getting enough.

Cleft palate

One of the most difficult problems preventing babies from breastfeeding is a cleft palate. A cleft may be complete or partial. It may involve both sides of the midline or just one.

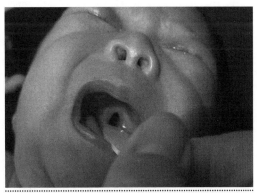

This baby has a cleft of the soft palate, which was not diagnosed in hospital. A baby with this type of cleft may take the breast into his mouth, but each time he sucks he makes a smacking sound. When a baby doesn't latch on and makes smacking sounds, one should look at the palate.

CREDIT: JACK NEWMAN

Usually the cleft palate is visible in an ultrasound done during the pregnancy. Sometimes, however, it may not be noticed until the baby is at the breast. In our clinic, we have seen at least five babies in a single year whose cleft palate was missed in hospital and during the well-baby examination. Teresa has also sent a few mothers back to their doctors to have a cleft palate diagnosed after watching the baby at the breast. When these babies suck, they are not latched on (they slip off the breast easily) but make a clicking noise with each suck. If this clicking noise is heard, in conjunction with not latching on (some babies that are latched on may make the sound, but that doesn't imply a cleft palate) the baby's palate should then be promptly checked by a doctor or a nurse.

A baby with a cleft palate has great difficulty latching on and if he cannot latch on, he cannot get milk well from the breast. Some, maybe a tiny minority of babies, can actually manage to get a good amount of milk from the breast because the mother's milk supply is so abundant. Unfortunately, many cleft palate programmes insist the mother not even try to breastfeed because the baby can't, but I think this is the wrong approach.

First of all, the baby might just be one of the rare ones who does get enough milk. Furthermore, I believe it is important that mothers try so that if it doesn't work, at least they can feel they did try. See on our YouTube website the video of a baby with a cleft of the soft palate who breastfeeds with a lactation aid at the breast (http://youtu.be/9UJD-C3WHY8s).

Maybe if we tried to get babies with cleft palates to latch on instead of dismissing the possibility out of hand, we would find more techniques that work. In our clinic, we have not had huge success with cleft palates, but we often see the baby only after he has been bottle-fed for some weeks. Indeed, the one time I diagnosed a cleft of the soft palate like the one in the photo on page 255, the baby was doing well because of the mother's abundant milk production, but the cleft palate programme had told the mother to take the baby off the breast, so blinkered were they in their approach that "babies with cleft palate need to be bottle-fed."

Some palate clefts can and should be repaired immediately after birth, and then the the baby can breastfeed much more easily.

In some centres, babies with cleft palates are fitted with obdurators. These are plastic devices that fill in the cleft. They are not used frequently in North America, but I hear that they are used in Switzerland and that babies can, apparently, latch on and breastfeed when these are in place. I cannot verify this personally, but it makes sense to try, especially since they apparently help the baby's speech develop better.

Not that long ago, breastmilk was not considered important for babies with cleft palates, but when studies came out that showed that babies with cleft palates had fewer ear infections when fed breastmilk rather than formula, attitudes began to change.

When a baby is born with a cleft palate, the mother should start expressing her milk as soon as is practical, within two to three hours of the baby's birth, but for the first hour or two, the baby and mother should be skin to skin. There is no rush to separate mother and baby if the baby is otherwise well. This time is important for the mother and baby to bond with each other, especially since the baby's appearance may be unusual and this bonding time can help the mother connect to and accept her baby. And who knows, maybe the baby will latch on as he crawls to the breast?

Expressing milk can help develop an abundant milk supply, so that if the baby allows the breast into his mouth or latches on at all, he'll get milk. Even when bottle-fed, many babies with cleft palate do not gain weight well. It is worth giving breastfeeding a chance. In the first few days, babies need very little milk. By "allowing" breastfeeding in the first few days, it is possible that the baby might learn how to adapt to the mother's breast. Breast compression may help the baby get more milk. Any additional milk he might need can be given by lactation aid at the breast or by cup or spoon.

If, even with good skilled help, it is impossible to get the baby breastfeeding, he can still get breastmilk. There is an additional reason for this: some of the milk the baby drinks will invariably come out of his nose. Formula is quite irritating to the nasal passages; breastmilk is not. Also, the baby will often choke and milk will sometimes go down the wrong way; it this happens, it is much better for it to be breastmilk than formula. In some centres, the cleft palate is fixed early, within the first couple of weeks. It is not too late in such cases to get the baby to the breast. Unfortunately, plastic surgeons often tell mothers that they cannot put the baby to the breast for several days to several weeks after surgery—two weeks is typical. But the mother's breast is much softer than a nipple made of latex or plastic, and it should not affect the suture line.

Cleft lip without cleft palate

Babies with a cleft lip alone should not have real difficulty breastfeeding. Many go to the breast easily and breastfeed well. The mother can position the baby so that her breast covers or fills in the cleft in the lip. Thus, if the cleft is on the right side (it is rarely in the midline), the mother can feed the baby on the left side using a cross-cradle hold with the baby leaning slightly upward, which is a good position anyway. On the right side, the mother can use the football hold. Or she can use her finger or some non-allergenic tape to seal the cleft. Once the alveolar ridge (where the teeth will eventually be) is involved, the situation becomes more difficult but not impossible. See photo opposite.

Getting the baby to breastfeed after surgery for cleft lip or cleft palate

It is usually difficult to get a baby who has been bottle-fed for months because of cleft lip or cleft palate to breastfeed, but it is worth a try. If, however, the baby was breastfeeding before surgery, he can continue afterwards. In the past, surgeons were concerned that breastfeeding might result in poor wound healing or damage to the stitches, but there is no evidence of this and no reason to expect it. Today, most surgeons do not advise mothers to stop breastfeeding after surgery, or if they do, it is for only a day or two. Undoubtedly, the baby's pain will be more significant in the first 24 hours.

But what if the baby is 10 months old, has been bottle-fed until now and has finally had the cleft palate repaired? Is it possible to get him breastfeeding? Well, it might be. This is discussed in greater detail in the chapter "Induced Lactation and Relactation," but here are the steps:

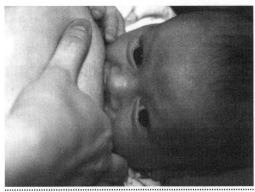

A baby with a cleft lip latched on and breastfeeding. A cleft lip without an accompanying cleft palate should not, in itself, cause difficulties in latching on. This baby latched on easily.

CREDIT: JACK NEWMAN

1. Stop all bottles and use an open cup to give the baby liquids, particularly your own milk.

2. The baby can also have liquids mixed with solids, which presumably by 10 months he is taking. The baby will still want to suck, and with no bottles may be more willing to take the breast.

3. Keep the baby as much as possible in skin-to-skin contact, with your breast available. In the night and during naps, cuddle in bed with the baby, with him in just a diaper, and your upper body exposed. (There is no reason this type of skin-to-skin contact could not be initiated from birth, well before the repair is done.) Of course, safe co-bedding should be the rule; see the chapter "Sleep: Yours and Your Baby's." You can also use a carrier or a sling to carry your baby around.

Even if your milk supply is more than adequate, increasing it will often give the baby a reason to latch on. Domperidone can be particularly useful at this time. We start with a dose of three tablets (30 mg) three times a day.

Phenylketonuria

It is not possible in a book this size to discuss every possible illness a baby may have or develop, but I wanted to include this rare disease as an example of how breastfeeding solutions can often be found even when mothers have been told it is impossible.

Phenylketonuria (PKU) is what is called an "inborn error of metabolism," which means the baby is lacking or has an abnormal enzyme necessary to metabolize something in the body. In the case of PKU, the problem is with phenylalanine, an amino acid that is normally converted to another amino acid, tyrosine. When the enzyme converting phenylalanine to tyrosine is absent, or insufficient, phenylalanine builds up and may cause seizures and severe developmental problems.

Babies in all jurisdictions in North America and Western Europe are screened for PKU with a blood test soon after birth. If a low phenylalanine intake is instituted early enough, the problems associated with PKU can be prevented or at least diminished significantly.

For a long time, it was felt that breastfeeding could not be allowed. Since "normal" formulas contained too much phenylalanine and "normal" formulas were based on breastmilk, there had to be too much phenylalanine in breastmilk. Once again, this turned out to be false; breastmilk contains significantly less phenylalanine than "normal" formulas. Since everyone needs some phenylalanine—but not too much—experts in this field began to believe that the baby with PKU could get at least some breastmilk.

At the Hospital for Sick Children in Toronto in the 1980s, a new approach to feeding babies who had PKU was instituted. The dietetic's department would calculate how much low phenylalanine formula the baby would require, based on his initial blood levels and adjustments made for the effect of treatment.

The amount of phenylalanine in breastmilk was now taken into account. An estimate of the amount of breastmilk and special formula the baby needed was calculated and mothers instructed as follows:

1. The baby would be weighed before a feeding (a scale was provided).
2. The baby would breastfeed on each side for 10 minutes and then be re-weighed.
3. The rest of the feeding, based on the weight gain, subtracted from the total calculated to be given to the baby, was given as low phenylalanine formula.
4. By following the baby's phenylalanine levels weekly, adjustments could be made to the amount of formula given.

Anyone who has read the chapter "Increasing Breastmilk Intake by the Baby" in this book should immediately understand why this didn't work. Aside from the inconvenience to the mother of carrying around a scale everywhere she went and weighing the baby before and after breastfeeding, the baby eventually got used to the bottle and refused to take the breast. Mothers were nervous about feeding 10 minutes on each side, worrying that if they went to 11 minutes, the baby would get too much phenylalanine. Breastfeeding rarely lasted more than two weeks.

Taking into account some basic breastfeeding principles, I was able to suggest the following changes to the approach:

1. The dietitians calculated the amount of special formula the baby needed.
2. The entire amount of formula was given at the breast with a lactation aid *at the beginning* of the feeding.
3. The baby breastfed until he did not want any more.

There was no problem with the baby refusing the breast and the baby was able to suck at the breast as long as he wanted rather than being "ripped from the breast" at a certain time. No need for weighing or timing or bottles. The babies' phenylalanine levels were well controlled.

As a result, during the first year of the programme using my approach, at least one baby breastfed 18 months, and several breastfed for six months. One baby who had atypical PKU, which is uncommon, was able to breastfeed exclusively.

Women with PKU who are pregnant has now become an issue. Most children who need to be on the special low-PKU diet are able to go to a normal diet as adults but when women with PKU become pregnant, it is recommended that they go back on their diet to keep phenylalanine levels getting to the baby from being too high. The baby is unlikely to have PKU unless the father is a carrier of the gene. If the father has PKU, the chances for the baby having it are 100%. When breastfeeding, mothers should stay on the low-PKU diet even if the baby does not have PKU. Whether this is necessary or not is unknown, since if the baby has the enzyme to metabolize the phenylalanine, there should be no problem, but it is considered prudent.

Breastfeeding before surgery and after

Until recently many babies needing surgery were forced to fast beginning at midnight on the day of the operation. This approach is disappearing with the knowledge that breastmilk exits rapidly from the stomach and that aspiration of breastmilk is far less harmful than the recommended "clear fluids" allowed until two or three hours before surgery. There are still some hospitals that impose long periods of fasting on young babies before surgery. This is not good for the baby, and it's unnecessary. Parents should find hospitals where this is not the rule. Even fasting for six hours is a terrible hardship for both the breastfeeding mother and her baby. Many babies won't take a bottle or even a cup or spoon of the apple juice that is recommended. Many still wake up frequently in the night and react strongly if not fed, sometimes crying for hours. The situation is worse when surgery is delayed, as it often is. Six hours of fasting often becomes eight or even more. The whole process becomes torture for the baby and his parents.

Some children's hospitals are more enlightened: Boston Children's and Philadelphia Children's now allow breastfeeding up to three hours before surgery. Unfortunately, most Canadian hospitals have not yet caught up.

Incidentally, especially for the toddler, it would be much easier if surgery were scheduled for the afternoon instead of the morning. It's easier to distract a toddler from breastfeeding during the day, even if the fasting period is unnecessarily long.

After the surgery, if there is no reason to restrict oral feedings, the breastfed baby can go to the breast as soon as he is awake. It is a great comfort for the baby to be able to breastfeed. Surgery is a frightening business for an adult who has some idea of what has happened; a baby or toddler doesn't understand any of this. Many hospital protocols require the child to drink a clear fluid before being permitted to go to the breast in case of aspiration. This is yet another example of thinking that formula is basically the same as breastmilk; if the baby aspirates, the anti-inflammatory factors in breastmilk will minimize any reaction. Also, unlike bottle-feeding, breastfeeding is an *active* process. If the baby is awake enough to breastfeed, he has the gag reflex necessary to avoid aspiration. Bottle-feeding is more passive; a baby can drink without being completely awake and with little participation.

If the baby is hospitalized

Some hospitals do not encourage or even permit parents to stay with their children. This is a ridiculous policy. Even if hospital policy "allows" parents to stay, many staff discourage it. Mothers are often told they need to go home and rest, that they will do the baby more good if they get a good night's sleep, that their presence is making the baby "unsettled." This can be really difficult for the mother to deal with because likely she is tired both physically and mentally.

The hospital may permit parents to stay with the child but will not provide any sleeping facilities so the mother has to sit beside her child in a hard chair.

Usually if mothers go home as they are encouraged to do, they don't sleep anyway; they worry about the baby and have to get up to express milk. The mother with other children at home finds herself torn between her baby, who needs her comfort and her breast, and her family, who also need her.

Support from partner, family and friends is critical in making this situation bearable. Be firm with hospital personnel about how important breastfeeding is for you and your child. Your child needs breastmilk and breastfeeding more when he is ill, not less. Maybe your partner or a friend can stay with the baby while you nap, and come to wake you if the baby needs to breastfeed. If you have other children, maybe you can arrange to have them brought to the hospital for visits. Some enlightened hospital policies include family rooms near the pediatric or neonatal unit or have a small residence near the hospital for parents who live some distance away, and the entire family can come and spend most of the day near the mother and the sick child.

If you can't stay at the hospital, express your milk while you are separated. Bring what you get to the hospital for your baby. Keeping up the milk supply will make it easier when the baby is ready to take the breast again full-time.

The bottom line

Most rules for not breastfeeding sick children are based on nothing more than a lack of knowledge and understanding of how breastfeeding works. If there is a will to keep breastfeeding, a way can often be found. It takes commitment on the part of the mother and good support. Unfortunately, good support is not always available.

For information on breastfeeding the premature baby, see the chapter "The Preterm and Near-term Baby."

17 | Induced Lactation and Relactation

Myth #1: If a woman has never been pregnant, she cannot produce milk for an adopted baby.

Fact: Not true. A woman with a functioning pituitary gland and breasts can produce milk.

Myth #2: Most women inducing lactation will not produce all the milk the baby needs, so it's not worth trying.

Fact: Some women *will* produce all the milk their babies need. In fact, we've had a few mothers who induced lactation for twins and produced plenty of milk for both babies, and I have a report of a mother who induced lactation and exclusively breastfed triplets. However, breastfeeding is so much more than breastmilk. Even if the mother cannot produce all the milk the baby needs, she *can* still breastfeed, and both she and her baby will benefit.

Myth #3: There are many reasons why mothers must stop breastfeeding: medications, illness, the baby not getting enough milk, the mother having sore nipples, etc.

Fact: This is almost never true. The vast majority of medications are compatible with continued breastfeeding; most maternal illnesses do not require a mother to stop breastfeeding; the baby not getting enough milk from the breast should be managed without taking the baby off the breast; sore nipples can be fixed without taking the baby off the breast. It is much better to help mothers with these issues without taking the baby off the breast and therefore without requiring relactation.

Myth #4: Once a mother has stopped breastfeeding, she cannot go back.

Fact: Many mothers have gone back to breastfeeding, sometimes four or five months or longer after the baby has been completely on the bottle and formula. The sooner the baby is put back to the breast, and the greater the milk supply, the easier it is to restart breastfeeding. Skilled, knowledgeable, hands-on help can make all the difference.

Terminology

For the sake of convenience, throughout this discussion I will use the terms "adopting mother" for the mother-to-be who is adopting a baby, "carrier mother" for the mother who is pregnant with the baby, and "adopted baby" for the baby born to one mother and raised by the "adopting mother," recognizing that some babies are born through surrogate carriers who are pregnant with the ovum of the adopting mother and the sperm of the adopting mother's male partner and are thus not technically "adopted." Although "biological mother" is often applied to the woman who is pregnant with the baby, in the case of a surrogate carrier, the sperm and ovum are actually from the "adopting" parents and thus the mother "adopting" the baby is actually also the "biological mother."

This chapter takes a different approach than that of the Newman-Goldfarb protocols published in 2003. I believe this different approach is less complicated. Of course, every mother's situation is different. For example, in some cases women over the age of 40 or 45 may be reluctant to take estrogens and their doctors may be reluctant to prescribe them, but such issues should be approached case by case. After all, some adopting mothers in this age group may be on estrogens as part of hormonal replacement therapy and should be able to continue the hormones, although the way they take them may be different (see below).

Why should a woman adopting a baby or getting a baby by surrogate bother breastfeeding?

For the same reasons that *any* mother wants to breastfeed her baby. Breastfeeding is good for the baby and the mother. There are risks to artificial feeding. It is true that many adopting mothers will not produce all the milk the baby needs, but some milk is still valuable.

Also, studies show that babies who are adopted, even adopted from birth, are more likely to have difficulties with adaptation and attachment. Breastfeeding can help them overcome some of these difficulties.

The woman who has not been able to get pregnant has other reasons to breastfeed as well. Being able to breastfeed successfully, even if the mother is not able to produce all the milk the baby needs, compensates, in some measure, for feeling that her body has "failed" her for not birthing a baby. For an adopting mother, breastfeeding her adopted baby means a close physical relationship that makes it much easier for her to see that baby as truly hers. The first time the baby latches on, mothers describe feeling accepted by the baby and this enhances attachment. Breastfeeding can be very powerful in strengthening the mother-baby relationship.

For some mothers only a full supply of breastmilk will do; for others, simply getting the baby to take the breast is success. It's important to keep expectations realistic. Most women who have never been pregnant will *not* produce enough milk for the needs of the adopted baby. Even if they have previously breastfed one or more babies successfully, there is no guarantee of a full milk supply. Nevertheless, even if the mother needs to supplement, the baby is still getting some milk from the breast. As the baby begins to eat sufficient amounts of solids, supplementation can often be stopped and the baby can be breastfed and eat solids until mother and baby decide to wean.

So what's the approach?

There really are two facets to inducing lactation:

1.   Making milk
2.   Getting the baby to take the breast

In my opinion, getting the baby to take the breast is by far the most important part of all this. Once the baby takes the breast, the mother is breastfeeding, and as a result, milk production is likely to increase, because a baby suckling *well* at the breast stimulates milk production much better than a pump. Furthermore, if the baby is at the breast and breastfeeding, the mother is encouraged.

As a general rule, we discourage pumping *once the baby is breastfeeding*. Why?

1.   Pumping is expensive (it requires renting or buying a machine).
2.   Pumping can be tiring and time consuming.
3.   Pumping diminishes the mother's enjoyment of breastfeeding.
4.   Pumping, if not done properly, may cause sore nipples.
5.   Pumping does not accurately tell the mother how much milk she is producing or what the baby can get at the breast. Mothers too often look at what they pump and get discouraged.

6. Pumping is like compression, but with compression the mother can express into the baby instead of a bottle.

And sometimes, mothers concentrate more on pumping than breastfeeding. However, in the case of induced lactation, we do want the mothers to express or pump *before* the baby is born. See below.

Making milk
"Simulating pregnancy"
The basis of our approach to inducing lactation is to make the mother's body believe it is pregnant. During pregnancy, hormones prepare the breasts for breastfeeding by increasing the numbers of milk-producing cells and ducts. These changes begin within days of the embryo implanting on the wall of the uterus. By about 16 weeks the mother is starting to produce colostrum.

Estrogen is said to stimulate the growth of the duct system, while progesterone stimulates the growth of the milk-producing cells. Probably their functions overlap. Prolactin also is released in large amounts from the pituitary gland. Prolactin stimulates the production of milk, but its action is inhibited during pregnancy by progesterone and estrogen.

Preparing the breast with medication
It is not necessary to take medication in order to breastfeed the adopted baby. Some mothers choose not to use the medication, and I certainly respect that. It is likely that they will produce less milk without them. However, some mothers who take medication still don't make much milk. The goal, as I see it anyway, is breastfeeding, not necessarily a full supply of breastmilk.

Some women cannot take progesterone or estrogen for various reasons such as clotting disorders, recurrent migraine headaches, high blood pressure or a history of breast cancer. The adopting mother should check with her family physician before starting any treatment. Some physicians are reluctant to prescribe these hormones for women over 40. In our breastfeeding clinic, we insist that women who take estrogen and progesterone be followed by their own family doctor to make sure, before the medication is begun, that:

1. The adopting mother has no contraindications to taking progesterone and estrogen.
2. The adopting mother has a pap test done before starting the hormones.
3. The adopting mother understands the risks of taking these hormones (though we discuss them as well in the clinic).

Progesterone and estrogen
A combination birth control pill gives the mother both progesterone and estrogen. The blood concentrations achieved with the combination birth control pill are undoubtedly lower than if produced from the placenta, but still seem to work. There are various theories about the ratio of progesterone to estrogen that should be used, but I am not convinced it makes much difference as long as the adopting mother gets both. Some physicians or lactation consultants who are concerned about the mother taking estrogen may prescribe only the progesterone, and there is likely still some benefit. Is the effect as great as if the mother takes both hormones? I don't know, but I would assume that it is not.

The longer the adopting mother can be on the hormones, the better for milk production. Ideally, she should stay on them for nine months, but generally we ask her to stop them six to eight weeks before the baby is due. The adopting mother should take the pills every day, without a break (no placebos) so that her hormone levels are kept high, just as if she were pregnant. If the adopting mother is taking only progesterone, she could have vaginal bleeding (breakthrough bleeding). Any bleeding while taking the hormones should be checked out with her doctor.

When the adopting mother stops the hormones, she will have vaginal bleeding, perhaps heavier than usual. At this time she should start to express her milk.

Why take the hormones only until six to eight weeks before the baby is born?

1. The mother uses this time to express her milk and increase milk production, so that when the baby is born she has a good supply. If the baby is born prematurely, the mother still may have had enough time to get her milk production going.
2. Although it may take two or three weeks to get even drops of milk, the adopting mother can find this very reassuring.

I prefer that the adopting mother be on the hormones, if she decides to take them, for at least three months. But what if the baby is due in a much shorter period of time? In this case, I usually suggest the mother not take the hormones at all, but proceed with taking steps to build her milk supply.

Domperidone

Domperidone is a drug used to improve the symptoms of reflux in children, including babies, and adults, and to improve the emptying of the stomach in people with gastroparesis (stomach weakness). However, domperidone also interferes with the action of dopamine on the pituitary. Dopamine, made in the hypothalamus of the brain, inhibits the release of prolactin from the pituitary. Therefore, domperidone indirectly stimulates the release of prolactin from the pituitary.

We start with a dose of three tablets (30 mg)

three times a day (nine tablets a day). Others suggest starting with a lower dose and building up to prevent side effects, but side effects are uncommon. If there is plenty of time before the baby is due, then building up is fine, perhaps starting with one tablet (10 mg) three times a day and then increasing the dose over the next two or three weeks to three tablets (30 mg) three times a day. With less time, it is better to start with three tablets (30 mg) three times a day. We have gone up to four tablets (40 mg) three times a day (12 tablets a day) and sometimes four tablets (40 mg) four times a day (16 tablets a day). **US residents note:** If the domperidone is being made up in a compounding pharmacy, the pharmacy may make up pills that contain 20 or 30 mg of domperidone, unlike the manufacturer's 10 mg pills.

We recommend the adopting mother start taking domperidone at the same time as the birth control pill, if she is taking it, and to continue after she stops the hormones. Often the adopting mother needs to stay on domperidone for the entire time she is breastfeeding. She might be able to reduce the dose once the breastfeeding is well established, but we recommend she maintain the dose that works best at least until the baby is well established on solid foods. Even then, she may need to continue the domperidone.

See more information about domperidone and its possible side effects in the chapter "Increasing Breastmilk Intake by the Baby."

The non-pregnant member of a gay couple wants to induce lactation

At first, when couples began asking me about this, I was uncertain. I am reluctant to use medications unnecessarily, and I worried about treating the non-pregnant partner with medication that could potentially cause significant side effects even if they are rare. After all, the pregnant mother should be able to breastfeed the baby exclusively. The non-pregnant partner can put the baby to her breast, calm him and bond with him. She might even produce some milk simply because the baby suckles at her breast. I worried that inducing lactation in the non-pregnant member was the same as the father giving the baby a bottle so he can bond with him. I disagree with this approach even if it is breastmilk in the bottle.

I posted the question about gay couples on Lactnet (a lactation listserve where several thousand people, mostly lactation consultants, write about various breastfeeding issues). I was surprised by the almost complete agreement of the posts that, despite the possible side effects of the drugs, they would not hesitate to induce lactation in the non-pregnant partner (or "other" mother). Basically, I was told that women are different and their reactions to babies are different from men's. The need to put the baby to the breast is powerful; not being able to do so causes great distress in many women. If the non-pregnant partner in the relationship could not put the baby to the breast, she might feel extremely disappointed, even devastated.

I knew this, too, from reading so many emails from mothers describing their unhappiness and distress at the thought of not being able to continue breastfeeding or to latch the baby on, or even because they were using a nipple shield. These reactions are not due to breastfeeding advocates scaring them with stories about "bad bad formula" but come from a deep physical and emotional need to nurture their babies at the breast. Family and physicians are often amazed by how mothers continue to breastfeed despite excruciating pain in the nipples or continue trying to latch on a resistant baby; they continue to breastfeed or keep on trying, knowing nobody would blame them if they stopped.

I think the notion of the father helping by giving the baby a bottle is a misguided notion encouraged by formula marketing. It seems so reasonable! Surely it is important that the father bond with the baby, isn't it? Of course, but there are many ways that a father can bond with a baby. Caring for a baby is not just about feeding him. When a baby cries, helping him calm down makes the father to realize how much he means to the baby. And when the baby falls asleep in his arms, what a pleasure it is for the father! On the other hand, feeding a baby a bottle reinforces the false notion that bottle-feeding and breastfeeding are essentially the same. They are not, and in fact even feeding the baby breastmilk in the bottle changes our image of breastmilk into just another formula—a better formula for sure, but a product just like any other. What a father can do to help is discussed in greater depth in the chapter "Breastfeeding and Family Relationships."

Nipple confusion is real. How many emails have I received outlining the progression from "one bottle in the evening" to two bottles and then three because the baby doesn't seem to be satisfied any more at the breast? Many! And soon, pumped milk is not enough and the mother must now give the baby formula. And it goes downhill from there. I get daily emails from mothers who say "I am now exclusively bottle-feeding my baby. Can you help me get him back to the breast?" There are many reasons why mothers end up in this situation, but the "give the father a chance to feed the baby" is the thin edge of the wedge for many. Specialized bottle nipples that claim to be designed not to cause nipple confusion have not been independently validated.

Also, of course, where the partner is a woman, the baby gets the breast, not a bottle. He still has skin-to-skin contact, in this case the "other" mother.

So I agreed to help the non-pregnant mother

induce lactation. I am convinced it was the right decision.

The non-pregnant mother in this situation can continue the hormones, if she wishes, until the baby is born, if there would not have been sufficient time on the hormones to prepare the breasts adequately. On the other hand, if she's had more than five months, she can stop some time before the baby is born and begin expressing milk again to help build up a reserve.

One last thought. I worried about the "other mother" putting the baby to the breast for another reason. New mothers are often very possessive of their babies. Though they are sometimes happy to get help holding the baby for a while, they can also resent it. I can see how sharing could potentially create tension between two mothers. Does it? We have not heard.

The baby is born. What now?

Of course it is best if the adopting mother can put the baby to the breast immediately after the birth. In privately arranged adoptions or when there is a surrogate carrier, this may not be an issue. The sooner the baby goes to the breast, the less likely he is to refuse. Among the adopting mothers I have dealt with (several hundred), only two babies ever refused the breast. In one case, the baby did take the breast after a couple of weeks and went on to breastfeed for over 18 months. In another case, the baby did not latch on, but the mother's family was very negative about the whole process and very strongly discouraged her from trying. She did stop trying very quickly.

Why do we see so many babies born in hospital who refuse to latch on and not see this when the mother is breastfeeding an adopted baby or a baby born by surrogate? I find this very interesting and I think it speaks to the practices around labour and birth that make it difficult for the baby to latch on. See the chapter "How Birth Affects Breastfeeding."

Should the gestational carrier or the biological mother breastfeed?

The biological mother (or gestational carrier) will have colostrum and it would be good if the baby got the colostrum from the woman who carried him. This does not mean that only the biological mother should breastfeed during the first few days. The adopting mother should also be breastfeeding, which actually gives the baby a double advantage: the immunity of the carrier and the adopting mother. If the carrier mother breastfeeds for more than a few days, and the baby breastfeeds well, it will prevent her from getting painful engorgement on the third or fourth day after birth. In some cases, the carrier mother has expressed milk for several weeks and donated it to the adopting mother so that she can give it to the baby by lactation aid at the breast.

On the other hand, we cannot ignore the fact that breastfeeding results in a very close association between mother and baby and may make it even more difficult for the carrier mother to separate from the baby; it can be a heart-wrenching experience. However, none of the adopting mothers who have come to see us have reported a carrier mother who breastfed and refused to give up the baby.

Once the baby is home with the adopting mother, the approach is the same as if he were not adopted. If supplementation is needed, it should be given with a lactation aid at the breast. Here is the approach, already outlined in more detail in the chapter "Increasing Breastmilk Intake by the Baby."

1. The mother gets the best latch possible, an "asymmetric" latch. See photos on pages 67–70.
2. The mother observes the baby at the breast to see whether he is actually drinking. See the videos at www.breastfeedinginc.ca.
3. Once the baby is mostly nibbling, or drinking only a little, the mother uses breast compression

to keep him drinking. When compression no longer works, the mother switches the baby to the other side and repeats the process.

4. If the baby feeds from both sides and still needs milk, the mother supplements with a lactation aid at the breast. She does not give him a set amount, but lets the baby drink as much as he wants.

5. I do not think the mother should pump her milk to increase her supply or to supplement the baby. Once the baby is breastfeeding, it becomes a burden to keep pumping. Breastfeeding can be and should be a pleasure for the mother, not work. In any case, compression is like pumping, but doesn't require a pump and the milk goes directly into the baby.

What if the baby is not a newborn, but six months or even older?

We see this often in international adoptions. The approach to preparing the breast and making the milk is no different, but getting the baby to the breast may be more of a problem. The approach is more like that of getting the baby back to the breast when the mother wishes to restart breastfeeding after having stopped for some time (see Relactation, page 268). Especially with international adoptions, it is possible the baby was breastfed previously. So:

1. If the mother makes a fair amount of milk, that's good. If the baby goes to the breast and gets milk, he may stay there.

2. The baby should not receive any more bottles. A baby of six months or more can drink from an open cup or have milk mixed with his solids. If he is eating plenty of solids, the milk mixed with the solids can be whole milk. There is no "need" for formula for a year or more. If the mother is producing some milk, the baby can receive it from an open cup. He will smell the same odour when he is near the mother's breast. If the baby drinks from a sippy cup, he is more likely to smell plastic than breastmilk. A sippy cup is essentially a bottle. It is also better for the baby not to get a pacifier.

3. The mother (and father) should keep the baby skin to skin as much as possible during the day and he should sleep in the same bed with them; the mother should be undressed from the waist up. The baby should be in a diaper only. In their "half-sleep" some babies will latch on. Taking baths with the baby can also be helpful.

4. Trying to force a baby to take the breast will not work and should be avoided. It is better to go slowly and accept that the baby may take some time to realize he can get milk from the breast.

An issue sometimes comes up when a baby is put into foster care (generally with a view to later adoption). For reasons that are not clear to me, child protection services in some jurisdictions are dead set against the foster mother breastfeeding the baby. There are, I suppose, three possibilities: the baby will remain in care permanently and move through the adoption process; the baby will return to his biological family after some period in foster care; or the baby's future is uncertain. In the latter two cases, the parents could be asked permission for the foster mother to breastfeed the baby. In the first case, why would child protection services care? Unfortunately, like most of society, child protection workers rarely know much about breastfeeding and the many ways it can protect the baby's health.

Relactation

Mothers are told to stop breastfeeding for invalid reasons. If the mother stops because she is in terrible pain, this is understandable, but often the need to take the baby off the breast could have been prevented or resolved if she'd gotten better help. I get emails almost every day from mothers who regret having stopped breastfeeding and want to restart. These mothers often feel that they have lost something very important when they no longer breastfeed. Or perhaps they find that their babies don't tolerate formula well. Many mothers don't know that relactation is possible, and neither do their doctors. So they may be told just to change to another formula, which is no solution, rarely being told about restarting breastfeeding. **It is better not to stop breastfeeding than to relactate!**

Why do mothers stop breastfeeding?

1. The mother is put on medication and told that it is dangerous to continue breastfeeding while on this medication. Many health professionals also believe that, after breastfeeding is interrupted, starting again is really no problem. In fact, "interrupting" breastfeeding too often leads to stopping altogether. See the chapter "Breastfeeding While on Medication."

    • Most medications do *not* require a mother to stop or interrupt breastfeeding. When there is a real issue, it is sometimes possible to find another medication that treats the mother but does not pose risks to the baby.

    • In the vast majority of cases the tiny amount of drug that enters the milk is much less potentially harmful than putting the baby on infant formula.

2. The mother's nipples are sore.

    • Taking the baby off the breast for nipple soreness should be a last resort only. Unfortunately, too often it is recommended almost immediately, and after a few days off the breast, the baby may refuse to latch on. Or he returns to the breast with the type of latch and suck he uses for a bottle, and the soreness begins again.

    • Much can be done to treat sore nipples before taking the baby off the breast. See the chapter "Sore Nipples."

3. The mother is told by her health provider to take the baby off the breast and pump her milk because they are worried he is not getting enough milk from the breast. This is not the way to deal with the problem. What do we learn from knowing that the baby is now getting, say, 90 ml (3 oz.) of breastmilk from the bottle? It is not possible to compare breastmilk to formula. They are different, and 90 ml of breastmilk does not equal 90 ml of formula.

    • Perhaps the health provider believes that by pumping they know how much the baby is getting from the breast. But this is not true. What a mother can pump says nothing about what the baby is getting from the breast. A baby who is well latched on can get more than the mother pumps, especially if she is using compression to keep up the flow. A baby who is latched on poorly will get less than the mother can pump. If, as is often the case, the mother is able to pump what one "expects" the baby to get, a whole investigation for "failure to thrive" may be instituted even if the baby starts to gain well on the pumped milk. The obvious conclusion—that the baby is not getting what is available to him and the reason is a poor latch and poor breastfeeding "technique"— is not considered.

    • Perhaps the health provider believes that pumping will increase the milk supply. I suppose it can, but there are other ways of dealing with "not enough milk" and pumping the breasts and feeding the baby by bottle is not the way that makes sense to me, especially if the end result is that the baby stops breastfeeding altogether.

4. Mothers are advised to give bottles to supplement the baby. This can eventually result in the baby refusing the breast.
    - See the chapter "Increasing Breastmilk Intake by the Baby." If it is necessary to give the baby supplements, it is best to do so with a lactation aid at the breast. In this way, the baby does not refuse the breast.

5. The mother or the baby is sick.
    - It is not necessary in the vast majority of instances to feed by bottle either because the baby or the mother is sick. It is true that a sick mother may find it difficult to take care of a baby but often she can take the baby into bed with her and just let him suckle. If a baby is too sick to suckle, alternative means of giving him milk are preferable to bottle-feeding. If a baby can drink from a bottle, he can also drink from a spoon or cup. If he can drink from a cup, then he is probably not too sick to drink from the breast (unless he is refusing to latch). Feeding a baby by spoon or cup is not difficult, but the technique needs to be learned. Most nurses in pediatric hospitals know how to feed even a premature baby by cup.

6. Parents find bottles more "convenient."
    - There are many reasons bottles are given for "convenience." The mother wants to go out and leave the baby with her partner or another caregiver, or she is uncomfortable breastfeeding in public, so she brings a bottle. Or parents have been convinced that it's important for the father to give bottles so he can bond with the baby or give the mother a break. Whatever the initial reason, one bottle a day often leads to two bottles a day and then to three bottles a day. And soon the mother is not able to keep up with the pumping because the baby, even when he's at the breast, does not drink as he should, having gotten used to sucking on a bottle. So milk supply decreases. And soon the baby is also receiving formula in the bottle.
    - If mothers took their babies with them when they went out and breastfed in public, other mothers would also do it. Compared to what we see in advertising, a little skin is nothing to worry about. There is nothing more beautiful than a mother with her baby at her breast. If others find this vision offensive, let them avert their eyes and make no comment. Note that human rights commissions in Canada have always supported the right of mothers to breastfeed their babies anywhere they are legally allowed to be, including legally "private" places such as shopping malls.
    - I was always amused by the line "let's go out for a romantic dinner without the baby," usually proposed by the father. The mother agrees, sometimes reluctantly, sometimes enthusiastically, and Grandma or a friend is called into service to take care of the baby. A bottle of breastmilk is prepared. The mother does not find the dinner that romantic because she keeps thinking about her baby. As the time when the baby often feeds approaches, the mother starts to feel uncomfortable, and her breasts may start to leak. They may, if the baby is young, be engorged and painful. In addition, the mother is worried about the

baby. How is Grandma making out? Is the baby crying? She phones home and probably is reassured, but only for a while before phoning home yet again. The mother, at least, realizes, if she hadn't already, that things are not going to be as they always were. There's a new normal. It takes fathers longer to realize this.

- Really, how convenient is it to pump milk even once a day? It's a big deal, actually, getting ready, doing the actual pumping and then cleaning the pump afterwards and storing it away and also storing the milk. It's much easier to put the baby to the breast. In fact, even if the father gives the baby a bottle of breastmilk, the mother still finds it necessary to express her milk, her swollen and tender breasts waking her up from the sleep she so greatly desired. So we have the bizarre picture of the father feeding the baby expressed breastmilk in a bottle while at the same time the mother is expressing her milk.

- Many women in Canada are lucky. We have 52 weeks of parental leave and if the mother is employed in a full-time, permanent position, the law requires that she get that maternity leave. If a mother is able to take all or most of that time, then she never has to express her milk or give bottles or even formula (it is nice if the father can take some of that parental leave, not to feed the baby a bottle but to support the mother through the first few weeks, which can be challenging). In other words, the commonly heard advice "make sure the baby takes a bottle by six weeks of age or he never will" just does not make sense and is irrelevant anyway. It is true that not all women feel they can afford to take the time off an outside job; it is also true that not all women are eligible

for parental leave. The system is not perfect. A woman who works for herself does not qualify (unless she pays into the program in advance), but if she works for herself, she is the boss. She doesn't need anyone's approval to take her baby to work, which may be in the next room. I have heard of physicians and other people managing businesses who have taken their babies to work. The caretaker is in another room with the baby. If the baby needs to feed, the caretaker brings him to the mother and she breastfeeds him. Some physicians have breastfed while getting a history from the patient. And why not? It's time people in positions of authority do what they can to normalize breastfeeding. See the chapter "Breastfeeding and Mother–Baby Separation."

A problem arises when women are back to their outside jobs and have to go on a business trip for several days, even a week or two. The mother no longer has the protection of the 52 weeks' maternity leave since the baby is now older than a year. This is a very big problem, since a 14-month-old, say, whose mother is away for two weeks may not take the breast again. But more importantly, the stress on the mother, but particularly the baby, can be very significant. I think there are two options.

- The mother could seek alternatives to taking the trip. Refusal may be seen as a lack of serious commitment to her work, though, and may affect her career. Not all employers are happy with year-long maternity leave, and if "problems" continue to arise because of what may be perceived as over-commitment to family and under-commitment to work, this could affect her job and future opportunities.

- The mother could find a way to take the baby with her. Travelling for business with a toddler is not easy. What does she do with him when she is in meetings? I would think that child care could be arranged in advance. If the mother has a nanny, she could bring her, or perhaps another family member could join them for the week to care for the toddler. The mother can breastfeed him during any down time and during the evening and before work.

- If neither option is possible, the mother should express or pump her milk while away to maintain the milk supply and then hope the toddler will return to the breast. The child should not get bottles during this time. A one-year-old can drink from an open cup and/or have liquids mixed with his solids. An acquaintance of mine was put in this position when she had to go overseas for her mother's funeral. The baby did not have a passport so he could not go with her. The mother expressed her milk and, happily, the baby returned to the breast when the mother returned to Canada.

How to get the baby back to breastfeeding

If the baby will take the breast at all, everything is possible. Avoiding bottles is critical. If the baby takes the breast and suckles, the mother can supplement the baby with her breastmilk or formula by a lactation aid at the breast. This will work much of the time, though the older the baby, the less likely he is to accept the lactation aid. Most babies under two months will accept the lactation aid at the breast easily. After three or four months it is less likely but if the baby does, that is very helpful, even if he takes a supplement at the breast only once or twice a day. At times when the baby refuses to take the breast, calming him down with finger feeding for a minute or so (if the baby is under eight weeks) or

giving him a little milk by cup or spoon may make him willing to take the breast if he is not ravenous. If worse comes to worst, a small amount, say 30 ml (1 oz.) given by bottle will do the same thing, but I would advise this be done only when all else has failed at that feeding.

Essentially, the mother follows the Protocol to Increase Breastmilk Intake by the Baby, which is discussed in the chapter "Increasing Breastmilk Intake by the Baby."

If the baby is four months or older, adding solids can be a good stratagem. Instead of giving a bottle, the mother gives solids, with her milk (preferably) or formula added to the solids. The parents should allow the baby to eat as much as he wants, as frequently as he wants, without forcing. This means fewer bottle-feedings and also decreases the need for the lactation aid at the breast if the mother finds this difficult.

Expressing milk can be useful for increasing milk supply but is not always easy to fit into this whole process. If the baby takes the breast, it is better to work on the breastfeeding than to pump.

As in the situation when the baby won't take the breast, domperidone can be useful. Furthermore, faster milk flow will prevent the baby from pulling off the breast so quickly. Basically, the more milk the mother has, the more likely the baby will start breastfeeding again.

If the baby absolutely refuses to latch on, the approach should be the same as with any baby who refuses to latch on. Expressing milk in this situation does make sense, both to provide the baby with some breastmilk and to increase the milk supply.

In addition, the mother should give the baby lots of opportunity to find the breast. For example, she should take the baby into bed at night, with the baby in a diaper only and the mother undressed from the waist up. See the chapter "Sleep: Yours and

Your Baby's." During the day, the mother can carry the baby around in a sling, with the breast available, uncovered. Trying to force the baby to the breast is futile and it is best for the mother not to try to hurry the process along.

It can help mothers to know that there are steps along the way to breastfeeding that many babies follow. At first, they may touch the breast and nipple with their hands. Then they may lick or nuzzle the nipple, without latching. Many mothers feel frustrated at this point—they want the baby to latch!—but this is a part of the sequence, and the baby may do this several times before taking the nipple in his mouth and perhaps sucking briefly. This then progresses to actually latching on. So, though it's easy to get discouraged, patience and seeing these steps as part of a progression may make it all work.

What to expect?

It is true that this process *may* take several weeks, but usually the mother will see the baby beginning to breastfeed sooner. It is worth the time and energy. Here is one email among many I have received on this topic. Note that the information I gave the mother was through email:

"Just wanted to let you know that I have successfully managed to get my *five*-month-old to take the breast after three months of bottle-feeding."

18 | Breastfeeding "Devices"

This chapter discusses several gadgets that are sometimes used by breastfeeding mothers. Some can be useful, some are useful only under special conditions and some, I believe, do more harm than good and should not be used. Not all lactation specialists would agree with me on the use of these devices, but my approach is *not* to use any of them unless it's absolutely necessary. Unfortunately, some devices, such as nipple shields, are being drastically overused. We see dozens of mothers at our clinic every month to get off the nipple shield.

The baby bottle

The baby bottle is undoubtedly the most common device mothers use. Indeed, it is almost universally used for the following reasons:

To give the mother a "break." This has been discussed in the chapter on relactation. Mothers frequently feel they are "trapped" by breastfeeding because nobody else can feed the baby. A large part of this problem is that many mothers feel they cannot go out with the baby because they aren't comfortable breastfeeding in public. But if the mother goes out without the baby, she worries about him. Her breasts fill with milk and she gets uncomfortable. Perhaps one solution would be for the parents and baby to go out together so that if the mother wants a little time for herself, the other parent can take the baby off to a spot nearby, ready to bring him back if he gets fussy.

I would urge all breastfeeding mothers to go out with their babies and feed them in public. The more people see it, the more natural it will seem to everyone. Why should bottle-feeding mothers feel free to take out the bottle in the middle of a shopping mall and feed their babies, yet the breastfeeding mother not feel free to put her baby to the breast in that very same mall? One shopping mall in Toronto has a sign saying that there is a breastfeeding room beside the entrance. I think that sign should say "Feel free to breastfeed your baby anywhere in the mall. If, however, you wish privacy, there is a breastfeeding room beside the entrance." Perhaps the best place for the shy mother to start is at a movie theatre. The lights go down, the mother plugs the baby in and nobody knows. Obviously if the baby is fussy this won't work but if he's a calm baby willing to spend time on the breast, it can work very well. The mother has just breastfed in public. Some cinemas have special soundproof rooms (soundproof for the other patrons) for mothers and babies, and in the presence of other mothers and babies, women might feel more comfortable breastfeeding.

To give the father a chance to feed the baby. I discuss this at length in other parts of this book. I don't believe this is a good idea. The problem is that babies learn to prefer a bottle to the breast. Also, in many cases, mothers feel that expressing is just too much work, and formula becomes the bulk of—even all—the baby gets in the bottle. Now there is a nipple, which, according to the company making them (also a large pump manufacturer), does not cause nipple confusion. But the baby who gets bottles, even using a "special nipple," is at risk of going only to bottles. And of course the mother, if she wants to give breastmilk, will need to pump.

The baby is not getting enough from the breast. See the chapter "Increasing Breastmilk Intake by the Baby." Often this problem can be addressed and corrected by helping the mother understand what can be expected of the breastfeeding baby. Too often the mother believes that a baby who is feeding "too frequently" (say, 12 times a day), is not getting enough, when, in fact, he is getting plenty. Too often the mother believes that the baby who is "not feeding frequently enough" (say, five times a day), is not getting enough, when, in fact, he is getting plenty. The same for the baby who is on the breast "too long" or "not long enough." Babies are all different and so are their mothers. What is important is not how often or how long the baby is on the breast but rather how well he drinks at the breast. See the video clips at www.breastfeedinginc.ca.

If the baby truly needs to be supplemented, it should be done with a lactation aid at the breast, not with a bottle.

There are now bottles and nipples that supposedly don't cause nipple confusion. I truly doubt that. I think the first bottles that have been advertised this way had wide-based nipples that were supposed to keep the baby's mouth more open, as if he were on the breast. Anyone observing a baby sucking on a wide-based nipple can see immediately that he isn't actually keeping his mouth open any wider than he does on a "regular" artificial nipple.

Now we have a company advertising a nipple that supposedly mimics the flow from the breast. I

doubt it will prevent nipple confusion either. But it will cost more, both in money and in the length of time the baby breastfeeds.

No matter what people invent, a baby on a bottle is not on the breast, and no new gimmick will change that.

The baby is not latching on. Too many mothers end up exclusively bottle-feeding breastmilk because the baby will not latch on at first. Most babies can learn to breastfeed. Getting good hands-on help can make all the difference in the world. Being advised to use a nipple shield is not good hands-on help. See the chapter "When the Baby Does Not Yet Take the Breast."

The mother has sore nipples. In my opinion, taking the baby off the breast is a poor approach to helping mothers with sore nipples. Taking the baby off the breast and giving him a bottle should be a last resort, but with early and good help it should not be necessary. When I hear that a mother has been advised to take the baby off the breast when he is only three days old (it happens often), I cannot believe everything else has already been tried. The issue of sore nipples is discussed in the chapter "Sore Nipples."

The mother is returning to work outside the home. In Canada, this should not be a huge problem for most women. With 52 weeks of maternity leave, it is completely unnecessary for a baby to drink from a bottle. At the age of one, almost all babies should be drinking from an open cup (many babies can manage by seven months, often earlier), not a bottle. Incidentally, a sippy cup is essentially a bottle. If necessary, milk can be added to a baby's solids instead of given by bottle.

Not all mothers can take the full 52 weeks off, for various reasons. Some cannot afford it. Some work for themselves and may have a hard time

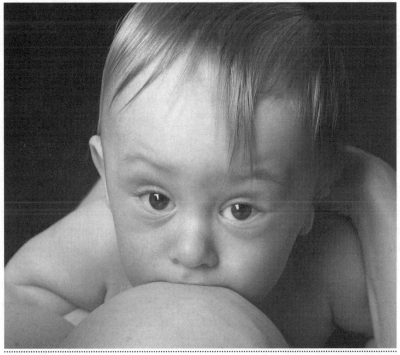

CREDIT: JÁN VEREŠ

shutting their work down, although new laws allow self-employed women to pay into EI so as to be eligible for leave. Still, if possible, mothers should take at least seven months so that the baby is starting to drink from a cup and is on solids when she returns. Then he can eat and drink when they are apart, and breastfeed when they are together. See the chapter "Breastfeeding and Mother–Baby Separation."

The lactation aid used at the breast

As I mentioned previously in this chapter, I believe that if supplementation needs be given to a baby, this is the way to do it.

However, some mothers do have difficulty using the aid, whether it is the manufactured version (Supplemental Nursing System or SNS) or our improvised version. I think that the improvised version works better much of the time. Some mothers have difficulty getting the tube in the right place, especially when they are already having difficulty latching the baby on and/or they do not have help using it. Help from another person, at least the first few times, can make all the difference. With time, it becomes easy as the mother gets the hang of it. So what do mothers complain about with regard to the lactation aid besides making it work?

It takes too long. This is a variation on not being able to make it work at all. The tube is in the baby's mouth and the baby is on the breast, yet the mother says it takes him an hour to get 30 ml (1 oz.) of supplement. This makes for a very long feeding and I agree that something is not working well. Incidentally, using a 38 cm (15 in.) tube, instead of a 91 cm (36 in.) one, also makes this whole operation awkward. So why is it taking so long?

- The baby is either not latched on well, the tube is not well placed, or both. The chapter "Increasing Breastmilk Intake by the Baby" discusses latching on and how to insert the tube. We also show how to insert the tube in the videos at www.breastfeedinginc.ca.
- The mother tries to use the tube only after the baby has completely "emptied" the breast. Though I can understand her reasons for trying to squeeze the last drop out of the breast before inserting the tube, the problem is that the baby will often be sleepy and slipping off the breast if the mother waits too long to insert the tube or, in the case of the SNS, to open the valve that lets the supplement flow. It is not necessary to try to get every last drop out of the breast before using the lactation aid. Indeed, I would recommend the mother use it sooner rather than later, though not from the very beginning of the feeding. The mother feeds the baby on the first breast until the baby is drinking only occasionally, even with compression (see the chapter "Increasing Breastmilk Intake by the Baby"), and then changes sides. When the baby is drinking only occasionally on the second side, even with compression, the mother inserts the tube. If the baby pulls off the breast, she can try latching the baby onto the breast and the tube at the same time. The baby, if latched on, will continue to get milk from the breast even as he is being supplemented at the same time. A baby who breastfeeds really well for 10 or 15 minutes on each side (not to be measured, just as a sort of "benchmark") will not usually need a lactation aid at all. If the baby drinks well for three or four minutes, say, and then drinks occasionally for another three or four minutes, he will be on the breast without supplementation for only about 10 minutes and then gets the supplement. The whole feeding should

not take more than 30 to 45 minutes, maybe an hour, but certainly not two.

- Mothers often shy away from using the lactation aid at the breast when out in public. Nobody is surprised if a baby is fed a bottle while the parents are at a restaurant or at the mall, for instance, and rarely is a mother ever asked why she is bottle-feeding her baby. It's normal to feed a baby with a bottle, right? But if a mother is using a lactation aid, she worries about being a spectacle and being asked why she is doing that and why isn't she just giving a bottle? Many mothers who manage the lactation aid at home very well have refused to use it in public. But I think this is a very good way to educate others about the importance of breastfeeding and keeping the baby at the breast. Mothers can tell anyone who asks: "I need to supplement him and because bottle-feeding is not what I want, I am supplementing him this way in order to keep up the breastfeeding and prevent him from refusing to latch on." Furthermore, it is easy to set up the lactation aid so that the container is hidden and only a very little of the tube is noticeable, and even then only at close range.

The lactation aid is preventing the mother's milk from increasing. I must say I don't understand this conclusion. The baby is still on the breast when using a lactation aid and thus still drinking the mother's milk, even if only small amounts, and this has the potential of increasing the milk supply. True, the baby may now nurse less often, but this may not be a bad thing—it may be because he is getting more milk now.

The teaching "the more the baby sucks, the more milk there will be" is not true. The truth is that the more milk the baby drinks from the breast, the more milk there will be.

The lactation aid used to finger feed the baby

This technique can be very useful, particularly to prepare a baby to take the breast when he does not latch on. Finger feeding wakes up a sleepy baby; finger feeding calms a baby who is upset. If done properly, it also teaches a baby to suck as he would on the breast, wrapping his tongue around the finger and drawing backward, just as he should wrap his tongue around the breast tissue and draw backward. When preparing the not-yet-latching baby to take the breast, it is rarely necessary to finger feed more than a minute or two to get him sucking as he would on the breast, especially if he is younger than five or six weeks. He might then, if brought to the breast in the ideal manner, actually latch on. See the video clip "Finger Feed to Latch" at www.breastfeedinginc.ca.

However, if the baby is latching on to the breast, using finger feeding to supplement makes no sense. The lactation aid should be used *at the breast* to supplement.

Finger feeding is sometimes used with a syringe on the end of the tube and the mother is advised to push the milk into the baby's mouth as he sucks. This is contrary to the whole idea of what finger feeding is for and does nothing to improve breastfeeding as far as I can determine. The syringe is encouraged with the notion that one has to get more milk into the baby without using a bottle. It is rare that the situation of the baby's intake of milk from the breast is so poor that one has to push milk into his mouth. If the baby is latching on, supplementation can be given with a lactation aid at the breast. If the baby is sleepy to the point of concern, waking him up with finger feeding will work, but then the baby should go to the breast. If the baby wakes and is ready to feed but doesn't take the breast, using a cup or spoon to feed him is better than pushing milk into his mouth.

What I say here about pushing milk into the baby's mouth can be said about the syringe or dental syringe as well. And perhaps the syringe is even worse than a bottle. It is hard, not flexible. The baby doesn't even have to suck to get milk, he needs only to swallow; with a bottle the baby does suck, even though the sucking is different from sucking on the breast.

See the chapter "When the Baby Does Not Yet Take the Breast."

Using a cup or a spoon to feed a baby

Small cups, shot glass size, are now being used to feed babies much younger than we used to think possible. In the text books of pediatrics, it used to be said that a baby couldn't drink from a cup until he was about seven months old, sometimes older. Experience has shown that even premature babies can drink from a cup. (Note that I mean an open cup. A sippy cup is essentially a bottle.) However, some mothers have used tumbler-sized plastic cups and one mother even sent me a photo of her baby drinking from a wine glass (breastmilk, not wine!).

Using a cup is a way of feeding a baby milk when he won't take the breast or when the mother is not present. It should not be used when the mother is present or if the baby takes the breast; in this case, if the baby needs supplementation, it should be given by lactation aid at the breast.

There has been concern expressed that the cup is a danger to the baby because he may aspirate the milk. There is no evidence that this is true. I suppose it could happen if the technique used to cup-feed the baby is very sloppy. The baby should not get milk poured down his throat from the cup. The baby should be in a more or less upright position or *slightly* tilted backward and the cup should be brought to his lips. The lower rim is in contact with his lower gum and the cup is tilted gently until the baby starts to feel and taste milk on his lips. The baby's natural reaction will be to start lapping up the milk and thus he is in control and drinks and stops when he does not want any more. See the video clip "Cup Feeding" at www.breastfeedinginc.ca.

Babies, even very young ones, can drink quite quickly from a cup and this is one reason some nurses prefer it. Some lactation specialists believe that the way the baby uses his tongue is conducive to learning to breastfeed. At least a cup is better than a bottle.

A spoon is really just a small cup. In the first few days, when the mother is normally producing only small amounts of colostrum and can express only a few millilitres, a teaspoon (which holds approximately 5 ml) can be easier to use than a cup. A baby will lap up the milk from a spoon just as he would from a cup. However, with the small amounts in a teaspoon, slowly tipping the colostrum into the baby's mouth will work well.

Syringes

Syringes are used to push milk into the baby's mouth while finger feeding, either with a tube attached to the syringe or not. Where a tube is not used, lactation consultants often suggest using a dental syringe, which has a curved end. While the baby is sucking on the finger, the mother or lactation consultant pushes milk into the baby's mouth. In theory, the push of milk into the baby's mouth should occur when the baby is sucking well, but often the baby gets a gush of milk even when his sucking is disorganized. This technique, though it feeds the baby, does not improve his breastfeeding.

As noted above, finger feeding with a tube attached to a syringe can also be misused. If the milk in the syringe is pushed into the baby's mouth with the plunger, the baby does not learn how to suck. Furthermore, using a lactation aid attached to a container sitting on a desk by the mother or in

her shirt pocket is a lot easier than manipulating the syringe and the baby and the tube.

Some argue that the baby is able to suck the milk out of a syringe without depressing the plunger and while this is true, it does not make using the syringe any better. Used this way, with the baby sucking the end, the syringe is essentially a bottle.

I think many lactation consultants and nurses like syringes because they appear more "medical," more scientific. They're not. Using syringes is not necessary and can cause problems.

Nipple everters

When a mother has "inverted" or "flat" nipples, a nipple everter is recommended. This gadget can be made from a 12 cc or 20 cc syringe by cutting off the end that holds the needle and then putting the plunger in the "wrong" way to prevent the jagged end from coming into contact with the mother's breast. This can work very well to pull out the nipple temporarily, but often it sinks back in once the everter is removed. When the mother is trying to latch a baby on, she may have only a couple of seconds to get the baby onto the breast with the now protuberant nipple.

There is at least one company making nipple everters which, unlike our gadget, can be worn for extended periods of time during the pregnancy. Whether this helps or not, I'm not sure, but I don't think it can hurt. The company states the product should not be used during pregnancy but it seems to me this would be the best time to use it. I doubt very much that its use would precipitate premature labour.

Nipple shields

I have a real problem with nipple shields. I believe they do very little good and most of the time they do much harm. I can think of very few situations when I have been convinced that the nipple shield actually helped a mother or a baby. Yes, some mothers who have had a baby refuse to latch on have breastfed through a shield for months, but they managed this only because they had an abundant milk supply. If any other medical device caused as many problems as the nipple shield, with as little benefit, it would be withdrawn from the market. In effect, the nipple shield turns the breast into a bottle. Manufacturers may claim that today's nipple shields are much better and don't interfere with breastfeeding, but that's just marketing. Our clinic experience says otherwise. The mother experiencing breastfeeding problems needs good help, not a nipple shield.

Nipple shields usually cause a decrease in milk supply. Sometimes if the mother has an abundant supply, the baby can still gain weight and be content; nevertheless, her supply will decrease. Some lactation consultants will recommend the mother express her milk after feeding to prevent a decrease in milk supply. But what a pain!

A baby on a nipple shield is not actually latched on to the breast (or, at best, poorly latched on), and a baby who is poorly latched does not get milk well. Once the milk supply has decreased, it becomes more and more difficult to get the baby latched on.

Just one email of hundreds of similar ones I've received: "I started using a nipple shield when the baby was a few days old, after my milk came in... It seemed to go okay, but somewhere around three weeks I began to notice she didn't seem to be sucking properly and by her one-month check-up she'd only gained an ounce." The mother did not say why she started using the nipple shield, but I would suggest whatever problem she had could have been approached differently and with more success.

Why are nipple shields used?
The baby is not latching on. See the chapter "When the Baby Does Not Yet Take the Breast."

The single most important factor that determines whether a baby will latch on is the mother's development of an abundant milk supply. When a mother uses a nipple shield, it is very likely the milk supply will decrease, making it more and more difficult to get the baby off the nipple shield.

I would prefer that a mother whose baby is not latching on express her milk and give it by bottle than to use a nipple shield, because the milk supply is usually better maintained when the mother expresses her milk. Some lactation consultants agree that nipple shields decrease the milk supply, so they have the mother pump after feeding the baby through the nipple shield. I don't see that this is an improvement. In the first case, the mother expresses and then feeds the baby the bottle. In the second, the mother feeds the baby through the breast-made-bottle (with a nipple shield) and then expresses. But there are other approaches recommended in the chapter "When the Baby Does Not Yet Take the Breast."

Very often the baby will latch on easily, especially if the mother gets good help, when her milk "comes in." For this reason I consider using a nipple shield before the mother's milk comes in to be contraindicated. A little patience, please! The problem, of course, is that if the mother starts a nipple shield on day one or two, something that happens all too often, she may consider her problem solved and not realize there is a new problem until she notices the baby has not gained weight well. Often it's so easy to get a baby to latch on when the milk comes in!

Several studies now show that babies learn to find the breast by smell. The Montgomery glands (those little bumps on the areola out of which sometimes milk actually comes out) emit compounds that attract the baby to the breast and help him latch on. This is why washing the nipples early on is not a good idea. I am not saying "never wash," but the old rule about washing the nipples before putting the baby to the breast was wrong for many reasons. Furthermore, washing the nipples removes secretions that actually protect them. So washing does the opposite of what it is purported to do. Finally, it's a nuisance to wash the nipples many times a day.

The point of mentioning that babies are attracted to the nipple and the breast and are helped to latch on by smell is that a nipple shield does not smell like the nipple or the breast or the milk. It smells of the chemicals used to make it. If the baby gets to associate the smell of the nipple shield with *getting* milk, the smell of the nipple/breast/milk may no longer attract him.

The mother has sore nipples. I believe that this is yet another reason not to use a nipple shield. Aside from decreasing the milk supply, it often does not decrease the mother's pain. Many mothers have contacted me saying the nipple shield makes the pain even worse. Here is part of an email from a mother using a nipple shield: "The lactation consultant also provided me with a nipple shield, but the pain was even worse when I used it. It was extreme pain and a burning sensation and it lasted for a while after feeding, so I stopped using it." Some mothers do feel some pain improvement but they still are not pain-free and so they figure they should continue using the nipple shield.

Here is another email from a mother: "I developed several cracks on my right nipple which were excruciatingly painful because my baby would not latch on to my left breast." (*This is not true. A baby does not cause the mother sore nipples simply because he is feeding more on one breast.*) "I used an Avent nipple shield for a week to help speed up the healing process, with poor results. Initial latch would make me cry even with the shield. My breasts felt on fire, which I thought was due to engorgement." (*It is quite possible that the mother became engorged*

by using a nipple shield. With a nipple shield, the baby does not drain the breast adequately and engorgement may result.)

I admit that I have also heard from mothers who said that if it hadn't been for the nipple shield they could not have continued breastfeeding. Some even managed to feed the baby exclusively on a nipple shield. But these mothers are the exceptions, not typical at all. And even in their cases, attention to how the baby was latching on, using our all-purpose nipple ointment, releasing a tongue tie and other approaches, especially if started early, would have allowed the mother to continue pain-free without using a nipple shield.

The baby is premature. Some studies show that premature babies get more milk through a nipple shield than directly from the breast. I cannot understand why this should be the case, unless perhaps the babies who were on the breast directly simply were not latched on well.

If mothers and babies were actually together in Kangaroo Mother Care, not just an hour or two a day, babies would get more milk when they are on the breast.

The problem of "pseudo" Kangaroo Mother Care is compounded by the fact that in some hospitals in North America, and many in Europe, babies are not allowed to be put to the breast until they are at least 34 weeks gestation and are then fed on a three-hour schedule. In fact, we know from information published in Sweden that babies as young as 28 or 29 weeks gestation are able to take the breast. And though I have said this before, I will state again that babies, even premature babies, learn to breastfeed by breastfeeding, not by being fed by gastric tubes or a bottle. See the chapter "The Preterm and Near-term Baby."

But even if occasionally a nipple shield *might*— and I emphasize "might"—be useful to encourage

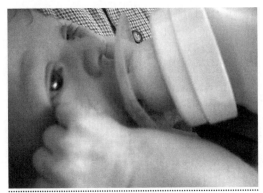

CREDIT: JACK NEWMAN

the premature baby to take the breast, there is often no effort to take him off the nipple shield and so the baby and mother eventually go home on a nipple shield.

What should we make of the photo above? This baby was not latching on. The mother is feeding the baby with a bottle through a nipple shield. The only explanation I can think of for doing this is that the mother was convinced by someone that feeding through a nipple shield was very much like breastfeeding. The mother naturally concluded, I believe, that this is the way to teach the baby to latch on. Unfortunately, too often mothers are given the impression that using a nipple shield is just like breastfeeding and so it is good.

Breast shells or breast shields

Breast shells are different from nipple shields. Nipple shields are designed to be worn while breastfeeding. Breast shells or breast shields are meant to be worn between feedings. There are two conceivable purposes for the use of breast shells.

1. To help form nipples that are suitable for breastfeeding. This is not a reason to use breast shells. They have never been shown to work and they can also be a pain to wear.

2. To keep sore nipples away from the mother's clothing and from wet breast pads, which can make the pain worse. They do sometimes help in this situation, but not always. They tend to make the mother leak more milk, and that can be inconvenient. They can also cause pain if they don't fit properly. On the other hand, they may help collect milk in the small space in the bottom of the shell.

Breast pumps

Although the vast majority of mothers in Canada will not need a breast pump, many get them anyway. In fact, a breast pump seems to be a favourite baby shower gift, suggesting that pumping the breasts is normal and that the baby will need to receive bottles sometimes.

However, even if the baby needs to get expressed milk, the mother can learn to express her milk by hand. It's a lot more convenient if she is at work to express by hand than to lug a breast pump around with her, and with a little practice most women can express a considerable amount quite quickly.

I do not recommend specific breast pumps. I try not to recommend any brand name of anything, on principle. Furthermore, there is no "best breast pump." Women are all different and some breast pumps seem to work well for certain women and not so well for others.

Our website, www.breastfeedinginc.ca, has an information sheet on expression of milk.

Breastfeeding pillows

Another common baby shower gift, the breastfeeding pillow, can be useful but is usually unnecessary for the vast majority of mothers. To breastfeed, a mother needs a breast and a baby. Although pillows can help support a baby when the mother is learning to breastfeed, there is usually no need for a "special" breastfeeding pillow. Well-placed regular pillows can be used.

Once the mother has learned breastfeeding 101, she will find a pillow unnecessary. The problem with the pillow is that if a mother believes she cannot do without it, she may not go out with her baby very much. Who wants to drag an awkward pillow to the park with the baby?

Some pillows are actually not very helpful, and some are worse than not very helpful. The baby may be too high with some pillows, making breastfeeding uncomfortable, or too low with others, requiring the mother to lean over and possibly get back pain in order to feed the baby. Even mothers of twins can manage to support both of them with ordinary pillows and, once they get the hang of it, can do without a pillow. While some mothers say they find pillows useful, I think breastfeeding can be comfortable and enjoyable without them, and certainly more convenient if the mother doesn't have to drag a big u-shaped pillow around.

If you really want a pillow, don't buy one before the baby is born—you need to make sure it fits both you and the baby. Look for one that is firm but not hard and that will support your arm as you hold the baby (don't lay the baby on the pillow!)

This is where the cradle hold comes into its own. We teach the cross-cradle hold to mothers who are learning to breastfeed and trying to get the baby to latch on with an asymmetric latch. This position usually works well, but once the mother is comfortable with breastfeeding, she can switch to the cradle hold. With a cradle hold, the mother does not need a pillow.

19 | The Breastfed Baby and Solids

Myth #1: Babies need to eat solids by a certain age because breastmilk no longer contains all that a growing baby needs.

Fact #1: While there is some truth to this, eating is also a social behaviour for babies about six months old just as it is for adults. A baby of six months is much more aware of what is around him than, say, a baby of three months. He wants to be part of the family and do things as the rest of the family does, and that includes eating solids. That's why I think giving babies special "baby foods" is not desirable. Babies want to eat what the rest of the family is eating.

But the idea that there is a set age at which every baby should start eating solids does not make sense. Parents worry that a baby who is not eating by seven months, for example, is in danger of nutritional deficiencies or that a baby who clearly wants to start eating at five months should not be given solids until six months. A baby should start eating solids when he wants to start eating solids.

Myth #2: After six months or a year of age (take your pick) there is no nutritional value to breastmilk.

Fact: This nonsensical statement is so completely incorrect, I hardly know where to start. Breastmilk contains appropriate amounts of protein, fat, carbohydrate, vitamins, minerals and other elements for nutritional needs. It also contains growth factors that help the baby's brain, immune system, gut and other organs to mature. And breastmilk still contains the immune factors that continue to protect the breastfeeding toddler from infection, especially if the child is in daycare. Infections in daycare centres run through the children at incredible rates and although breastfeeding does not protect the child 100%, it certainly offers considerable protection, as several studies show. Let us not forget either that breastfeeding is a lot more than breastmilk. It is a relationship, something very special between mother and child, that doesn't go away just because the child is 8 months or 18 months or 3 years, for that matter.

So why do children start eating food? They do need to take in other foods in order to prevent deficiencies in certain nutrients. Breastmilk provides everything to the full-term healthy baby from birth to roughly six months, but eventually babies need to eat other foods. This is not to take away anything from how very special breastmilk is but there comes a time when adding complementary foods is appropriate. The fact that breastmilk does provide everything for so long is truly amazing and should fill us with admiration for this incredible liquid.

Why do babies need to start eating other foods around six months of age?

1. Calories. Many mothers can breastfeed exclusively for longer than six months while the baby continues to be satisfied and to grow well. However, in some cases the baby does not seem to get enough and other foods should be

added. In fact, for those mothers whose milk supply decreases after three or four months and all measures to increase it have been tried, adding solids may help the baby grow normally and eliminate the "need" for formula.

2. Iron. Most babies will have sufficient iron stored up at birth to keep them iron sufficient for about six months, sometimes longer. If the cord was not clamped and cut immediately after birth, the baby will have more iron stored up. Breastmilk does not have large quantities of iron, but the iron it has is very well absorbed. A study a few years ago on babies breastfed exclusively up to nine months showed that only 15% were iron deficient and none was anemic. However, if the mother was anemic during the pregnancy, it is quite possible the baby did not get a full complement of iron during the pregnancy and could be at risk for iron deficiency.

3. Zinc. Zinc deficiency is also a possibility in a baby who is breastfed exclusively for more than six or seven months. Again, there is not a lot of zinc in breastmilk, and deficiencies can result in diarrhea and a typical rash on the face. These symptoms plus, in some babies, loss of hair due to zinc deficiency is called acrodermatitis enteropathica. It can also be a genetic disease and used to be common in premature babies who were not breastfed before zinc was added to their feedings. Another example of "Oops, we didn't know about that." Little research has been done on this question of zinc in breastfed babies but it should be a consideration when recommending when breastfed babies should begin taking solids.

Eventually, of course, all babies need to start taking solid foods. It's not surprising that breastmilk alone won't *always* be all the baby needs.

Babies show signs they are ready to eat solids

Babies, especially breastfed babies, are pretty amazing. It doesn't matter how long they generally sleep, they frequently wake up and want to breastfeed just when the mother, but not necessarily the father, sits down to eat. This happens even if the mother and father are not eating at the same time. How do the babies know this? Is there some sort of chemical signal that the mother sends out that says, "I'm just about to put the fork into my mouth"? I suppose it's possible. If pheromones can induce humans to be sexually attracted to each other, why not maternal pheromones that say, "It's time to eat"? There is no scientific proof for this, but the experience of mothers is important and we should listen to mothers more often.

In any case, the result is that babies are often sitting on their mother's or father's lap when one or the other is eating. By about four months of age, the baby becomes very interested in what is going on. He will often watch attentively the mother's fork or spoon as it moves from the plate to her mouth and back again. By five or six months he not only watches, he may try to grab food out of the plate and put it into his mouth. In fact, I have seen babies put their hands into the mother's mouth to try to get the food. It seems to me that a baby doing this is ready to eat solids, whatever his age. Of course, a two-month-old won't behave like this, so there is no question of him being ready to eat solids. And if the baby is ready for solids at five months and two weeks, why not start feeding him solids when he's so interested?

What solids should the baby get when he's ready? I think it makes sense that the baby of five months and two weeks who is trying to grab the piece of steak out of the mother's plate be allowed to eat it. Okay, it can be cut to a reasonable size or shredded, but the baby can eat the same food as the parents eat, with few exceptions.

Which exceptions? Round, slippery food, such as whole grapes or peanuts, are dangerous. They are often just the size to block the baby's trachea (breathing tube). Hot dogs present a similar risk. Popcorn has been cited as a food that can be aspirated into the trachea. Very hot spicy food are better avoided for a while since burning the baby's mouth is probably not a great way to encourage him to eat solids. But that's about all. Of course, making sure the food is not too hot is just common sense. There's often no need to cut the food into small pieces: a baby can hold a broccoli floret in his hand and gnaw away at it or pick up a pear with two hands and chomp on it.

But I have heard the argument that a baby of five or six months will put anything into his mouth, even stones and toys, if he has the opportunity. Yes, this is true, and since the parents are usually there when a six-month-old baby is putting a plastic toy into his mouth, they will usually quickly and anxiously pull it out. The baby will learn that toys are not food, or at least are not to be put into the mouth, though they will keep trying from time to time until they really learn. I would suggest that if a baby puts a piece of chicken into his mouth and the parents react in the same way to the chicken as they would to a stone, the baby will learn that maybe chicken is not food either. Perhaps he's a little confused because the parents are eating chicken, but somehow this food the parents are eating is not for him. I believe a lot of pickiness about food comes from "special foods" for babies and the reaction parents have to the baby eating foods other than the ones specially made for them. Here are some examples.

Commercial cereals

I have never been a fan of commercial cereals for babies. In the same way as most pediatricians, I learned in my training that babies' first solids should be commercial cereals. We were told that they are easy to digest, they are made from a single food product (such as rice or oats) and thus can make it easy to spot an allergic reaction, and they provide added iron. None of these reasons, however, stands up to scrutiny.

Incidentally, cereals have been promoted so aggressively by pediatricians and public health, not to mention baby-food companies, that many parents do not consider them solids. Several mothers, when I asked them whether the baby was taking solids, answered "No, but he is getting rice cereal." Somehow, undoubtedly due to marketing, some parents believe that cereals are in a category by themselves.

"Easy to digest"? Commercial cereals, because they are high in iron, cause many babies to be constipated. Breastfed babies do not need to worry about digesting their solids in the same way as artificially fed babies. Breastmilk contains enzymes—proteases to help digest protein, amylase to help digest starch and lipase to help digest fat.

The whole notion of giving only one single food a week and then adding another for a week and so on when babies are starting out eating solids doesn't make sense to me nor does it seem very practical. Who would want to eat only one food for a week? At this rate, you have only four foods in the child's diet by the end of a month, and only eight at the end of two months. The notion of one food a week goes against the whole idea of feeding the child "family foods," which is being strongly emphasized by the WHO Code and Health Canada. I believe a relaxed approach to eating is important so it is enjoyable for the baby and the family.

But what about allergies? How can parents know if the baby is allergic to a food? Here are just a few signs that parents believe indicate an allergy.

1. The baby gets hives, a skin rash that is often associated with allergy. But there are many causes of hives besides food allergies. Many physicians believe that the most common cause of hives is a viral infection. Is it possible the baby got a viral infection when he started eating fish and that accounts for his runny nose and hives? It is quite possible, but this baby may then be labelled allergic to fish, perhaps for the rest of his life.

2. The baby gets a red rash around his mouth. This occurs typically with acid foods such as tomatoes or strawberries. But the rash does not necessarily mean the baby is allergic. It may just be the baby's delicate skin is reacting to the acid in the food. Many babies are labelled allergic to tomatoes or strawberries for this reason, which is really too bad because these are very tasty foods and a pleasure to eat.

3. The baby vomits the food. Vomiting may be a reaction to eating a food to which the baby is allergic. It is useful to know that vomiting, diarrhea, coughing and choking on food are protective mechanisms to eliminate something that may not be good. Vomiting is an effort to eliminate something in the stomach the body recognizes as possibly harmful, such as a food to which the person is allergic. But babies also vomit for other reasons, including viral or bacterial infection of the gut (gastroenteritis), and the fact that the baby got strawberries that day for the first time does not mean he is allergic to strawberries. Furthermore, when babies don't like a food, they often vomit it.

4. The baby gets diarrhea. Diarrhea may occur when he gets a food for the first time. It doesn't mean, as above, that the diarrhea is an allergic reaction. Diarrhea occurs frequently with any sort of infection, even the common cold.

5. The baby's diaper contains undigested food. In fact, this is normal and common even into the second year of life. There is no reason to believe that undigested carrots found in the baby's diaper have anything at all to do with allergy.

As for iron, which is one of the major reasons for recommending commercial cereals, this doesn't stand up to scrutiny either. Most of the iron in commercial cereals is not absorbed by the baby. It ends up in his diaper. There are many foods that provide better absorbed iron, including some meats and whole grains. I am hearing more and more that mothers are being told not to start meat before nine months of age. If the baby is interested, and the parents also eat meat, there is no reason to wait until the baby is nine months old to start meat. Where do these ideas come from?

Cereals, as mentioned earlier, tend to be constipating for the very reason they are recommended, the high iron content. They also don't taste very good. They are, at best, very bland. Imagine eating the same bland food three times a day every day for a week.

Finally, commercial cereals are not rich in nutrients, except for iron. In other words, parents are paying a lot for very little when they buy commercial cereals for infants.

I followed the rules with our first baby. At six months we offered him commercial cereals. After he spit out the cereals three times in a row, we got the idea. And the first food he grabbed from his mother's plate was a strip of steak I had just cut for her. He grabbed it, put it into his mouth and chewed on it for a long time. Eventually he spat out the pulp of what had been a strip of steak. So he probably didn't swallow much, but he got the juice and probably a fair bit of iron. After that, we offered him the same food we ate and he never had a problem eating anything. We respected his preferences if he had any, not trying to push "good foods" such as vegetables, but allowing him to decide what he wanted to eat. I don't remember any fights about eating in our household.

But don't some babies start to use up their iron stores before six months of age? Yes, some probably do, but I believe that these are the babies who will become very interested in eating before that "magic" age of six months. Our body tells us when we need something. For example, if your blood sugar drops, your body will make efforts to increase the blood sugar by breaking down glycogen (a complex sugar stored in the liver) to provide you with glucose. It will also start breaking down fat to provide you with free fatty acids, lactic acid and ketone bodies (see the chapter "The First Few Days," the section on hypoglycemia). But these processes take time and what your body also tells you is "I'm hungry." So you try to find something to eat.

I believe that this sort of "feedback mechanism" works for other nutrients, including iron. A baby whose iron or zinc stores are starting to drop will begin to show an interest in eating food.

If instead of cutting the umbilical cord as soon as the baby is born, we waited until it stopped pulsating, the baby would get more blood; therefore he would get more iron and perhaps a lot of iron deficiency would be prevented. It is true that more blood may cause higher levels of jaundice, but if the baby is breastfeeding well and red blood cells are not being destroyed at a faster than normal rate (hemolysis), there is no issue.

Starting solids

If a baby shows his parents that he wants to eat, there is no reason to hold back starting solids because he is not yet six months of age. He should start eating and the parents should let him have food. How much should he get? He should get as much as he wants to eat, as often as he shows interest in eating, without being forced to eat. There is no need to limit the baby to one food per week or to have a certain order to the introduction of the food. The baby should have, essentially, the same diet as the parents. If the parents' diet is a concern, they should be advised that, for the sake of the child, maybe this is the time to look at healthy eating habits.

But if the baby of six months has not shown any interest in eating food, there is also no reason he *must* start. If he starts at seven months, that's okay also, if he is otherwise well and gaining on breastfeeding alone. Is he all right to start at eight or nine months if he is otherwise well and gaining on breastfeeding alone? I would say yes. Too many parents have been made extremely anxious because health professionals have frightened them with dire consequences of not starting solids by six months.

There is now a push to return to starting solids at between four and six months in both Canada and the United States. Perhaps by the time this book is published, it will already have happened, though as a member of the group advising on the revision of the infant feeding statement for Health Canada, I will fight this move. As it turns out, the new infant feeding statement, published in 2012, reiterated that babies should be exclusively breastfed to six months. In Europe they moved back to starting solids at four to six months in 2011. And what has happened in Europe? We see it already. Instead of four to six months as the starting age for solids, which the European Community is recommending, it has become four months as a rule.

A word about puréed foods

Parents are exhorted to start babies on puréed foods first. This is not really necessary if a baby is starting solids at around six months or later. It is simple enough to mash foods slightly with a fork, or give the baby foods he can hold and chew on.

"Babies should start eating foods in a certain order"

This has been taught in medical schools for years. First of all, the baby is offered commercial cereals in this order: first rice for a week, then oats for another week, then mixed cereals for another week. Then vegetables are started, first yellow vegetables, then green vegetables. I'm sure I learned the reason for yellow vegetables before green somewhere in my pediatric training but I forgot. Or maybe I missed that class. It was also important to give vegetables before fruit because fruits are sweet and if the baby is given fruits first, he won't accept vegetables.

Well, that is very interesting about fruit. Why would a baby not accept vegetables because he ate fruit first? Breastmilk is one of the sweetest foods around, and the fact that a baby is breastfed exclusively for six or seven months does not usually prevent him from eating commercial cereals (which are anything but sweet) or meat (which is not sweet either).

Here is another interesting point about breastmilk and formula. Formula is supposed to have about the same amount of sugar (lactose) as breastmilk. But formula does not taste sweet; breastmilk tastes very sweet. How can that be? By the way, soy formulas contain plain ordinary table sugar (sucrose) instead of lactose. Lactose may be important for the growth of the brain. Think about that for a bit.

In any case, vegetables at this point are nice but *not* necessary from a nutritional point of view, and many babies will reject them anyway, even if offered before fruit.

One of the reasons breastfeeding is valuable is that babies get the tastes of whatever the mother is eating through the milk. So if the mother is eating vegetables, her baby is learning the tastes of vegetables. And, in fact, researchers have found that breastfed babies are much more likely than formula-fed ones to accept any foods, including vegetables and fruit (unless their mothers didn't eat those foods) when they start solids.

Choking

Parents are frequently worried about the baby choking on food. As a parent myself, I know that the sight of a baby choking on food can be very frightening. However, choking is the body's way of preventing something that has gone down the "wrong way" from continuing down into the lungs. Babies have a very strong gag reflex and that's a good thing. The baby should be encouraged to feed himself and parents should trust that he'll be okay. However, babies shouldn't be left alone when they are eating. If, on the other hand, on the rare occasion that a baby doesn't recover quickly and chokes and coughs, and especially if he has difficulty breathing or turns blue, an infant Heimlich maneuver should be done and the baby taken to the emergency immediately.

"Making a mess"

It can't be helped. Babies will make a mess as they learn to eat solids. Parents can turn eating into a

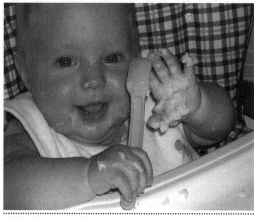

CREDIT: **GRAZIA DE FIORI**

nightmare if they try to make sure the baby never makes a mess. Putting an old shower curtain or newspapers around the high chair while the baby eats can decrease the worry about food on the floor. Food on the baby's face and hands is not so easy to avoid. But babies are washable. And this baby in the photo is obviously enjoying himself eating.

How much food should the baby eat? I think that's easy. As much as he wants. We should not try to force babies to eat more than they want or try to limit the amount they eat. Just as adults, babies will sometimes want more at one meal and less at another. It's not a tragedy if he eats less at a particular meal than usual, though many parents see it as some sort of reflection on themselves if the baby is not that interested in eating at a particular time. True, a baby who is sick may not be interested in eating, but if the child is obviously well and just not interested, well, that's okay.

Won't the milk supply decrease when the baby is eating solids?

Undoubtedly, if the baby is eating ample amounts of solids, he may take less breastmilk. And if he drinks less milk from the breast or less frequently from the breast, the milk supply will likely decrease. But this is how it works and it was meant to be this way. As long as he breastfeeds well and is obviously taking in milk, it's all good, no problem.

There is one thing we need to watch out for. If the baby was exclusively breastfed but the milk supply decreased for some reason, or if the mother was restricting breastfeeding in order to keep to a schedule or not "spoil the baby," he might be very enthusiastic about eating solids and eat very large amounts, which may further restrict how much he breastfeeds. Likely the baby was hungry when breastfeeding exclusively, even if he was gaining weight well. If the mother continues to restrict breastfeeding or schedule feedings

(which is essentially the same thing), her milk supply may decrease very rapidly. In this situation, the baby should be offered the breast before solids any time he seems interested in food.

Some babies don't want to eat even at a year or later!

This is true. What is going on when this happens? From my experience, there are two groups of babies who refuse to eat solids after six months of age.

Babies who are gaining weight well. I don't know why babies a year old or older are not interested in eating. It is possible, I suppose, that his signals that he is ready to eat were missed because parents thought "well, he puts everything in his mouth." But I doubt it. I think the baby is just not ready. Why is his body not telling him to start solids? Maybe he doesn't need them. I remember two 14-month-olds whose mothers said they were breastfeeding only. Both were slender, it is true, but not terribly so and they were gaining reasonably well. But when we did iron studies on these two children, they had normal levels and neither was anemic! This seems impossible, based on what we know about what iron stores babies have at birth. I have no explanation for this and will not attempt to give one.

These babies need to have food put in front of them when other members of the family are eating so that they can start eating when they are ready. Pushing them will not make them eat and can, in fact, turn them off eating. Nobody likes to be forced to eat, not even babies. I am aware of many babies who did not start eating until nine or ten months and then, once they started, they soon ate as much as other babies their age. These babies need only be monitored to make sure they continue to gain weight. Iron or zinc deficiency can be treated with medicinal supplements.

Babies who are not gaining weight well or are even losing weight. This group can be divided into two again: babies who are on the breast for only very short periods of time and babies who spend very long periods of time, often much of the day, on the breast. Some babies alternate these behaviours at different feedings.

These babies are often of great concern to both parents and health providers. Mothers are often urged to stop breastfeeding so that the baby will start eating.

I think the reason the first group is not gaining weight is that the mother has actually had a significant decrease in her milk supply. See the chapter "Late-Onset Decreased Milk Supply."

The second group of babies spend long periods on the breast, often hours at a time with little time between feedings. Often the physician states that the baby is not gaining because he is drinking "too much milk" and filling up on breastmilk and thus not interested in eating solids. This is completely backward, actually. It is false to conclude that since the baby is spending so much time on the breast, he must be drinking a lot of milk. If the physician actually watched the baby at the breast and knew how to evaluate the adequacy of the breastfeeding, he would see that the baby is hardly drinking at all. The problem is not that the baby is filling up on breastmilk, but rather that he is hardly drinking any milk at all.

Physicians often tell the mother that they have to stop breastfeeding completely, or in the case of the baby who is on the breast for long periods only at night, that they have to stop at night. This *might* work to get the baby to eat food and gain weight, but it doesn't always.

I have seen a baby who was breastfeeding but eating very few solids, only some Jell-o, who neither gained nor lost weight for about six months. The mother was told she had to stop breastfeeding so the child would start eating food, which she did (against my advice). However, the child wouldn't eat food and started to lose weight. Even if the baby had started to gain weight after being weaned he has lost the breastfeeding, which is a big loss. If there is another approach that does not sacrifice breastfeeding, should we not go that route? Is there a way? There is.

If I am correct in saying that this situation arises when the baby or toddler is at the breast for long periods of time but not actually drinking from the breast, we do have a solution. We should *increase* the mother's milk supply.

First, we must try to determine why the mother's milk supply might have decreased. This question is discussed in the chapter "Late-Onset Decreased

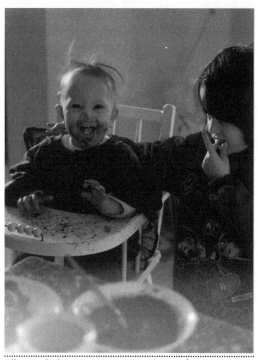

Allowing babies to enjoy eating is part of preventing feeding problems.

CREDIT: **GRAZIA DE FIORI**

Milk Supply." For example, if the mother is on the birth control pill, she should stop it. If there is no reason to avoid domperidone, I would start the mother on it so the baby gets more milk from the breast. Once the supply is cranked up, the baby/toddler might even start to eat solids.

Why would he start eating solids if he starts getting more milk from the breast? I'm not sure, but I know it happens and I will offer a hypothesis. First of all, sucking at the breast is pleasurable for babies and toddlers. I think anyone who has seen a baby at the breast can see this without the need for scientific studies to "prove it." I think these babies/toddlers are sucking at the breast for the comfort and pleasure it gives them, but because they are not getting many calories, they are likely to be in a state of ketosis and do not feel hunger. (Popular diets use the approach of making the dieter ketotic.) With increased intake of milk from the breast, the baby/toddler is no longer ketotic and starts to feel hunger again and may start eating solids.

Some people have hypothesized that zinc deficiency can cause a loss of appetite in babies/toddlers. I don't know if this is true, but perhaps a period of zinc supplementation is worth a try. Others hypothesize that iron deficiency may result in a loss of appetite. I'm not sure how that would work, but in any case, both iron and zinc can be given in liquid form with an eyedropper, eased into the corner of the baby's mouth as he suckles at the breast.

How to get around the problem of the child not eating solids?

1. *Increase* the milk supply with domperidone and do *not* limit the baby's intake of milk from the breast. However, the baby should not be allowed to nibble indefinitely on the breast. Once the baby is only nibbling and not drinking, even with compression, he should then go to the other breast and the process can be repeated. See the chapter "Increasing Breastmilk Intake by the Baby."

2. Once the baby has fed from both sides, he can be taken off the breast and offered solids, sometimes off a parent's finger. The baby should not be pushed to eat, as this can increase his resistance to taking food.

3. Sometimes, though not often, offering food before the breast might work.

4. Taking a child even as young as eight or nine months to a community centre where babies and toddlers gather (a drop-in centre, for example) might encourage him to eat solids. Seeing other children eating might encourage the reluctant eater to copy them.

5. Sometimes having someone other than the parents offer the child food (not try to force feed, but *offer* food) may work. But babies of eight or nine months are very independent-minded and may resist being fed and prefer to feed themselves, even if they get very little into their mouths. These babies will often suck their hands if they are taken off the breast, again, for pleasure and comfort. It might be possible to have them take liquefied food with an eyedropper. As they eat more, they may begin to like it.

6. I hesitate to propose this possibility, but I saw this situation in Africa. Babies or toddlers who refused food were admitted to hospital if their lack of weight gain was truly worrisome. A tube was put through the nose into the stomach and liquefied food was given. The mothers continued to breastfeed. As the children started to gain weight, they actually took an interest in eating normally and, according to the doctors, the problem was solved. I would suggest this only when necessary, but it is a possible solution if nothing else is working. Note that a

baby with a tube in the stomach does not need to stay in hospital.

What about the baby/toddler who spends only a very short period of time on the breast?

These babies/toddlers will often accept food very easily. They spend a lot of their time sucking their hands. If they are offered food, they will usually take it. The milk supply should still be increased.

Is it possible to prevent such a situation? I believe that if we helped mothers get a good start with breastfeeding from the very first days; if mothers knew how to tell when a baby is getting milk from the breast (and thus how to tell when a baby is not getting milk); if we did not give mothers inappropriate information such as "you must feed the baby on only one breast at a feeding"; if we avoided giving mothers medications that interfere with their milk supply; if we encouraged mothers to start solids when the baby is showing signs of being ready to eat—if we did all this, the problem of late-onset decreased milk supply would not arise and the problem of food refusal would not occur.

A few special situations
Exclusive breastfeeding for more than six months as a deliberate decision on the mother's part

Every so often I run into a mother who plans to breastfeed exclusively, without solids, for a year, and recently I met one mother who intended to breastfeed exclusively to three years, based on a biblical citation. Some women who want to avoid birth control will breastfeed exclusively as long as possible to suppress ovulation and space out their babies naturally. The usual reason I hear is that parents want to prevent allergies. In fact, there is *no* evidence that breastfeeding exclusively for more than six months prevents allergies at all. Indeed, one recent study suggested that it may actually increase the risk of allergies, though I didn't think this study was very well done. But there may be something to it. Studies from Sweden suggest that the risk of developing celiac disease in a child can be decreased by introducing gluten into the baby's diet while he is still breastfeeding. Celiac disease is, in some ways, similar to an allergic reaction of the gut. It is caused by gluten in the diet.

The parents are vegetarians or vegan

The American Academy of Pediatrics states that vegetarian and vegan diets are both appropriate for children and provide sufficient amounts of protein, calories and other nutrients.

Studies in both Great Britain and the United States found that children on proper vegetarian or vegan diets had higher intakes of fruits and vegetables than non-vegetarian children and consumed enough protein, vitamins and minerals with the exception of calcium, and, in the case of some vegan children, vitamin B^{12}. Parents should make sure that they include many calcium-containing foods, such as almond milk, tahini, tofu, etc., and provide supplemental vitamin B^{12} to their vegan children.

Vegetarian and vegan parents should emphasize more calorie-dense foods such as tofu, legume spreads with vegetable oil, yogurt, mashed avocado and dried fruits (but be careful: dried fruits can cause tooth decay: brush the baby's teeth after he eats them), as well as smooth nut and seed butters. Vegetarian and vegan children get adequate amounts of iron provided they eat enough whole grains, legumes, green leafy vegetables and dried fruits. To help iron absorption their meals should always include a source of vitamin C, such as peppers, citrus fruits, etc. Adequate amounts of protein can be obtained by eating a variety of legumes, nuts and grains.

There can be one issue if the mother is vegan and has been for several years. It is difficult to get adequate amounts of vitamin B^{12}, though some prepared foods (such as some brands of nutritional yeast) contain added vitamin B^{12}.

If the mother is deficient in B^{12} during the pregnancy, the baby will be born with inadequate stores and the mother's milk will also be deficient in B^{12}. This may result in severe irreversible neurological damage to the baby. To prevent this, vegans should have their levels tested and/or take vitamin B^{12} either as a daily supplement or by injection in larger doses.

When a baby is B^{12} deficient and has suffered neurological complications, the mother is often told she must stop breastfeeding, which makes absolutely no sense at all. Unfortunate as the situation is, a single injection of B^{12} for the baby and the mother will correct the deficiency in both, though not necessarily the baby's neurological problem.

Why would anyone suggest stopping breastfeeding? One reason is that the baby may also fail to gain weight well as a result of inadequate vitamin B^{12} intake, though this is not a reason to stop breastfeeding either. It is better to prevent the problem than to treat it. Vegan women intending to become pregnant should get an injection of vitamin B^{12} first.

With some planning it's quite possible to provide a vegan baby with all the nutrients he needs. Again, consultation with a breastfeeding-friendly pediatric dietitian can be very useful.

The baby was born prematurely

As far as starting solids, for the baby born only a little prematurely, say 35 weeks gestation, the approach would be the same as if he was born 38 or 41 weeks gestation. No issue as far as I can see.

The best approach is to follow the baby's lead. Unless he has significant neurological problems, the baby will let the parents know when he is ready to eat solids. It's not useful to try to decide if the baby should start solids according to his "corrected" age or "chronological" age.

Teresa's grandson Sebastian, who was born at 32 weeks, started solids when he was about nine months old—or seven months corrected age—because that was when he showed interest and was ready.

Do breastfed babies need vitamin D supplements?

We all need vitamin D. Without it, we develop bone disease. Children deficient in vitamin D before their bones are fully developed get a disease called rickets. Rickets is characterized by softening of the bones and deformities due to weight bearing on softened bones. Typically, the young child with rickets who is walking will often have exaggerated bowed legs. The child also can develop a "rachitic rosary," a line of lumps near where the ribs join the breast bone.

Adults who are deficient in vitamin D may develop osteomalacia, bones that have inadequate amounts of calcium and are thus prone to fracture. Adults with osteomalacia often have bone pain as well.

Until modern times, the need for vitamin D supplements did not exist. People were outdoors much more than they are now. Exposure of the skin to sunlight (ultraviolet rays) results in skin cells manufacturing active vitamin D. The body does not need long exposure to sunlight to make the necessary amounts of active vitamin D. A few minutes a day is enough, even in winter. Vitamin D is fat-soluble, so if the person has extra, it is stored in the liver. Thus, it is not necessary to get outside exposure every day. Furthermore, even on cloudy days, some ultraviolet radiation gets through and helps produce active vitamin D.

However, things have changed. We have become positively sun phobic. Of course, overexposure to the sun is not good, but complete avoidance is not a good idea either. Parents cover their children with sunblock for even a very short exposure to the sun. On top of that, smog, common in cities and more and more common even in the country, cuts out some of the ultraviolet rays. If the mother is deficient in vitamin D stores during the pregnancy, the baby will be at risk of having inadequate stores of Vitamin D as well.

Why would a mother not have enough vitamin D?

1. If she is dark skinned, she will absorb less of the ultraviolet rays to which she is exposed.
2. If she is in the habit of covering most of her body, as is common in some religious groups (Hasidic Jews, Muslims), she may not get adequate skin exposure to ultraviolet radiation.
3. Milk in North America is fortified with vitamin D, but many people, especially recent immigrants from Africa and Asia, do not drink milk.
4. Many immigrants from hot countries dread northern winters and do not go outside much from fall until spring.
5. Prenatal vitamins contain small amounts of vitamin D, but if the mother is already deficient, this amount may not bring up her stores adequately.
6. In many cities with significant smog problems, even being outside more may not improve the adequacy of the pregnant woman's stores of vitamin D.
7. Advice to use sunblock whenever going outside means that even women who are outdoors every day or go to sunny climates in the winter may not make much vitamin D.

Thus, there may be good reasons for breastfeeding mothers with insufficient amounts of vitamin D in pregnancy to give vitamin D supplements to their babies. Just as important, women who are at high risk for vitamin D deficiency should also supplement their own diet with vitamin D, preferably *before* they become pregnant, but also during the pregnancy to build up stores so that the baby is born with enough.

We used to say that there was not very much vitamin D in breastmilk and that the amount in the milk could not be changed by taking more vitamin D. However, there are a couple of studies that show if the mother is taking 5,000 International Units of vitamin D a day, her milk will actually provide enough vitamin D to protect the baby.

So, should we have a blanket statement (as most pediatric societies in North America have) that says: "All breastfeeding babies should receive vitamin D supplements"? I think the statement should be different. It should be: "All babies need vitamin D supplements in the first 6 to 12 months of life. Artificially fed babies will receive vitamin D that is added directly to their formula, since this vitamin is missing from cow's milk. Exclusively breastfed babies should get vitamin D supplements as medicinal drops."

I have to admit that part of the reason for my reluctance to accept the "need" for medicinal vitamin D is that it is not natural and that vitamin D can be had by outside exposure. At one time, vitamin D supplementation ads used the need for vitamin D to imply that breastmilk was not complete, but formula was. Many women do not breastfeed even if they believe that breastmilk provides everything that the baby needs. The notion that the need for suplemental vitamin D makes breastmilk less than perfect is just not true, and may discourage mothers from breastfeeding.

The bottom line

Starting babies on solid foods should be easy in the vast majority of cases if the parents abide by certain principles.

1. Respect the child. A child should start eating solids when he is ready. A child will vary how much he eats at any particular time, just as an adult does. There are times he may not want to eat at all. There are times when he might eat like a horse. When he wants to feed himself, he should be encouraged to do so, even if he does make a mess. One learns by doing.

2. There is no need to follow a particular order when starting the baby on solid foods.

3. There is no essential food except breastmilk. A baby doesn't have to like fish or pasta if he eats a variety of other foods.

4. "Nutrition" has become a sacred cow in North America. Too many people eat nutrition, not food. Just as breastfeeding is more than breastmilk, eating is more than nutrition. Mealtimes should be fun, not a struggle between parents and children.

5. For the child it is also a milestone to start eating solid foods. It means he's taking part in this family activity.

PART IV:

You and Your Breastfed Baby

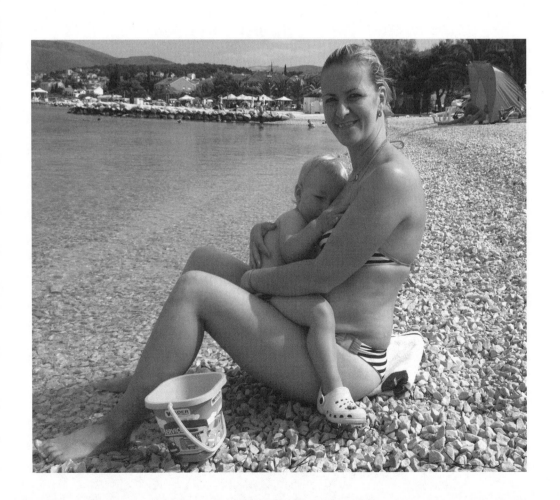

20 | Life with a Breastfeeding Baby

Breastfeeding, bottle-feeding—it's just about getting milk into the baby, right? Shouldn't make much difference in your life with the baby. Well, it does. And it can be challenging at first to figure out how to fit breastfeeding into your already busy life.

Maybe the most important thing to remember about life with a baby is that it gets easier. Those first few weeks with a new baby are overwhelming no matter how you are feeding him, and it's even tougher if you are also recovering from surgery or other birth interventions. So it's pretty much inevitable that the early weeks will be somewhat chaotic and stressful as you figure everything out.

Some mothers are prepared for that. They get some help with breastfeeding, get all the positions and techniques down pat, but life is still challenging, and at around six weeks they start to think, "Why isn't life back to normal?" Maybe friends and family are starting to complain a little bit because they aren't getting the attention they used to.

The truth is that life is never going to be back to "normal." You have a new normal that, taken in the right frame of mind, can be very good. Having a baby and breastfeeding are life-changing experiences. All of a sudden going to a movie on the spur of the moment is not so important anymore. You are now parents of a breastfeeding baby, and you *can* make it work. Here's how:

Make it easy to breastfeed at home

In the beginning, you probably need to sit or lie down or recline to breastfeed, and you'll probably be in that position for a while. You don't want to have to head back upstairs to your bedroom every time he's hungry, especially if you have a C-section incision that's just healing. So try to find (or create) several places in the house where you can easily get comfortable to nurse the baby.

Once you pick those spots (maybe your bed, the living room couch, a recliner in the family room or a comfortable armchair in the basement), you can decide what supplies you'd like to stock nearby: pillows to support you and the baby; a water bottle and some snacks; extra diapers and receiving blankets, just in case, and anything else that you find helpful. If you have a toddler or preschooler as well as your new baby, add some books or toys to entertain the older child while you nurse. You won't need these nursing stations forever, but they can make the first weeks easier as you recover and get things underway.

Another way to make breastfeeding easier at home is to recognize that it may take a lot of time at first, so there will be less time for other things. Some mothers deal with this by lowering their housekeeping standards. If the toilets don't get cleaned this week because the mother was nursing 12 times a day, then the toilets don't get cleaned, and if dinner is whatever the pizza guy delivers, then that's okay too.

But if you have the money or if you have friends who want to give you some gifts for the baby, you can pay to have someone do those things you don't have time for. Teresa knows one mother of twins who hired a personal chef for a day while she was pregnant. He discussed with her what foods she liked, went shopping and in a marathon cooking session prepared enough food to stock up her freezer for weeks. Some women have requested that people coming to their baby showers bring home-cooked meals to stock up their freezer or pantry rather than tiny outfits. You might have friends who would pay for a cleaning service for you for a few weeks so you can spend more time with your baby. There's no better baby gift!

Is your challenge finding the time and energy to entertain a toddler or an older child? Maybe you can hire a teen to come in for a few hours every day after school, not so you can go out (unless you want to), but so you can nap with the baby, catch up on emails or have a shower all by yourself. That's been a sanity saver for many mothers.

No generous friends to buy you some help, and you don't think you can lower your standards any more than you already have? Set some priorities: what things will make the most difference for you? For some it's having dishes clean and put away every night, for others it's having a clean bathroom, for still others it might be having healthy, nutritious meals every day. Focus on those priorities, and let the others slide as much as you need to.

There's one thing that only you can do, and that's breastfeed your baby. Get as much help as you can with all the other things so you can focus on breastfeeding. And remember what we said earlier—it gets better. Your baby won't always breastfeed this often or need so much time and attention at each feeding.

Have a "babymoon"

If you've been working full-time, when you are pregnant your maternity leave may look like a vast expanse of free time. Sure, you know you'll have to take care of the baby, but hey, those babies on TV sleep most of the time, don't they? You're excited about having time to go out with friends, shop on weekdays and avoid the weekend crowds or go to the theatre. You make plans and fill up your days, and then discover that the baby has his own plans.

The idea of a honeymoon dates from the time when husbands and wives didn't live together before they got married. It was meant to be a time for them to get to know each other better and get used to life together, without all the usual demands of work and family and friends. Parents of new babies need something similar. You need to get to know your baby's unique personality and needs, and he needs to get to know you. The work of building that relationship and establishing breastfeeding is going to take up much of your time for the first few weeks.

So if you can, block out the first six to eight weeks after your baby's birth for your "babymoon." Don't make too many plans, especially plans that require you to leave the baby behind. These weeks are an investment that will repay you many times over: you are establishing a good milk supply and, just as important, building a close relationship with your child that serves as the foundation for the future.

Forget about schedules

At first thought, it seems like scheduling feedings would make life easier. We like to have our days organized, with meetings and project times slotted in at predictable hours, so feeding the baby on a schedule seems appealing, too. But the truth is, not scheduling breastfeeding actually makes life easier.

Why? Well, first because breastfeeding works so much better when you're not trying to stick to a schedule. Stretch out the time between feedings to some arbitrary number of hours, and you're likely to be dealing with a cranky baby, uncomfortably full breasts and difficulties maintaining a good milk supply. You would need to find ways to soothe your baby (who really just wants to be at the breast), and you may have to take additional steps (such as pumping or taking supplements) to boost your milk production. You're not really gaining anything by trying to impose a schedule on something that just doesn't work effectively that way. It's surprising how many breastfeeding problems can be solved simply by feeding the baby in response to his cues.

Second, scheduling makes breastfeeding about *feeding* and not about the whole relationship that is involved. Breastfeeding isn't just about getting milk into the baby; it's about all the closeness, comfort, skin-to-skin contact, suckling, cuddling and hormones that go along with having a baby at the breast. Sometimes the milk is more like a nice little bonus. You wouldn't make up a schedule that said: "4:00 kiss baby; 4:45 cuddle baby; 5:30 comfort baby who was just startled by a loud clap of thunder." Breastfeeding does all those things and more for your baby, and focusing on it just as a method of feeding deprives both you and your baby of something special.

Third, when you schedule breastfeeding it's more likely to be a big production. You sit in your special nursing chair, maybe with a nursing pillow, and plan to sit there for 20 to 30 minutes while your baby feeds. Of course, it's fine to relax in a comfortable chair while you feed your baby! But if you are feeding in response to your baby's signals, you don't have to sit down every time. Once you've gotten past the early days of learning, you can nurse while you walk around, get a snack out of the fridge for your toddler, work on the computer, stand up and talk on the phone, lie down in bed for a little rest and maybe watch some TV or sit cross-legged on the floor to fold laundry. And each of these nursings may last only a few minutes or so. They would barely interrupt what you're doing. It's all these quick, casual nursings that

help keep up your milk supply and help keep your baby satisfied and happy—two things that make breastfeeding and mothering easier.

Another bonus: if you're feeding in response to your baby's cues, breastfeeding is easily interruptible. You don't have to be stuck on the couch for 30 minutes (unless you want to be because you're chatting with a friend or watching TV!). Let's say you are nursing the baby and suddenly remember you need to get the trash to the curb in time for pick-up. No problem—slip your finger into the corner of your baby's mouth to break the suction, put him down (or bring him with you) and carry that bag of garbage out to the road. When you come back in, offer to nurse again. He may be interested, he may not be. If he didn't take a full feeding, he may just nurse a little sooner next time.

You can also initiate a feeding if you want to, even if your baby isn't acting hungry. Maybe you have a doctor's appointment soon or you really want a shower, but your baby is contentedly batting at his baby-gym toys. Go ahead and offer to nurse. He might refuse, but many babies are quite willing to nurse even if they're not all that hungry—and this may prevent him crying miserably in the car or while you're in the shower. When you don't bother with a schedule, breastfeeding can be quite flexible and adaptable.

Get comfortable with breastfeeding in public

La Leche League did a survey a few years ago to find out why mothers opted not to breastfeed, and one of the most commonly cited reasons was that they didn't want to breastfeed in public. That's understandable, given some of the unpleasant comments and harassment breastfeeding women have sometimes had to endure, but it's a very sad statement about our society. Breasts as sexual objects are

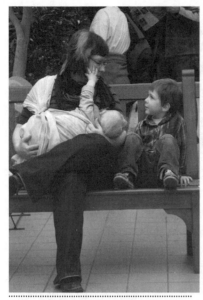

CREDIT: THOMAS BEAUCHAMP

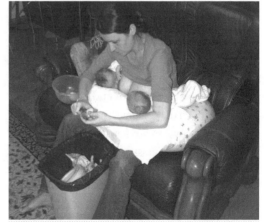

Breastfeeding can happen anywhere, anytime. Just make sure the baby is safe.

CREDIT: GREGORY D. MCMILLAN

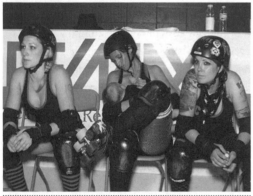

CREDIT: RUSS DESAULNIERS

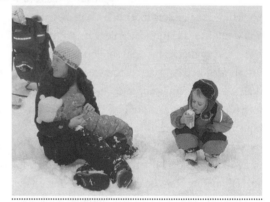

CREDIT: ANDRIES MELLENA

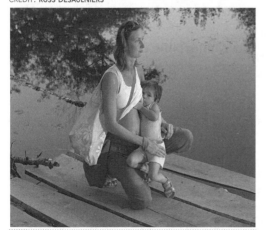

CREDIT: ANDREA POLOKOVA

CREDIT: ANDREA POLOKOVA

used to sell everything from cars to beer, but when breasts are used to feed babies, it's outrageous. Yet some mothers do get the thumbs-up from passersby. Accept the positive and forget about the unpleasant comments. Your baby's need to breastfeed is more important than some stranger's prudery.

The importance of breastfeeding is widely recognized these days, yet women who do so in public are still often told to "cover up" or leave to feed their babies. This continues even though human rights commissions in every Canadian province where this issue has come up, as well as explicit laws in most U.S. states, clearly state that women have the right to breastfeed wherever they and their babies have the right to be.

Knowing your rights is important because your life as a breastfeeding mother will be much easier if you can feel comfortable breastfeeding in public. The alternatives are either to stay home most of the time, leaving only for short periods (and worrying that you won't get back in time or that your breasts will leak while you are out), or to plan ahead for every outing by finding some extra free time (and remember how hard this can be!) so that you can pump and bottle-feed your milk. (These suggestions are sometimes made in comments to online articles about mothers breastfeeding in public. They are generally made by people who don't have babies.) If you can breastfeed your baby anywhere, you have the freedom to go anywhere and do what you need to do. In fact, it's much easier to be out and about with a breastfed baby than with one who is bottle-fed: no need to pack bottles and formula or worry about keeping it at the right temperature.

Many women are quite comfortable breastfeeding in public right from the start, but others may not have seen it happen very often so they feel anxious about it. If you're nervous about breastfeeding in public, here are some tips to make it easier:

- Practice latching your baby on at home in front of a mirror. You'll soon see that there isn't as much breast visible as you imagined, and watching in the mirror will help you see how to adjust your clothes or position for maximum modesty, if that's what you are looking for.
- If you wear a loose top or T-shirt that you can lift up from the bottom (rather than a shirt that you pull down from the top), your breasts will be less exposed. If you are wearing a button-up shirt, leave the top buttons done up and unbutton from the bottom.
- An unbuttoned shirt or jacket over your T-shirt will help cover even more.
- Sometimes it's not so much about exposing your breasts as it is about the embarrassment of revealing your postpartum tummy when you pull up that T-shirt. You can get an ordinary tank top and cut out openings for your breasts, then wear this tank under your shirt so the fabric covers your belly when you lift up your shirt to breastfeed. Some nursing tops are designed in a similar way. Or if you used a belly band when you were pregnant, you might want to dig it out again for nursing in public.
- Many babies will nurse well in a sling or wrap carrier, and the fabric of the sling can be pulled up slightly to cover you and the baby. Your tummy will be exposed, though, and you may want to wear something to cover that body part—see the previous point.
- Getting the baby actually latched on is the trickiest part in terms of how much breast is exposed, so you may want to see if you can turn away from any onlookers for a moment or two during that part. In a restaurant, for example, see if you can sit with your back to the rest of the room. Once the baby is nursing, you can move to a more comfortable position. In our society,

exposing breasts is considered audacious at best, actually obscene at worst. Remember, though, you are doing nothing wrong.

- In a previous chapter, I mentioned getting comfortable breastfeeding in public by taking the baby to the movies and breastfeeding when the lights go down.

What about breastfeeding cover-ups? I do not like the message they send—that breastfeeding needs to be covered up in public. Some women love them, but many feel they just announce: "Breastfeeding is going on here! But it's embarrassing, so we've had to use this big obvious cover-up!" And often they create more problems than they solve. Especially in the beginning, it can be hard to latch the baby on without being able to look at him. And, not surprisingly, many babies hate them. Would you like to eat a meal with a blanket over your head? Of course, a cover-up can be useful if someone makes a negative comment about not wanting to see you breastfeeding your baby. Just hand him the cover-up and suggest he can put it over his own head. Problem solved!

There's no denying that it can be very upsetting to be approached by someone and told to "stop doing that" or "go to the washroom." Here you are, giving your baby the best possible nourishment in the most natural way, and someone is suggesting that what you are doing is wrong, disgusting or even obscene. Many women have been reduced to tears in such situations, and even those who are normally confident are surprised at how vulnerable and embarrassed it can make them feel. But you have every right to feel confident about what you are doing. You are *not* in the wrong. The person harassing you—and yes, it is harassment—is wrong, and the law supports you. In every single case we know about where a breastfeeding mother has gone to court or to a human rights commission, or even just to the management

of the company where the incident occurred, she has been proven right and given an apology. Take courage from that.

And remember that by nursing in public you are doing something very important for the next generation of breastfeeding mothers. Some little girl may see you lovingly feeding your baby and file that away as something she wants to do someday. Some teenager who had the idea that breastfeeding "wasn't for her" because it would tie her down too much may realize that she can, in fact, have a life and go to lunch with her friends even if she's breastfeeding.

Of course, if you find you are really uncomfortable with breastfeeding in public, using a cover of some kind is better than feeding your baby with a bottle when you go out or not going out at all. We still think the message it sends is a negative one, and that many babies don't like them and will try to push them off. Do try practising nursing at home in front of a mirror without that cover-up and you'll probably find you can do without it.

Here's an email from a close friend: "I agree with indiscreet breastfeeding even though I would normally be shy about many things in public. Breastfeeding in public somehow always seemed normal to me, and I would breastfeed in public all the time; never once did I have any comments from anyone. I wonder why that is. There was a group of us breastfeeding mothers who would go to restaurants and parks and other places and breastfeed very indiscreetly, and no one said a word. Actually, the first time I heard this was an issue was when I heard you talk about it at a conference. I do not think it takes courage—I am not a courageous person—it is just that the baby must feed and if he doesn't, he is going to scream, and I thought that would bother people a lot more. So by keeping my baby quiet on the breast I thought I was doing everybody a service. I do not like the idea of breastfeeding covers, and the list of things you must do to prepare for breastfeeding in public seems to me to imply that you must think very carefully before you do it, and that is a pity."

Keep your baby close

It's easier to figure out your baby's cues and respond to them quickly when you have him close by. Sure, you can leave him in a crib in another room with a baby monitor to pick up his crying, but by then you might have missed the early signals such as his finger going to his mouth, or his squirming and trying to suck on his blanket. Crying is a late sign of hunger, and a baby who is upset and crying hard may not nurse well (and has probably swallowed air as well).

Keeping your baby close to you has many other benefits besides making you more aware of his feeding cues. Your baby's brain is growing and developing quickly during these early years. His experiences affect how his brain is wired and connected. Keeping him close to you means he's getting exposed to all kinds of new things, even when he's sleeping in your arms or in a sling—the sound of your voice as you talk with your partner, the smells of the food you are cooking, the feel of the wind on his cheek when you go outside—and all those things register in his brain. And he is also sharing germs with you, and that is a *good* thing. A baby lying in a crib in a quiet room is not having all those important experiences.

If you use a sling or a wrap or a soft baby carrier to keep your baby with you, there are even greater benefits. With your baby positioned upright, tummy against your chest, the small movements he experiences as you walk around act like a gentle massage. That upright position can help with reflux (the bent-in-the-middle position babies are forced into in car seats tends to make reflux worse). Canadian researcher Dr. Ron Barr found that breastfed babies who are carried in slings or infant carriers cry less than half as much as babies who are not, and gain weight better.

But wait! you say. I need a break. Sometimes I want to go out, do something for myself, just not have to worry about the baby for a while. Is that possible if I'm breastfeeding?

Sure it is. And it's important to take care of yourself when you have the big responsibility of caring for a baby. It helps to figure out what you really need. Maybe you don't actually need to be away from your baby—maybe all you need is a change of scenery. Your sling or carrier makes your baby very portable. You might find that doing some of the things you always enjoyed in the past (dinner with friends, visiting a museum, walking on the beach) with your baby along for the trip will give you enough of a change that you feel refreshed.

Maybe what you need is not time away from the baby but more help with other tasks. It might feel easier to deal with a fussy, frequently nursing baby if you could get help with laundry, dishes and food preparation. Or maybe you just need more time with friends or with your partner to get some emotional support and reassurance that you are doing a great job.

Maybe you need just an hour or two to relax. That can usually be managed pretty easily, too: feed the baby first, then head off for your massage or pedicure, or just lock yourself in the bathroom for a bubble bath and some time to read a novel while your partner or Grandma or another caring person tends your baby. By the time your baby's hungry again, you'll be refreshed and ready to jump back into motherhood.

Really desperate for a longer break?

Remember that you are much more to your baby than a milk provider. He is attached to you, the most important person in his life, and he may not be happy about being apart from you. If you can find ways to meet your needs with your baby there as well, both you and he will be happier. The time when your baby needs you so intensely is really very short, and soon he'll be waving good-bye as he goes off to spend the day at a friend's house.

Sleep close to your baby

Sleep tends to be an obsession for new parents, and we have an entire chapter on sleep. But here's a summary: babies need to nurse during the night. How often they nurse, and when they will outgrow this need, depends on a number of factors, including your milk storage capacity, the baby's rate of growth and probably his temperament (remember, it's not just about the milk). Night feedings are important to maintain your milk supply and delay the return of your menstrual cycle (because prolactin levels are higher during night feedings).

But you're *tired. Exhausted*, even. And you hear that babies sleep longer and better if they get formula. Not true. Several recent studies have shown that mothers breastfeeding exclusively get *more* sleep than those who give some formula or those who bottle-feed exclusively. That's right, *more*. But a key factor is sleeping close to your baby, whether it's sharing your bed or with the baby in a crib or bassinet right beside your bed.

Here's where the ease and convenience of breastfeeding is most obvious. There's no need to get up in the night to warm up a bottle or go to another room to get the baby. Your baby may not even be fully awake when you lift him from the bassinet to the bed or simply snuggle him closer and help him latch on. He'll drink all he needs and drift back to sleep again, and you can too. Your sleep was barely interrupted, and the act of breastfeeding has produced plenty of relaxing hormones to help you go back to sleep as well.

Experiment with sex

Talking about sleeping with your baby tends naturally to lead to another topic: What about sex? If the baby sleeps in your room or in your bed, is your sex life over?

It doesn't have to be, but you may find at first that your interest in sex is fairly low anyway. This varies among women, but some find that while they are breastfeeding, sex is low on their priority list. The hormones of lactation may mean less vaginal lubrication and a lowered sex drive. And, when you're as tired as most new mothers are, you don't have much energy for sex. If you're going to be in bed, you'd like to be sleeping.

But this can actually be a great time to experiment. If you're worried about waking the baby, sneak out of the bedroom and try another location. Get creative! You may need more "warming up" before you have enough lubrication for intercourse to be comfortable, and that's another opportunity to be creative and discover just what does "turn you on." You may need to try different positions to find those that are most enjoyable, especially if you had an episiotomy or if your breasts are tender. And yes, you may leak a little milk at times. Try feeding the baby first so you're not too full, and, as a bonus, the baby will be less likely to wake up and need you.

Remember, you are getting lots of physical contact and affectionate touching from your baby all day long, especially if you are using a sling or carrier. Your partner isn't getting nearly as much and is probably counting on you to help make it up. A massage, a warm hug or some cuddling on the couch will help your partner's mental health and ultimately help the relationship—and, who knows, you may find you feel like having sex after all.

Expect change

Here's the thing about babies: they grow and change very rapidly. Your tiny, almost helpless newborn may be walking and talking only 18 months later. That means every time you think you have him figured out, he changes. Some things will get easier, some may get harder. You'll go from having to carry your baby everywhere to having a mobile child who can get himself where he wants to go. So some things become easier—your arms aren't as tired. Other things become harder, because the baby who can get around on his own can get into everything, and you have to be constantly on alert to make sure he doesn't walk off the end of the porch.

Of course, that's change on a bigger scale. Babies also change from day to day. Maybe you had a houseful of visitors yesterday and your baby was overstimulated, so today he's fussier and clingier than usual. Or he picked up a virus and is sniffly and cranky and nursing constantly for a couple of days. He may not actually get sick, because the antibodies in your milk have helped to protect him, but you may have a couple of days when you seem to do nothing but nurse. That's what helps him stay healthy.

There will also be days when your older baby or toddler is learning new skills and exploring the world and gets so distracted by all these discoveries that he practically forgets to nurse. Or he'll nurse, but after a minute or so he may catch sight of a bird outside your window and let go of the nipple so he can check out this new, exciting creature. You'll try to coax him back to the breast but he hears a truck revving up on the road and wants to see what's making that noise. Often during this stage the baby starts waking more at night, making up for those interrupted and missed feedings.

The more flexible you are, the easier it will be to incorporate all these changes. Life with a baby is always going to be rather unpredictable, and being able to follow your baby's lead will make breastfeeding easier.

Wean only when you are ready

Mothers don't often come to our clinic for help with weaning. They usually come because they want help continuing to breastfeed. But they do call Teresa and other La Leche League leaders quite often with questions about how to stop breastfeeding.

The ideal, I think, is to let the baby wean himself. Baby-led or child-led weaning tends to be very gradual, and this is easier on both the mother and the child. However, it should be noted that eight-month-old babies do not "wean themselves." Indeed it is unlikely that any baby younger than two years old will wean himself. See chapters on "Late-onset Decreased Milk Supply" and "The Normal Duration of Breastfeeding."

However, there may be times when baby-led weaning isn't possible. Sometimes there are medical reasons: a mother needs chemotherapy or must take another medication that is simply not compatible with breastfeeding, though the vast majority of drugs are (see the chapter on "Breastfeeding While on Medication"). There may be situations in which mothers need extra support so they can continue breastfeeding or make the changes necessary for breastfeeding to work. Breastfeeding is a relationship between two people and creative ways can often be found to ensure that the needs of both mother and baby are met. It might be helpful for mothers to know that breastfeeding is not an all-or-nothing proposition, and especially when the baby is over six months, adjustments can be made so that breastfeeding can continue.

An LLL leader will usually try to explore a mother's concerns with her, since very often mothers are told they have to wean before it's necessary. The medication the mother needs to take may, in fact, be perfectly compatible with breastfeeding. There may be options the mother hasn't thought of that might make it possible to continue at least partial breastfeeding after she goes back to work.

Many mothers are surprised when, even though they want or thought they wanted to stop breastfeeding, they have an unexpected emotional reaction to stopping. I used to get emails from mothers who were on domperidone and who stopped breastfeeding, usually "cold turkey," and found they were anxious and had panic attacks. In some cases they couldn't sleep. I worried that these reactions were due to stopping the domperidone, but I've heard from other mothers since who had never taken domperidone or other galactogues but had the same strong reaction to weaning. One mother told me that she had decided to wean her son, and had cut back to two feedings per day. She'd noticed physical changes—such as her period returning—but said the most difficult part was emotional. She'd been experiencing anxiety and panic attacks and found the feelings very unpleasant and unpredictable. Yet she also felt weaning was necessary because she had ongoing chronic health problems. This mother's health problems were attributed to breastfeeding and everyone was telling her to stop, including several doctors, naturopaths and others. A public health nurse told her to "bribe" the three-year-old with candy and ask her GP for an antidepressant for the "'hormonal' component." An antidepressant to solve her reactions to not really wanting to wean the child? Bribe the child with candy? What interesting ideas! Yet this mother was now feeling worse than she had before she started the weaning process. This woman had three young children. Taking care of children is not easy work, but breastfeeding should not be exhausting. Everyone always blames

breastfeeding for mothers' problems, including, in this case, this woman's doctors, her naturopaths, public health nurses and probably her family. It's not the breastfeeding!

The point is that sometimes mothers do not know how much they care about breastfeeding. Often they think they want to stop because others feel they should. When her life is not perfect, others tell her it's the breastfeeding that's at fault. Actually, this seems to be very common even if everything is going well for the mother and baby. "When are you going to stop feeding her? It's not normal," is a common theme. But, at least for this mother (and many others, I may add) the problems aren't because of breastfeeding. On the contrary—it would appear that breastfeeding kept her on a more even keel. Here is what she wrote me, after I expressed these feelings: "Thank you! I am almost crying tears of relief."

Trust your baby, trust yourself

As a new mother, you'll get plenty of advice on how to take care of your baby. But you are the one who knows yourself, your situation and your baby best. While at first it can be hard to figure it out, you'll soon learn to read your baby's signals and know when he's hungry or tired, needs some entertainment or just wants to be close to you. You'll figure out your own needs and priorities and find ways to make breastfeeding fit your situation in whatever way works for you.

21 | Sleep: Yours and Your Baby's

Myth #1: Formula-fed babies sleep better than breastfed babies.

Fact: Even though everyone (even many breastfeeding advocates) may say this, it is not really true, or not necessarily true.

Myth #2: If you bring your baby into your bed at night, you are starting a bad habit that will create on-going sleep problems, or you are putting your baby at risk of death by SIDS or smothering.

Fact: Breastfeeding babies have slept with their mothers for thousands of generations, and there is absolutely no evidence that this is harmful, especially when the baby is breastfed exclusively. The studies that seem to "prove" that babies sleeping in parents' beds are at greater risk do not usually distinguish whether the baby was breastfed or not. They don't usually distinguish between babies in a safe co-sleeping situation or an unsafe one, such as the baby who is overdressed, covered with a duvet or sleeping on a water bed.

Talk to parents in any country in the world and you'll hear the same thing: babies wake up at night. They wake up to feed, but also perhaps to reassure themselves that they are safe and have an adult close by to protect them. Some babies wake up quite frequently at night—others, only once or twice, and of course the pattern changes over time.

Many breastfeeding mothers find it easy to manage feedings at night if they keep the baby in bed with them, or if the baby sleeps in a bassinet or crib right beside the bed. Then it's a simple matter of moving over a little and breastfeeding the baby when he wakes in the night, or picking up the baby and breastfeeding. Research has shown that the "family bed" or bed-sharing arrangement is associated with breastfeeding for a longer period of time.

Does this mean you *have* to have your baby in bed with you to breastfeed? No, not at all. Each family needs to figure out what works best for them. There certainly are parents who have managed to breastfeed successfully with the baby in a crib in another room at night. (Having the baby sleep in a separate room increases his risk of SIDS. If you or your partner smoke, even if you never smoke in the bedroom, the baby is safer sleeping at some distance from you. If you don't smoke, it's safer to have the baby sharing your room.)

There has been an active campaign in the United States, Canada and some other countries suggesting that it is very dangerous for parents to bring their babies into their beds. One advertisement shows a bed with the headboard turned into a tombstone. (Many babies die in cribs but you don't see ads showing the side of a crib as a tombstone.) Another ad shows a baby sleeping in bed with a meat cleaver. Outrageous.

These campaigns are based on research that is not reliable. Infant deaths that occur anywhere but in a crib are often lumped into one category—so included in that group are babies sleeping in car seats, on couches and recliners (both known to be very dangerous for entrapment), on water beds, left alone on an adult bed, sleeping with teenaged babysitters, with parents who have been drinking heavily or taking drugs, etc. Some of these cases may have actually been homicides. Because the overall number of infants who die is quite low, all these confounding factors are significant.

Most important, these reviews almost never take into account how the baby is fed. We do know from research that babies who are breastfed are much less likely to die of SIDS. Research by Helen Ball, an anthropologist from Great Britain, has shown that breastfed babies are less likely to die of overlaying or suffocation because their mothers position themselves in the bed differently. In her study, in which she videotaped mothers sleeping with their babies, she found that breastfeeding mothers slept facing their babies with one arm resting on the bed above the baby's head. It is impossible to roll over on the baby in that position. The baby was also at breast height.

Bottle-feeding mothers, on the other hand, often slept with their backs toward the baby. In this position, the risk of rolling onto the baby is somewhat higher (although it is still unlikely). The bottle-fed babies were often placed in the bed with their heads near or on the pillows, increasing the risk of suffocation.

In a more recent study, Ball noticed that families from India and Pakistan living in England had much lower rates of SIDS than families she described as "white British" in the same town. She interviewed families from both groups about how they cared for their babies and found that those from India and Pakistan were much more likely to have their babies share their beds. They were also less likely to smoke and more likely to breastfeed exclusively.

Based on various studies, sharing a bed with a baby is safest if:

- the baby is next to the mother (not another adult or child), and the mother has not been drinking or taking any drugs that might make her too drowsy to be woken up easily;
- neither parent smoked during the pregnancy or smokes at present;
- the mother is breastfeeding the baby, especially exclusively;
- the mattress is firm, with minimal pillows and (ideally) open-weave blankets rather than a heavy duvet or comforter;
- the baby is dressed in light clothes, as overheating is linked to SIDS and can be a problem in bed-sharing;
- the baby sleeps on his back.

Lactation consultant Diane Wiessinger comments: "Use common sense. Just as parents and manufacturers have taken steps to make cribs safer, you can do the same with your bed or bedroom arrangement."

You can also try using a "co-sleeper," a mattress that attaches to the side of your bed and keeps the baby within arm's reach. Even if you decide to have your baby in a crib or bassinet next to your bed, there's no reason not to bring him onto the bed to breastfeed at night, and then gently move him back when he's asleep again—though this last part is really hard to do without waking the baby.

Keeping your baby close to you at night makes breastfeeding easier. It can be especially important in the early days. Another study by Ball took newborn babies in a hospital and divided them into three groups. One group slept in bed with their mothers, the second group slept in co-sleepers attached to the hospital beds and the third group slept in bassinets beside their mothers' beds. The first and second group of babies nursed more often and lost less weight than those in bassinets. The real story, though, is in the results four months later: only half as many of the bassinet babies were still breastfeeding, compared to the babies who shared their mothers' beds. The babies in the co-sleepers were slightly less likely to be breastfeeding than the babies who had bed-shared.

Dr. Jim McKenna observed babies when they slept with their mothers and when they slept alone and found that those who slept with their mothers woke more often to breastfeed and were stimulated to breathe by the mother's breathing and movements in her sleep. He concludes that bed-sharing can protect against SIDS.

Night feeding

Even those who don't push the idea that it is dangerous for a healthy, breastfeeding baby to be in its mother's bed will criticize the mother for nursing the baby through the night. I often hear this. Mothers are told that having the baby in bed and responding when the baby wakes at night will cause "unhealthy sleep habits," and that the baby who wakes at night and nurses back to sleep has a "sleep problem."

In fact, there is a whole group of pediatric specialists who deal with "sleep problems." Many of these specialists believe that babies should never be breastfed to sleep and that after a certain age— usually around four months, but definitely after six months—babies should not be breastfed at all during the night. The old tactic of letting the baby "cry it out" is back in vogue (though now it may be called "controlled crying" or "learning to self-soothe"). These specialists believe that a baby who wakes during the night after six months is not exhibiting "normal" behaviour and has a sleep problem. This becomes a newly classified medical problem and, unfortunately, many of the recommended "treatments" end up interfering with breastfeeding.

Let's consider, first of all, the question of the

baby waking at night to feed. Is this normal, or is it a symptom of a sleep problem with potentially harmful long-term consequences?

Our perceptions of sleep have changed considerably over the past century. Here is a quote from *Canada's Baby Book*, published in 1928:

> At birth the baby should sleep almost 23 hours out of 24.
>
> He should sleep at least 18 hours a day until six months old.
>
> At least 16 hours until one year old.
>
> At least 14 hours until four years old, part of which should be in the afternoon at a regular hour.
>
> The baby should sleep alone in a room or at least have a crib or a bed to himself. Never rock a baby to sleep. Never put a baby to sleep in your arms; it is a bad habit, tiresome for yourself and unwholesome for the baby.

Whose baby are they talking about? I have never heard of a six-month-old baby sleeping 18 hours a day, unless he was drugged. Not even at three months. Perhaps some babies sleep a lot in the first two or three days of life, but after that—23 out of 24 hours? That's actually not good if the baby is more than a few days old.

Think about this in terms of actually looking after the baby, even if the baby is feeding just once every four hours: that means six feedings in 24 hours. He has only an hour, total, to get in six feedings, so we're allotting 10 minutes per feeding. Apparently the baby is also expected to sleep through bath time and diaper changes.

Was this *really* true in 1928, or was this something that health professionals decided was "best for baby"? Probably the latter, as these commandments are not based on reality. The same is true in this new century, when sleep experts decide at what age babies should sleep through the night, among other "rules" for "normal infant sleep."

Let's look back to the time when our ancestors lived in tribal communities. Babies and their mothers slept together, usually with older children and fathers, too. It was safer that way. There was nothing easier for a lion or other carnivore to pick off than a single human sleeping alone. Gorillas and other primates sleep this way. And of course, it is still the norm in traditional human societies around the world.

Human milk has adapted to this situation—or perhaps it is the other way around: humans have adapted to their milk. There is a general relationship between the type of milk a species produces and how often the nursling goes to the breast. For example, some mammals, such as rabbits, feed their babies only occasionally and leave the babies alone in a nest or shelter for long periods of time; the milk of these animals is high in protein. It is a good strategy for rabbits, which are prey for owls and foxes, not to have to feed their babies too often in case they need to run. Other mammals have low levels of protein in their milk, and they feed very frequently and keep their babies close to them. Humans fit into the second group.

In traditional societies, babies sleep next to their mothers and generally feed on and off throughout the night. It is *normal* for babies to want and need to feed at night. Most adults are used to a certain number of hours of uninterrupted sleep, though most do wake up a few times and don't usually remember doing so. Babies do not have to sleep an uninterrupted number of hours at night, and are usually quite happy and content to wake up frequently *if they are comforted and fed.*

Just as in the case of colic, which eventually gets better, there will come a time when a child will sleep through the night. There will also be a time when he leaves the parents' bed. When he is 16 years old, those night feedings and night wakings will be a distant memory! I have, in my office, a drawing called "Night Feeding" by a mother who nursed five children. It is obvious that, at least from the distance of several years, those were not terrible times for her. Indeed, many mothers remember the night feedings as the best times they had with their babies—when it was just mother and baby, away from the rush and hubbub of the day.

Once mothers are reassured that night feedings won't lead to unhealthy sleep habits or an overly dependent child (or the other problems they've been warned about) they stop being concerned. When a baby sleeps next to his mother, their sleep and wake cycles match, so the mother is never jarred out of a deep sleep. She wakes up as her baby wakes up, they nurse and drift back to sleep together.

Nursing a baby to sleep is not harmful, either. I suppose it would be nice if the baby could also fall asleep without nursing some of the time, but he will eventually be able to do that, guaranteed. Maybe not at six months, maybe not at a year, maybe not even at two or three years—but eventually, it will happen.

Some physicians view nursing a baby to sleep as on a level with child abuse, yet are enthusiastic about letting a baby cry himself to sleep. Researchers at Harvard University found that when babies are left to cry themselves to sleep, they have high levels of cortisol, the hormone released when we experience stress. Is that surprising? Other studies have shown that even when the baby stops crying, his cortisol levels stay high.

One of the great pleasures of parenthood, in my opinion, is having a baby fall asleep in your arms. It makes you feel good. It makes you feel competent. "The little guy trusts me so much he will just fall asleep in my arms." And the heat he gives off when he just falls into sleep—what a pleasure it is to feel that! But too many parents are advised to make sure this never happens, because it will be spoil the baby and he will never sleep through the night. Not true; I don't know if this is a secret I'm sharing, but one day your child will indeed sleep through the night. Guaranteed.

Sleeping with your baby is not harmful for him, for you or for your partner. On the contrary, it is healthy for everyone. Many mothers and babies prefer sleeping together, and many fathers enjoy it, too. You are much less tired if the baby is sleeping next to you and wakes up for nursing. No need to get up and go to the baby. Yes, you must become more inventive with regard to intimacy—but that just adds to the excitement.

One mother told me that people commented all the time about how beautiful, sweet, healthy and friendly her son was. He was affectionate yet independent at just over a year old. The mother commented that this was very different from what she'd been told: people had warned her that her son would become clingy, anxious and spoiled because he nursed and slept with her at night.

In fact, this mother was told by a psychiatrist that her feelings of concern and protectiveness were not normal and that she should force herself to put the baby in a crib at night. This is an incredible statement for a psychiatrist to make. What could be more normal than for a mother to feel concerned and protective about her baby? When I hear advice like that, I believe it is more often the issues and "baggage" of the professional that are being revealed, because there is certainly no scientific research to support this. Another mother was told that putting the baby in a crib to sleep would help his verbal development, because when the little boy woke up in the morning alone, he would talk to himself. If the mother kept the baby in her bed, he would be deprived of this valuable experience. I burst out laughing when I heard this. What nonsense! The

Sleeping arrangements

Parents have come up with many ingenious methods to keep their babies close to them at night. The simplest, of course, is just to bring the baby into your bed. Here are some other strategies parents have used:

- A very young baby can sleep in a bassinet next to the bed.
- An adjustable crib can be pushed up against the bed, so that the crib mattress is level with the bed, with the side of the crib removed. Be sure there are no gaps or cracks the baby can fall into.
- "Side-car" beds attach to the parents' bed and consist of a small mattress with a railing around the other three sides.
- Mattresses can be placed on the floor—a queen-sized mattress for the parents plus a single mattress pushed up beside it for the baby and any other children, providing lots of space and no worries about falls.
- A bed or mattress in the baby's room has helped some families when the father finds he doesn't sleep well with the baby close by. The baby goes to sleep and is put in a crib in his room. When he wakes up, the mother feeds him in the bed in this room, and they both spend the rest of the night there.

baby who wakes up next to his parents has an actual person to talk to, and can have his babbling and early words responded to—a much better way to encourage language. It just goes to show that any argument, no matter how ridiculous, can be used to justify a strongly held belief. Too often parents believe such arguments, even if they make no sense, because the advice comes from an authority figure.

Research on long-term effects of co-sleeping

In a paper published in 2005 in *Pediatric Respiratory Review*, Dr. James McKenna summarizes work by a number of other researchers who looked at the long-term outcomes for children who slept with their parents when they were babies or preschoolers. Their results contradicted many of the dire warnings parents are often given. The studies found:

- Children who routinely slept alone were more likely to be fearful and have tantrums, and were described as "less happy."
- College students who had slept with their parents when they were young had significantly higher self-esteem and less anxiety.
- Children who had slept with their parents received higher evaluations from their teachers and had lower rates of psychiatric problems.
- Co-sleeping children grew up to have greater satisfaction in life and other positive traits.

Encouraging sleep

Would my baby sleep longer if he were bottle-fed?

This is yet another myth that arises from using the bottle-feeding baby as our model of "normal infant feeding." I believe this based on my understanding of breastfeeding, as well as based on the stories of mothers who say that their babies sleep better when fed by bottle. It doesn't matter what is in the bottle. The baby sleeps four hours, for example, after 120 ml (4 oz.) of formula, but also after 120 ml (4 oz.) of breastmilk. Yet he will sleep only two hours when breastfed. Why would that be?

The answer goes back to how mothers are taught to breastfeed. When babies go to the breast, rarely do they latch on in the most mechanically efficient manner for getting milk. This does not always matter because in the presence of an abundant milk supply, the baby can do fine. However, this often means frequent feedings and long periods on the breast. It also means frequent feedings at night. In most traditional societies, this is not a problem. Women in traditional African San (or Bushmen) society apparently feed as often as four times an hour, though obviously the feedings are short. If you are walking along, going about your work, and the baby nurses all the while, almost without your noticing it, it is no big deal. If sleeping with your baby and having him nurse periodically is what your society sees as normal, it is no big deal.

In North America, though, the baby who does not nurse effectively (for our "lifestyle," since the San baby is nursing quite effciently for his "lifestyle") will also want more frequent feedings. The baby may not get 120 ml (4 oz.) as he would from the bottle. He may get 60 ml (2 oz.) or even less and, not surprisingly, will sleep only a couple of hours or less. Or he may stay on the breast because he is not satisfied and eventually fall asleep at the breast. A few minutes after the mother eases him off, he may begin to cry.

If you want your baby to sleep longer between feedings, get the best latch possible. Use compression to increase the amount of milk he gets at the breast, and try to "finish" the first side before you offer the second. How do you know a baby is finished? Because he no longer actually gets milk, even with compression (see the video clips at www.breastfeedinginc.ca). But remember, even when a baby may not be getting milk for a few minutes, there may be another letdown of milk and he will drink again. So don't be in a big rush to take him off the breast.

If your baby drinks really well and gets plenty of the high-fat milk, he may in fact go several hours between feedings. As the weeks go by, he may stretch out the feedings at night, and eventually sleep through the night. I usually worry when a two-week-old is sleeping through the night, since this may indicate inadequate intake of milk, but I have seen exclusively breastfed, well-gaining babies who are, in fact, sleeping through the night at two weeks of age. There is nothing about formula that "makes" babies sleep longer. The determining factor is the quantity they get.

I realize that this is different from what you may have read elsewhere about breastmilk emptying out of the stomach faster than formula, or about certain amino acids in artificial milk that make the baby sleepier. There may be something to that, but essentially, babies will be hungrier faster if they get less milk at the feeding, whatever that milk is. Overall, the amount the baby gets may be more than enough, but if he gets it in little "snacks," he will feed frequently.

Babies don't wake up in the night only because they are hungry. Researchers have shown that whenever a baby is learning a new skill, for example (such as rolling over or sitting up or crawling), he's likely to start waking frequently during the night. The excitement of his new daytime accomplishments seems to make him restless at night. Breastfeeding is a great tool to have in these situations: it soothes the frightened or lonely baby, calms the restless one and helps everyone go back to sleep as quickly as possible.

So what to do?

You can work to increase the effectiveness of your baby's latch so that he gets the maximum amount of milk at each feeding, and this may encourage him to sleep longer. You can also continue feeding him at night as long and as often as he needs to with the confidence that this is not harmful or dangerous.

Researchers in Australia have found that mothers vary quite a bit in their milk storage capacity. Some women create and store up more milk in their breasts than others. Even though they all can make enough for their babies over 24 hours, those with lower milk storage capacities have to feed the baby more often. These mothers in particular may find the night feedings are essential to help their babies get enough milk.

Dr. Spock was wrong

This one is our own story—mine and Adele's—so names will not be changed to protect the innocent. Our first child did not sleep through the night until he was four years old. At one point, we had decided it was getting too difficult, and we tried letting him cry it out. This was when he was seven months old.

The first thing we found out was that the baby will cry longer than 20 minutes the first night. Dr. Spock was wrong. Even 20 minutes, to the ears of his parents, seems like about two hours. It is awful, and, truthfully, I don't know how some parents can survive it. Perhaps we should have been stronger, but we gave in. I think we were right; but we felt weak.

When our son was over two years old, we thought we would try it again. (We were slow learners, but our excuse was that we weren't getting much sleep.) We finally gave in, as we heard him cry from his crib, "This is your little boy, Daniel. Why are you doing this?"

We can learn a lot from our children. I think we both learned a lot through this issue of sleep. Daniel is 37 years old now. He is a great person (objectively speaking, of course). We survived the four years of frequent interrupted sleep. And we are glad we didn't let him cry it out. It wasn't easy to be awakened every night, night after night. But after all is said and done, it was for the best.

Despite what is said and written about the need to build "healthy sleep habits" by leaving babies to cry themselves to sleep, there is no evidence that babies and young children who sleep with their parents, or who are rocked to sleep and responded to at night, grow up to have any more sleep problems than those who are left alone to cry. I always found that my kids were great sleepers and could sleep anywhere—in hotel rooms, other people's houses, tents. And consider this—it is in North America, where crying to sleep has been the approach recommended for babies for some time, that people spend millions on remedies for insomnia and other sleep disorders.

A dog's life

On more than one occasion, I have seen dogs tied up to bicycle racks or lampposts while their owners are shopping or otherwise engaged. The dog whines, cries, and all sorts of people, obviously unknown to the dog, come up, caress and even hug the dog in order to comfort it. Some of the people telling you to let your baby cry it out are probably dog-comforters. Why do people see the dog's crying as a signal that it needs comforting and should be responded to, but do not respond the same way to a baby's crying?

All wait, no gain

I have seen babies who stopped gaining weight after being "trained to sleep." The pattern seems to be that the baby was left to cry and was perhaps given a pacifier or he learned to suck his thumb or two fingers to comfort himself and get back to sleep. This also became common during the day, and the baby would frequently be seen sucking on his thumb or pacifier. Mothers were pleased because in addition to getting rid of the night feedings, the baby seemed to be feeding less often in the day as well. It was only at the next doctor's visit that they discovered the baby had gained no weight, or very little weight. And then the mothers would call me for help. See the chapter "Late-Onset Decreased Milk Supply."

Teresa tells me that she spent some time at the home of one of these mothers and it seemed to her that having left the baby to cry had "desensitized" the mother to her baby's cues. This little girl, about five months old, would start to fuss or even cry and seemed hungry, but her mother would not respond. After a minute or so the child would pop her thumb in her mouth and either just sit in her seat sucking her thumb or actually go to sleep. Teresa had to spend some time getting the mother to see the child's cues and to offer the breast at those times.

I think that the crying-to-sleep method teaches babies that even if they are hungry, nobody is coming to feed them, so they'd better find some other way to cope with it. Some of them end up doing the same thing during the day. It also seems to desensitize mothers—if you force yourself to ignore crying at night, I think it's almost inevitable that you become less responsive to your baby's cries in the daytime. And I think that for some babies the result is that they don't get enough milk, and weight gain becomes a problem.

> The moment she had laid the child to the breast, both became perfectly calm.
>
> —Isak Dinesen, *Ehrengard*

There are many more families out there who share a bed with their babies than we know about. Many don't tell. Just as a child will eventually stop breastfeeding on his own if you and he allow yourselves the luxury of waiting until you are both ready, so will a child eventually leave your bed when he's ready and confident enough. When our last child finally left our bed, we were sad. But having children means adjusting to the fact that they will eventually leave you. It seems far off, but it happens much faster than you imagine.

Will giving cereal in the evening help?

Studies on this question are inconclusive, but there is actually no reason cereal should help a baby sleep longer. *If the baby gets enough to drink at the breast,* he should not need cereal. Some mothers swear that cereal has helped, though. Perhaps the babies who do sleep better once they get cereal in the evening are getting much less milk at their evening feedings. Using breast compression, switching back and forth or using herbs may help the baby get more milk. If the baby is definitely hungry in the evening or throughout the day, the milk supply may have decreased. See the chapter "Late-Onset Decreased Milk Supply."

Domperidone may help if there has been a significant decrease in milk supply. It is better to hold off on solids, if possible, because solids—incomplete foods—can replace the complete food: breastmilk. Why start solids early? The longer the baby is breastfed exclusively (up to about the middle of the first year) the better. Formula is also incomplete food.

To sum all this up, there may be things you can do to encourage your baby to sleep for longer stretches, like increasing the amount he gets at each feeding. However, many babies will continue to wake at night to breastfeed, and will be happiest in your bed. This doesn't mean they have sleep problems. It's normal behaviour for human babies. As Vancouver psychologist Gordon Neufeld said at a conference, "Babies and small children are not designed to sleep alone."

22 Breastfeeding and Family Relationships

Myth: When a mother breastfeeds, the father is left out of the relationship. He can help by giving a bottle at night, and this involves him with the baby.
Fact: There is lots the father can do to help with the baby and develop his own relationship with him. It is not necessary for him to feed the baby for this to happen.

Fathers and breastfed babies

Does breastfeeding mean that the father's relationship with his baby is hindered or diminished? Is it a good idea to give the baby a bottle or two a day from the very beginning so that the father can be involved in feeding? Are the benefits of breastfeeding outweighed by the benefits of having both parents share equally in feeding the baby?

All these questions have the same underlying assumption—that feeding a baby is the only way, or the primary way, to develop a close and loving relationship with him. Another assumption is that the father who gives the baby a bottle at night is sharing equally in the feeding.

The truth is that there are many things to do when caring for a newborn baby that promote bonding—changing his diapers, bathing him, sleeping with him, carrying him in your arms or in a carrier, singing to him, taking him for walks, massaging him, talking to him, burping him, and many, many more. All of these are wonderful ways for fathers (and mothers, grandmothers, siblings and other family members, too, of course) to interact with the baby without disrupting breastfeeding.

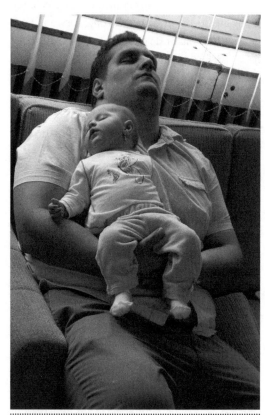

There is plenty that fathers can do to help. But giving a night bottle so the mother can sleep is sometimes the beginning of the end of breastfeeding.
CREDIT: JACK NEWMAN

The father who wants to be involved and share in parenting can bring the baby to the mother to nurse, change the baby's diapers, give the baby a bath, and take the baby for a walk afterwards. Not only is that baby enjoying time with his father, but he is getting all the benefits of breastfeeding as well.

And most fathers who really understand the benefits of breastfeeding want their babies to have "the best."

Aside from this hands-on involvement, fathers are extremely important in terms of supporting and

---

The idea of bottle feeding just to "involve the father" is one more instance of preserving the status quo at a price to the baby.

—Marni Jackson, *The Mother Zone*

---

encouraging their partners in breastfeeding. They can make the difference between forging on through challenging situations and giving up at the first sign of diffculty.

One mother told me how frustrated she was when her baby was just a few days old. He'd already woken up several times in the night to nurse, and she was tired and worried that she didn't have enough milk. She woke up her husband and asked him to drive to the 24-hour drugstore near their home to buy some formula. Instead, he held her in his arms for a while, told her how much he loved her and their new son and how happy he was that she was breastfeeding. Then he gave her a back rub and brought in some more pillows so that she'd be in a more comfortable position for the next feeding.

That mother said she could feel her milk letting down as her husband rubbed her back. She's convinced that if her husband had brought home the formula, she would have given up on breastfeeding, but his support and encouragement that night made all the difference.

This can often be a fine line for fathers to walk, though. It's tough to see your wife struggling with breastfeeding, perhaps crying because her nipples hurt or because she's so frustrated. Formula seems like a quick solution. And maybe that's what she really wants—no father wants to be the "bad guy" who is forcing his partner to keep breastfeeding when she's ready to stop.

But often what women need in this situation is not a solution but some empathy. Yes, breastfeeding and caring for a newborn is harder than it looks on TV. And boy, you never thought you'd end up with a Caesarean, did you? Fathers can also remind their partners of other possible solutions to the problem: calling a lactation consultant or a La Leche League leader, or making an appointment at a breastfeeding clinic. He can offer other alternatives—perhaps give the mother half a day in which she can just sleep or do what she likes and bring the baby to her when he needs to breastfeed.

Many mothers say they rely on their partners to "run interference" for them; to protect and defend them from the criticism of others, including family, friends and medical professionals. Having to always explain to people that the baby is getting enough to eat, that her breastmilk is good enough and that it's normal for a baby to eat this frequently can be exhausting for a new mother, especially if this is her first baby and she doesn't have a lot of self-confidence. If the father speaks up and is positive about breastfeeding, it takes some of that burden away from her and boosts her self-confidence.

Practical help is always appreciated. Breastfeeding a baby can take up quite a bit of time, especially in the early weeks while mother and baby are both learning. This is the time to master the art of washing dishes and doing laundry, to arrange for a diaper service or a cleaning lady, to make a nutritious meal (or order in pizza or Chinese food) when supper hasn't made it to the table.

In other societies, and in times past, new mothers could often rely on their own mothers or other relatives to take over the housework and meal preparation during the first weeks and months after a new baby. For many North American women, this isn't possible. Their own mothers are probably working full-time. Family members may live far away from the new parents. Becoming a mother—trying to cope with all the needs of a baby, as well as other household responsibilities—can be an isolating and overwhelming experience.

Fathers can do a lot to relieve that sense of being overwhelmed if they recognize that taking the time to get breastfeeding well established is time well spent.

When Dad's the best

Mothers are definitely best at breastfeeding. But fathers have their special talents, too: Dad's deeper voice is more soothing to the baby when he sings or talks to him. Babies seem to really respond and relax when they hear the deep, rumbling sounds of a male voice.

Dad's flatter chest makes a great place for the baby to nap. Lie down on the couch, drape the baby over you, and everybody gets a rest.

For the same reason (no breasts to get in the way), the father can often carry the baby in a sling or soft baby carrier more easily than the mother.

Breastfeeding and sexual relationships

One reason fathers are sometimes not as supportive of breastfeeding as they might be is that they see the intimacy of the mother-baby relationship as a threat. If my wife loves the baby that much, he may think, how is she going to have enough time and love for me?

It may take longer for the new father to take on his role than it does for the mother. After all, she's had nine months of dramatic and intense physical changes to prepare her. For the father, the baby may not have seemed quite real until he was born. Now he's asking, "Where do I fit in?" His connection to the baby will happen, in time, and he will find his place in the new family he has helped to create.

In some ways, it can seem as though the new breastfeeding mother is less interested in her husband than she was in those days "before baby." After all, she has a whole new responsibility here. And sex becomes less frequent. Certainly, there is research to show that new mothers have sex with their husbands less often than they did before or during pregnancy, and some studies have found this rate to be lowest for breastfeeding mothers (although others contradict this). Why does this happen? There are several reasons:

- Taking care of a new baby (whether or not you have given birth to the baby and whether or not you are breastfeeding) is tiring. Most people are less interested in sex when they are tired, whatever the cause. (To quote the mother of a six-week-old: "Frankly, I'd rather have a nap than an orgasm.")

- Recovering from pregnancy and birth is also tiring, and the physical changes the mother's body has gone through can certainly decrease her interest in sex. The mother may have stitches that make intercourse painful, for example.

- Nursing a baby may meet most of the mother's needs for physical contact and affectionate touch. In fact, some mothers describe feeling "touched out"—they've had so much physical stimulation from being in constant contact with their babies that they don't want anyone else to touch them.

- The hormones normally present during breastfeeding can cause vaginal lubrication to decrease. Even when the woman is sexually aroused, she will have less lubrication, and this may make intercourse uncomfortable or even painful. Using a vaginal lubricant can help.

- The breastfeeding mother's nipples may be tender in the early days, and then become less sensitive to stimulation as breastfeeding continues. If nipple stimulation has been an important part of sexual activity for the couple, this can be a problem.

- Both men and women react differently to full or leaking breasts during sex. Some men like the taste of breastmilk and don't mind a little leaking, while others don't like it at all. Women will sometimes have a strong letdown of milk when they reach orgasm. This bothers some women, and not others. If the milk is a problem, nursing the baby right before sex can help. Putting a towel underneath you helps, too.
- The mother's body is different after the birth. She may be embarrassed by her stretch marks, her blue-veined breasts and her sagging belly. Her husband may not be bothered by this, or he may be turned off by the changes he sees and hope that if she quits breastfeeding she can get her body back into shape more quickly. (In fact, breastfeeding helps the mother's body to return to normal more quickly. Her uterus will contract to its normal size more rapidly, and weight put on during pregnancy is usually lost more easily when the mother breastfeeds.)
- Sex is less spontaneous and more likely to be interrupted now that a baby is in the house.

While some of these factors are directly related to breastfeeding, others are simply part of being new parents. It is important, though, to recognize that a reduced libido is common and normal during breastfeeding, and that the mother's interest in sex will gradually increase again.

Intimate relationships are about more than just sex. During the early weeks after the birth intercourse may be uncomfortable for the mother, so what are other ways parents can express their love for each other and be intimate? This can be a great opportunity to expand your sexual repertoire. If the new mother is feeling "touched out," how can her partner help her feel more comfortable and ready to be close to him? (Hint: a chance to take a long bath, all alone, while the father takes the baby for a walk is usually much appreciated.)

Sex is more enjoyable for breastfeeding mothers if they accept that it will take them longer to become aroused and that vaginal lubrication will be less than normal, and if both partners can accept that they may occasionally be interrupted by the baby. Take your time. Enjoy the "warm-up." You can have some touching, fondling and stimulation, stop for a while to nurse the baby, and then resume what you were doing. (Your baby is small for only a short time, and there will be plenty of opportunities for uninterrupted, leisurely sex in the future.)

Sometimes couples decide to take a weekend away from the baby to be alone together again, hoping this will bring them closer. What usually happens is that the mother spends much of her time calling home to check on the baby and pumping her milk, only to find that she leaks all over the bed anyway. When they come home, the baby is miserable and clingy and has trouble latching on well after a whole weekend of being fed bottles. The mother may feel guilt and regret over leaving her baby and the father feels disappointed that the weekend away didn't really recapture the relationship they once had.

The truth is that your relationship will never be exactly as it was before you had a baby. The baby has changed your life. Your body is different, your emotions are different, your priorities are different. What you need to do is figure out, often by trial and error, how the two of you can have a close and loving relationship now that you have become a family. This is the "new normal." It can be much better and more satisfying than the relationship BB (before baby), but it will definitely be different.

Often these changes are harder for the father to accept than for the mother. After all, she's been through all kinds of hormonal realignments that

----

She pictured a child, her own . . . at her own breast, with her husband standing by and gazing fondly at her and the child.

—Leo Tolstoy, *War and Peace*

----

encourage falling in love with her new baby. This isn't a rejection of the father, although to some men it feels that way. Dr. Michel Odent, a French obstetrician, shows a series of slides in which a woman gives birth and later sits, holding her baby and gazing into its eyes. She is clearly entranced and falling deeply in love with her child. In the next slide, though, the baby's father has moved in between the mother and baby in order to kiss her—but Dr. Odent comments that what he is really doing is trying to "break" that intense, loving look between the mother and baby. It's as though he is saying, "Don't forget about me."

If fathers can understand how important that intense love is for the development of their children, they will encourage it rather than try to interrupt it.

Every couple will need to find their own way to keep their relationship strong while dealing with a new baby and breastfeeding. It will involve compromise. Some nights the mother decides to be sexual with the father even though she isn't feeling "in the mood" because she sees that it's important to him; other nights he decides to do laundry and prepare food for the next day, even though he'd rather be having sex, because he genuinely wants to help his wife get a little extra sleep. It might mean planning ahead rather than being spontaneous, or it might mean taking advantage of whatever moments there are ("Hey! The baby's asleep and just had a good feeding—let's do it!"). It often means doing things with the baby along, rather than just the two of you,

and that's good—picnics in the park, going to the drive-in, visiting friends, ordering dinner in instead of going out to a restaurant, renting a movie instead of heading to the theatre (although you can certainly take your baby to a restaurant or cinema if you want).

The rest of the family

Breastfeeding is likely to have an effect on your other family relationships as well. A lot will depend, of course, on family members' own experiences with breastfeeding and your previous relationships with them.

Often, though, a new mother decides to breastfeed even though her own mother used formula. The new grandmother may feel a bit resentful. Perhaps she thought breastfeeding was a bit "disgusting" or "animalistic" and feels uncomfortable seeing her daughter breastfeed. She's heard that "breast is best" but can't quite get past feeling that it's somehow "yucky." Or perhaps she wanted to breastfeed, but didn't succeed (thanks to strict schedules and unhelpful advice), and now that old disappointment resurfaces.

As well, she feels cut off from her eagerly awaited grandchild. She had looked forward to taking care of the new baby—perhaps for a nice long weekend while the new parents went away together—and certainly expected to be able to feed the baby. Now she has to hand the baby back to the mother every time he fusses. Her experienced advice on feeding schedules, methods of cleaning bottles and pacifier use is ignored.

Even if the new grandmother did breastfeed, she may have started solid foods very early, fed according to a schedule and weaned after just a few months. It's hard for her if she feels that her children have decided she did everything "wrong" and she may be concerned that the mother is breastfeeding too often and will damage her breasts or become exhausted, or that her milk will turn "bad" after three months. After all, that's what she was told when her babies were born.

It's a challenge for the new mother, who needs support, encouragement and practical help at this point in her life, but who may, instead, be massaging bruised egos and dealing with unhelpful criticism. Many mothers find it helps to say, "This is what my doctor advised me to do" when it comes to breast-feeding techniques or timing (even if it hasn't ever been discussed with the doctor). Most people will respect "medical advice." The mother can also offer books or other materials about breastfeeding, especially those that refute some of the still-prevalent myths. (Why not this book, for example?) It can also help to encourage grandparents to build connections with the baby in other ways—giving baths, taking the baby for a walk in a sling or carrier, singing lullabies, whatever appeals to them. Even if breastfeeding is not something they know much about, they have a lot to contribute.

23 Breastfeeding and Mother–Baby Separation

Myth: Mothers who work outside the home or go to school can't continue breastfeeding.

Fact: While breastfeeding is obviously easiest when mother and baby are together, many women continue breastfeeding even though they are separated from their babies. Not only is it possible, but most mothers feel it is well worth the extra effort.

When mothers must be away from their babies, breastfeeding can be very important to the baby's health. While the mother is away, someone else is obviously taking care of the baby. Unless this is his father or another person who lives at home, the baby is probably being exposed to a variety of germs that he wouldn't encounter if he were at home full-time. If he is being cared for in a daycare centre, with a large number of other children and several staff, he's likely to pick up all kinds of infections. Continued breastfeeding will go a long way to preventing illness or minimizing the severity of the illness, while speeding the baby's recovery if he does get sick. Studies have shown that working parents whose children continue breastfeeding take fewer days off work because their child is sick less often than parents whose children are not breastfeeding.

As well, breastfeeding is a great way to connect with the baby at the end of a long day of work. When the mother puts her baby to the breast, her body releases the hormone oxytocin, which encourages the milk to flow. Oxytocin and prolactin, another breastfeeding hormone, also have an important side effect—they are natural tranquilizers that help the mother relax. Many women say they can feel all the tension leave their bodies as the baby nurses. They also like the fact that breastfeeding is something only they, and not the babysitter, can do. Mothers separated from their babies during the day often find themselves caught in a dilemma: they want their babies to like the caregiver and to be happy while the mother is away, but they don't want to lose the vital bond and connection with their babies. They don't want the baby to become more attached to the caregiver than to them. Continuing to breastfeed can be very reassuring to mothers with those concerns because it maintains that special aspect of their relationship. The baby's obvious enthusiasm for nursing lets the mother know that she is still special to him.

Finally, the long-term benefits of breastfeeding, discussed elsewhere, continue to be important for the baby whose mother is away, just as they are for the baby whose mother is with him most of the time.

So how can mothers manage continued breastfeeding despite separation?
Preparation

Getting breastfeeding well established in the beginning is especially important for the mother who is anticipating returning to work outside the home or being otherwise separated from her baby. We have described mothers in Africa or other communities who carry their babies with them and nurse several times an hour. When there is that kind of continuous contact and very frequent nursing, it doesn't matter so much if the latch is not as good as it might be, or if the milk supply tends to be a little on the low side. For a mother who will be away from her baby, who may need to pump milk at least some of the time and whose baby may be getting bottles or sucking on a pacifier while at the caregiver's, learning to latch the baby on well and build up a good milk supply become essential. (Of course if the baby is six months old, he will not need bottles and even before six months he may not need them.)

The longer a mother can be at home with her baby before returning to outside work or school, the easier it will be to maintain breastfeeding. Not that many years ago, women often had to return to work before their babies were six weeks old, even earlier if the mother started her maternity leave before the birth. In Canada today, many women can take a full year to be with their new babies, and many companies will extend that leave (paid or unpaid, depending on the company) if the mother requests it. This allows mothers to have breastfeeding well established before they must be away. The situation isn't good in the United States (where maternity leaves may be as short as two or three weeks, in some states) and many other countries. On the other hand, it is much better in some European countries, where women can take up to three years away from work after giving birth.

Of course, even in Canada some mothers must be separated from their babies sooner than six months. Self-employed women, for example, may not be able to stop working for more than a short period of time, and women who are attending school may have to go back to class when the baby is younger than they would like.

During the mother's time at home with her baby, it helps if she can resolve any breastfeeding problems she might have. If her supply is low,

for example, this is the time to try some of the techniques suggested in the chapter "Increasing Breastmilk Intake by the Baby." If she leaves until she is back at work, she may find that her breasts are going without stimulation much of the day, her baby is getting milk from a faster-flowing bottle, and her milk supply will gradually decrease until the baby is weaned, long before she had planned.

It is not necessary to introduce a bottle early on so that the baby will take a bottle at the sitter's or the daycare centre. If the mother takes at least six months of maternity leave, her baby can drink from an open cup or have milk mixed with solids. If the mother needs to go back sooner and her baby resists bottles—and some completely breastfed babies do—there are many other ways the caregiver can give him food. She can use a small open cup, or a spoon, for example. If the baby is four months or even a little younger, he can be started on solids mixed with the mother's milk.

Finding the right caregiver

Part of preparation for breastfeeding and working outside the home is finding the right caregiver. Here are some things to consider:

If a mother can find a caregiver close to her work, rather than close to home, she can minimize the time she is away from her baby. She can nurse the baby when she drops him off, go to work, and then nurse again when she is finished work and before she starts for home.

If the daycare provider is close enough, she may be able to go over to the caregiver's location during lunch hour, or during breaks, for a nursing session. Or perhaps the caregiver can bring the baby to the mother during lunch or breaks.

The mother should discuss breastfeeding with the caregiver and ask about their policies. For example, some daycare centres will not allow women to leave breastmilk for their babies because they consider it a potentially dangerous bodily fluid. (If a mother runs into this policy, she should look for another caregiver.) The Center for Disease Control in the United States has issued statements making it clear that no special care needs to be used in handling human milk.

Some daycare centres insist that all babies over a certain age (usually a year) be given cow's milk (or alternative milk). In response to this stupid policy, the mother may choose to keep on breastfeeding at home but let the baby drink cow's milk at daycare. Or the baby can eat other foods during the day and not have any milk while at daycare. But what right does anyone have to insist someone else's baby drink cow's milk? Another issue is the fact that many daycare workers just don't know that a six-month-old or eight-month-old may not know how to drink from a bottle and insist the baby be forced to learn. They need to add some courses on breastfeeding in early childhood education classes! Explain politely that the baby can drink very well from an open cup or milk can be mixed with his solids.

Teresa has heard from mothers who have been told by their daycare providers that they can't breastfeed in the daycare centre where the other children might see them, or that breastfeeding a child over a certain age (in some places, as young as one year!) is inappropriate. This may be another issue to discuss with the caregiver in advance. If necessary, don't back down on your legal rights to breastfeed anywhere you are legally allowed to be. And remind the caregiver that the problem is not that the children might see breastfeeding, which would be a healthy learning experience, but the caregiver's reaction to breastfeeding.

The mother should discuss ways of feeding breastmilk without using a bottle, if that is what she wants to do to help avoid nipple confusion. She might have to demonstrate how to use the cup, and see if the sitter is comfortable with this. Another alternative is for the mother's milk to be mixed with any of the solid foods the baby is eating—there is no reason that liquids need to be taken separately from solids.

The mother might find she needs to make sure the caregiver knows how breastmilk looks. Because it is not homogenized, like cow's milk, it will naturally separate into layers when left in the fridge or freezer, with the "cream" on top. Sometimes people assume this means the milk is spoiled, but it isn't. It may also be different colours—more bluish or yellowish—at different times. The caregiver should also know that an exclusively breastfed baby's bowel movements are supposed to be yellow and very loose.

The mother should talk with the caregiver about how to handle situations when the baby is fussy and the mother is due back soon. It can be frustrating for the breastfeeding mother to arrive at the daycare with full breasts, only to hear that the baby was just fed.

The mother should plan with the caregiver what to do if the daycare runs out of expressed breastmilk. Some women opt to leave a supply of formula or cow's milk, depending on the baby's age. Others ask the sitter to give the baby some solid foods, or a little diluted juice, or something else until the mother gets there. The answer, of course, may depend on the age of the baby. There is no need for a baby older than six months, who is breastfeeding and also eating plenty of solids, to be given formula; homogenized milk will do just fine. In fact, there is *no need* for any extra milk to be given in this situation. Cheese or yogurt are good sources of calcium if the mother wants the baby to get extra calcium.

Planning at Work

What are the mother's options at work? Does she have regularly scheduled breaks and lunches that she could use for pumping? Does she have an office with a door that closes (and, ideally, locks), giving her some privacy, or will she need to express in a washroom or the office sickroom or some other location? Is the mother planning to leave the office and nurse the baby during breaks, or can she arrange to have the baby brought to her?

Women have found various ways to work outside the home and still provide milk for their babies. One mother who managed a golf course was able to arrange for a sitter to come and care for the baby in her office. Much of the time, she did paperwork in her office while the sitter and baby played nearby, and she nursed when needed. Sometimes the sitter would take the baby out for a walk through the quieter parts of the golf course. When the mother had to meet with customers or suppliers, she left the baby with the sitter and went to another part of the building. This made it easy to nurse her baby frequently throughout the day. You don't need to manage a golf course to figure out this way of continuing breastfeeding. Several physicians I know made this work for them; a store owner who did not have a caretaker and a massage therapist were able to manage a system similar to this.

Another mother arranged with her employer to come in half an hour early each day and stay half an hour later each evening. In exchange, she was given two half-hour breaks—one mid-morning and one mid-afternoon, as well as her normal lunch break. She used those breaks to go over to the daycare centre, just a block away, and nurse her baby.

The most difficult situations are those where mothers work long shifts and have no regular breaks. For example, nurses often work 12-hour shifts and may have no breaks if the ward is busy. Flight attendants may also be away from their babies for several days at a time, and while the plane is in flight they don't have many opportunities to express milk or any room to store it. For these mothers, one approach

Why your employer should support your breastfeeding

- Your baby will be sick less often, so you won't need to miss work as much to take care of him.
- Your baby's lower prescription costs will mean lower premiums for the employee medical plan.
- You will feel more positive about your work, and will therefore be more productive.

may be to build up a good stock of expressed milk in the freezer while they are on maternity leave. Then, during ordinary bathroom breaks, they can express just enough milk to relieve the fullness.

Incidentally, Canada is a signatory of the International Labour Organization's 1919 paper guaranteeing all nursing mothers who work outside the home two extra 30-minute breaks during the day, either to return home and feed their babies or to express their milk. Of course, the existence of a signed document doesn't mean the provisions will be followed. Most employers or government officials have probably never heard of this paper.

Breasts are surprisingly adaptable. Many women have managed to continue breastfeeding or providing milk for their babies despite long separations, irregular schedules and other challenges. Remember that it is common and typical for mothers who are breastfeeding toddlers or older children to find that they are nursing three times one day, eight times the next day, twice the following day, and four times the day after that. They may find their breasts are slightly fuller on some days, but it all works out.

Pumping or expressing milk

Some mothers who know they will be going back to work begin pumping their milk several weeks or even months before their maternity leave is over. They store the milk in the freezer, and having this extra supply gives them confidence that even if they can't keep up with pumping once they return to work, there will be milk for their babies.

Others store only a few extra containers of milk, and rely on daily pumping to provide the majority of the milk for the baby's needs while they are away. The method that works best for any individual mother will depend on her work and daycare situation, but it is true that milk that is frozen loses nutrients and antibodies. It is still better than formula, of course, but lacks some of the protection of fresh milk. That's less significant if the mother is also breastfeeding her baby frequently when they are together, but the ideal would be to pump milk one day and simply store it in the fridge for the baby to have the following day. The milk the mother pumps on Friday will keep just fine in the fridge for her baby to have on Monday.

The first step in pumping or extracting milk is to encourage the milk to let down. This is easy if the mother is pumping at home and has her baby with her, because the baby's suckling will cause the milk to flow. For this reason, some mothers will nurse the baby on one breast and pump the other at the same time. Others will nurse the baby first, and then use the pump. While at first the mother won't get a lot of milk pumping this way, in time her milk supply will adjust. Even if she gets just a couple of ounces, she can save that milk and later mix it with other milk. (Don't add warm milk directly to frozen milk in the storage container, though. Let it chill in the refrigerator first.)

If the baby is not with her, the mother might need to take some extra steps to get her milk to flow easily. Applying warm, wet washcloths to the breasts can help. Many women find that gentle breast massage helps. The mother can massage from the top of the breasts toward the nipples with gentle strokes.

Rubbing the nipple with the palm of her hand held flat can also stimulate the milk to let down, as can rolling the nipples between finger and thumb. Sometimes looking at a picture of the baby or smelling an undershirt the baby has worn will also help. In time you will figure out what works best for you.

Some pumps are now designed with variable speed control, and some mothers find it helps to pump at a faster speed at first—much like a baby nurses with a series of rapid sucks in the beginning—to encourage the letdown, and then switch to a slower speed as the milk lets down.

Hand-expressing

To express milk by hand, the mother should first encourage the milk to let down. Then she can cup the breast with one hand and use the other hand to hold the clean container for storing her milk. The mother can place her thumb near the top of the areola and have her forefinger in about the same position on the bottom of her breast. She then presses her thumb and forefinger together, at the same time pushing back toward her ribs. Finally, she squeezes forward. She doesn't need to do this so hard it hurts and she shouldn't slide her hand on the skin, which will irritate it. The mother may get just a drop or two of milk, or a spray. She can repeat the pressing movement a few times, and if the flow of milk slows down, move her hand around to another part of the breast and press again. The milk ducts are all around the nipple, so her goal is to keep moving her hand until she has squeezed all of them.

If, after a few minutes of hand expression, the milk stops flowing or slows down drastically, the mother can try expressing from the other breast. Then she can repeat the breast massage, nipple rubbing and perhaps smelling the baby's clothes before she goes back to the first breast to encourage another letdown of milk.

This process takes practice, but mothers soon learn how much pressure to apply to achieve the maximum flow of milk and then it's quick and easy. A mother can also, with a little practice, express both breasts at the same time. The procedure is the same as with one breast, but this will take half the time and may produce more milk.

The best thing about hand expression: it is free, and a mother can't forget to bring her hands to work! The mother is also in control of the process, and this makes bruising or other damage to the breast less likely than with a pump.

Using a breast pump

As interest in breastfeeding has increased, many manufacturers have come out with their own versions of the breast pump. Some are basically useless—in fact, they may be worse than useless because when the mother uses them and discovers she can't get any milk out, she may assume this means her milk supply is low. This is not true. There are many women who never managed to get much milk from a pump or by hand expression, who nevertheless exclusively breastfeed their babies without problems. A baby who is properly latched on and feeding well is much more efficient at getting milk from the breast than any pump.

The most effective pumps for mothers who are separated from their babies are the high-grade electric models. The best of these are designed to allow the mother to pump from both breasts at the same time, and allow her to adjust the pressure and speed of the pumping action. Some are designed to be used hands-free.

Each pump works differently for each mother as women's breasts are all different. What a mother needs is a pump that fits her breast, creating a good but comfortable seal, and produces the right amount of pressure for her. If the first pump she tries is not

working well for her, she shouldn't just assume that means she can't get enough milk this way. Maybe what she needs is a different pump, or a different size of flange for the pump.

She can also use breast compression while pumping, in the same way she would if the baby were on the breast (see the chapter "Increasing Breastmilk Intake by the Baby"), to get more milk.

Breast tissue is sensitive and can be easily bruised. The electric pumps have strong suction and can cause sore nipples if the breast is centred in the flange. If pumping hurts, the mother should stop right away. She can see if adjusting the position of the pump, switching to a larger flange or decreasing the amount of pressure will make it more comfortable.

Storing milk

Breastmilk is a fluid with living, interactive components. Even when left at room temperature, milk remains safe for the baby for many hours after expression because immune factors will kill bacteria.

Containers should be clean, but they don't need to be sterilized. The white blood cells in human milk, an important form of protection against illness, can stick to the side of glass containers, but not to plastic. However, some of the fats in the breastmilk will stick to plastic, but not to glass. The white blood cells are also destroyed by freezing. There are some special plastic bags designed for storing human milk that are more durable than the plastic bottle liners many women use. However, recommendations for the best containers for expressed milk change all the time, and there probably isn't a big difference. Personally, I prefer glass containers because plastic ones may leach toxins into food.

Expressed breastmilk keeps safely at room temperature for up to 12 hours and can be refrigerated for up to five days. (Actually, I think that as long as the milk tastes and smells good, it is good, and that usually means longer than 12 hours at room temperature and probably longer than five days in the refrigerator.) This is good news for mothers who don't have access to a fridge or freezer at work. The mother can express her milk and simply keep the container in her office or locker until she goes home. Then she can put it in the fridge for use in the next few days, or freeze it. In a deep freeze, expressed milk will keep for six months or longer; in the freezer compartment of a refrigerator, it will keep for two to four months. The mother should mark the date on each container so she'll use up the oldest milk first.

The milk can be thawed best by holding the container under warm (not hot) running water, then shaking it well. The caregiver should check the temperature before giving it to the baby. It is not a good idea to microwave breastmilk for two reasons. One, some of the antibodies in the milk can be destroyed by the microwaves, and two, the microwaves can produce pockets of very hot milk that could burn the baby's mouth.

Common concerns

Mothers frequently mention that they put milk in the refrigerator and two hours later it smells funny and tastes bad. Or they freeze the milk, and then when it is thawed it has an unpleasant soapy smell and taste. This is not due to spoiling, but is thought to be due to the mother having a lot of lipase in her milk. Lipase is an enzyme that breaks down fat, and in this case it breaks down fat in the milk. The by-products of the breakdown taste unpleasant to adults, but are not harmful to the baby. The milk is "predigested."

This is often a concern for women who have frozen significant quantities of milk and then notice this change in smell and taste. They worry that they may have to throw all this milk away. But the milk can definitely be given to the baby if he'll take it

(some older babies will not drink it), or mixed in with his food to mask the flavour.

Scalding the milk before freezing or refrigerating it prevents the lipase breakdown of the fat. The mother puts her milk in a saucepan or double boiler and heats it to just below the boiling point—she should see bubbles appearing across the surface but it should not actually come to a boil. Then the milk is removed from the heat, set aside to cool, and put into containers to store in the fridge or freezer.

If a mother has had a *Candida* (yeast) infection, she does not need to throw away the milk she collected while she had the infection. *Candida* is everywhere; you can't get rid of it. Usually we live in harmony with it. Furthermore, breastmilk contains immune factors that keep *Candida* in its non-harmful yeast form rather than its problem-causing hyphal form.

When should I stop pumping?

Some mothers don't pump at all after they return to work. If the baby is six months or older and already eating a wide variety of solid foods in ample amounts, this approach can work. The sitter can provide solid foods, diluted juice and water during the day, and the mother can breastfeed whenever she and the baby are together. Sometimes mothers in this situation will need to pump or express milk for their own comfort during the day, though.

Other women prefer to leave breastmilk for their babies, and will pump for as long as the baby consumes the milk they leave behind. If the baby is allergic to cow's milk it is a good idea to continue providing milk.

As the baby gets older, and the number of feedings at the breast naturally decreases, it becomes easier to manage breastfeeding and working. An older baby will be able to have a variety of foods and drinks at daycare, and yet still benefit from nursing when with his mother.

When the mother leaves

The baby's reaction when his mother goes back to work or school may catch everyone by surprise. Some babies seem almost unconcerned that their mothers are not around. But many breastfeeding babies will protest and cry when they realize their mother is gone. Even a very good caregiver won't have the mother's smell, her special way of holding the baby, her voice or her breast.

Some mothers leave behind handkerchiefs they have worn in their bras, or T-shirts they have slept in, to provide the baby with that comforting and familiar smell. Mothers who use a sling or baby carrier can ask the caregiver to use it while looking after the baby—another way to keep the familiar things as part of the baby's day.

Mothers are sometimes surprised by the baby's reaction when they return. It is not unusual for a baby who has been at daycare all day to ignore his mother when she comes to pick him up. Sometimes he will start crying when he sees her—not at all the reaction she was hoping for! Some babies will refuse to be held or picked up by their mothers, or will react with anger by hitting or kicking her when she does hold them.

This is another demonstration of the baby's intense love for his mother. He is telling her that he did not want her to leave him. Breastfeeding is one of the best ways to soothe both mother and baby after this kind of tense, stormy reunion. Often mothers can see the baby's whole body relax as she begins to make the familiar gestures that show him she is preparing to breastfeed: settling him on her lap, unbuttoning her shirt, moving him into the nursing position.

A mother can sometimes make this transition easier by starting with short separations. First, she can let her baby spend time with her and the caregiver together, either at home or at the daycare. Then she can leave the baby with the new caregiver for a short period of time—less than an hour, perhaps. Gradually, over a period of two or three weeks, the mother can increase the amount of time the baby spends with the caregiver. This will also give the mother a chance to practise pumping, see how the baby does with the caregiver and see if the baby will accept her milk from a cup (preferably) or bottle, and so on.

When the mother does go back to outside work (assuming she is working full-time), it helps not to begin on a Monday but perhaps a Thursday, so that she will have a couple of days of work, followed by a weekend during which everyone can get readjusted, and then five days of work. Some mothers have found it helps to adjust their schedules to work longer hours four days a week, so they can have, say, Wednesdays off.

Often mothers who are separated from their babies during the day find that the babies wake up more at night. They may even refuse most of their daytime feedings of expressed milk and make up for it by nursing very frequently during the evening and night. This can be tiring for the mother who now has no opportunity to catch up with naps during the day. Bringing the baby into the family bed may be the easiest way to help everyone get the sleep they need. With time, the mother will learn to latch the baby on and then fall back to sleep while he nurses. Sleeping with the mother also lets the baby enjoy the physical closeness that he might be missing during the day.

The baby's behaviour will also change as he goes through different developmental stages. Many babies of six months will not be terribly upset about being left at a sitter's. This can change drastically when the baby is about eight or nine months, and the mother may unexpectedly find herself dealing with a baby who clings to her and screams each morning. Another time of developmental change is around the one-year mark, when the baby becomes more active and mobile. Even when their mothers are home full-time, one-year-olds often skip many daytime feedings and then "crash" at night, wanting to be held and nursed as they recharge themselves after a busy day.

Common concerns about breastfeeding and working
Plugged ducts

Some women find that because they are missing feedings during the day, they end up with plugged ducts, although this problem is not as common as expected. If you have experienced plugged ducts when you were with your baby full-time, you may be more prone to them once you return to work. This problem is more common when mothers don't pump or express milk during the day.

If this is a problem for you, the solution is usually to express milk during your work day, even if you can't store it, to relieve the fullness. If you notice the symptoms of a plugged duct beginning—a sore, tender and hard area in the breast—try to take a break as soon as possible, apply a hot washcloth or run the hand dryer on your breast, massage the area and express some milk.

Some women with repeated plugged ducts have found that adding lecithin to their diets has been helpful (see the chapter "Sore Breasts").

Decreasing milk supply

If your baby is getting bottles of formula or even previously pumped and stored breastmilk, he will not be nursing as frequently, and you may find that your milk supply begins to diminish. If you are concerned, you can pump during the day to build your milk production back up. However, if your baby is over six months of age and eating a wide variety of foods in ample amounts, he needs neither bottles nor formula. The baby can drink from an open cup and milk can be mixed with his solids. The "need" for formula to a year or even longer is largely the result of formula

company marketing. In fact, formula companies have started to push formulas for children up to three years of age. Furthermore, if the baby is still breastfeeding, there is no need for other milk at all.

If your schedule is erratic—for example, if you work three 12-hour shifts, followed by four days at home—you may find that your milk supply is irregular. On your first day at home after a three-day shift, your milk supply may be low and the baby nurses very frequently. By the fourth day, your milk production will probably have caught up to the baby's needs—but then when you get back to work the next day, your breasts will feel very full.

Some mothers try to balance this out by giving the baby bottles on the days they are at home, just as if they were away at work. This seems a shame, though. Why give the baby fourth-best (after breast, cup or milk mixed with solids) when the best is right there? Your body will be able to adjust to this cycle, and your baby will benefit from nursing as much as possible.

Leaking breasts

Leaking breasts are usually not a problem by the time the baby is six months old. They are more likely to be a problem if you have to return to work when your baby is still very young. Sometimes just thinking about your baby, or hearing another baby cry, can cause leaking.

Wear good, absorbent breast pads, and bring enough that you can change them frequently (milk-soaked pads against your nipples will cause chafing and soreness). Try to express or pump milk before you get too full. If you do feel the tingling or "filling up" sensations that often signal you are about to leak, try pressing against your breasts with your arms folded across your chest. This will often prevent leaking, and can be done without anyone noticing. Wearing patterned blouses, perhaps with a loose vest over top, or sweaters with a T-shirt underneath, can help disguise any leaks—a plain silk blouse is not a good choice for the potentially leaky lactating mother at work!

Baby won't settle or sleep for the caregiver

If you have always nursed your baby to sleep, he may not fall asleep easily for your babysitter, and your babysitter may be used to babies who are just put down in their cribs alone to fall asleep, or who take a pacifier.

Here are some ideas that may help:

- Practise the way the sitter is going to put the baby to sleep before you start working.
- Have her try different routines so she finds one that will work for her.
- Have the caregiver try walking around with the baby in a sling or baby carrier or backpack carrier.
- Movement can be very soothing. Have your caregiver try taking the baby for a drive in the car (in his car seat, of course) or pushing him around in a stroller or pram. She can push the stroller around inside the house, if necessary. Rocking in a rocking chair might work. If your baby is young enough, she can try a wind-up baby swing.
- Give your caregiver a T-shirt or nightgown that you have slept in, and have her wrap it around the baby while she rocks him to sleep. The familiar smell may do the trick.
- Sometimes a repetitive white noise such as a fan or radio static will drown out noises that may be distracting the baby and keeping him awake.

Baby starts to prefer the bottle to the breast

In general, as we have said above, it is better to avoid bottles whenever possible. However, some daycare providers are adamant that they will use only bottles, especially with younger babies. Better to look around for someone else rather than hire a caretaker who won't appreciate the baby's needs.

This problem is more common if the mother's milk supply has begun to diminish, so that the baby finds he gets steadier flow from the bottle than from the breast.

Older babies sometimes like the bottle because they can carry it around with them and feel more in control, in contrast to breastfeeding, which is now inaccessible to them for much of each day. However, this is not a good reason to start or continue bottles.

Avoiding bottles altogether will prevent the baby from preferring the bottle, and stopping bottles, if possible, will help to solve the problem.

You can start reducing bottles by asking the sitter to hold your baby during every bottle-feeding and not allow him to walk around with a bottle. Then ask her to reduce the number of bottles by offering an open cup instead when the baby is thirsty. At the same time, you should take steps to increase your milk supply by expressing or pumping more frequently, or by using herbs or domperidone. This should increase his interest in breastfeeding.

Into the toddler years

As your baby gets older, separations become easier to manage. Breastmilk is a smaller part of his daily diet, and your milk supply is well established and easier to maintain. Many women who work full-time enjoy an on-going nursing relationship with their toddlers or older children. The caregiver may not even know that the child is still nursing, because breastfeeding may be limited to bedtime and first thing in the morning. Even though there are only one or two breastfeeds a day at this point, both mother and toddler definitely benefit.

Separation from the baby doesn't mean that breastfeeding needs to end.

Access visits

Some of the most heart-breaking calls we get are from mothers who are separated or divorcing, and the father wants to have extended visits with the breastfeeding baby. The mother is already under stress because the marital relationship is breaking up, and she feels that she is about to lose the breastfeeding relationship as well and is anxious about how her baby will cope with this abrupt weaning.

We'll discuss the situation with toddlers in the next chapter. But there are even cases where the parents may have split up during the pregnancy, and the father is asking for lengthy visits right from birth. There have been cases where a mother was ordered by the judge to wean her young baby so the father could have equal time, or was ordered to pump her milk and provide it in bottles for the father. (Breasts don't always pay attention to court orders and many mothers have difficulty getting much milk when they pump.)

I think it is a serious flaw in our legal system when the health and development of a child can be compromised in order to give parents "equal time" with the baby. The father who is really concerned about his child and wants the best for him can usually work out a plan to have plenty of time with the baby without destroying the breastfeeding. I know one father who would go to the mother's house for his visitation days; he'd spend the day with the baby, taking him for walks, playing with him, bathing him, and rocking him to sleep, but was always able to bring him to the mother when he needed to nurse. Not all divorced parents have the kind of relationship that would make that plan possible, but there are other ways to work things out. The dad could have shorter, more frequent visits, say two hours

each evening, three or four evenings a week. This is much easier on the baby.

If the mother is able to pump enough milk for the baby who is with the father for an extended period of time, this could be an option, but it would be better if the father is willing to feed the baby with a spoon or cup, rather than bottles. Otherwise, especially if the baby is with the father for a whole weekend (as is often what the court, in its wisdom, orders), he then becomes used to bottles and may not latch well at the breast when he comes home. The mother will also need to pump or hand-express while the baby is away, or risk problems with plugged ducts or dropping milk production.

The baby's intense need for breastfeeding really lasts for only a short time—a few years at most. Yet breastfeeding has a profound impact on his health and development, an impact that will last his whole life. Parents—and courts—need to recognize this and put the needs of the baby first, and figure out ways to foster good relationships between fathers and their babies that don't jeopardize breastfeeding. I have spoken with a family lawyer in the United States. At least in her jurisdiction, the "best interests of the child" is usually interpreted as the baby having a close relationship with his father as well as with his mother. Perhaps this is a good approach when the children are five or eight years old. But if we are talking about a breastfeeding baby or even a toddler, derailing the breastfeeding relationship is not in the best interests of the child. The courts need to understand that a breastfeeding infant or toddler is not the same as a bottle-fed baby or non-breastfeeding toddler. It's another example of how we take the bottle-feeding baby or early weaned baby as our model of normal.

24 The Normal Duration of Breastfeeding

How long is it "normal" to breastfeed a baby/child?

This is not an easy question to answer, especially when one uses the word "normal." Perhaps it would be worthwhile to look at how long babies are breastfed in places other than industrialized societies of the 21st century.

If we look at the few tribal societies that remain relatively untouched by the "modern world," it is obvious that most often children are breastfed until they stop on their own. At some point between three and five years of age, most children will decide they are ready to move on. In such societies, breastfeeding three to five years is not considered unusual; indeed, it is considered normal. On the other hand, many people in industrialized societies say that "Once they have teeth, it's time to stop," presumably because they believe that teeth will cause pain for the mother, which is not true. Babies do bite sometimes if the mother's milk supply has decreased and the flow of milk is slow. See the chapter "Late-Onset Decreased Milk Supply."

Presented with a child who is two or three and still breastfeeding, many people in industrialized societies will say "If he's old enough to ask for it, it's sick." (I use the term "industrialized society" but in fact we really live in a "marketing society," the "age of persuasion" as a CBC radio series calls it, where every aspect of our lives is subject to the marketing of products, lifestyle and attitudes.)

How did things change so radically? Sure, everything is different now and the tribal society and the marketing society are two completely different worlds. Very few of us hunt for our food anymore. We don't live in grass huts or teepees. We don't marry at puberty and we don't have our first child well before 20. So why should we feed our babies for so long?

Let me suggest that in most tribal (or as some would say, "primitive") societies, babies and young children are doted upon, loved, shown affection to a point many of us would find surprising to say the least. Many would call that bizarre as well. (Although it is interesting that a recent study found that children who had been doted on in this way—the researchers described the mothers as "extravagantly affectionate" as compared to those who were "normally affectionate"—had significantly better mental health outcomes as adults.)

Because our attitudes to children have changed so much, it is even *more* important that our children have this special relationship, the strong physical and emotional connection that is often called "extended" or "prolonged" breastfeeding, but what I would call "normal," or perhaps better, "usual duration breastfeeding."

Breastfeeding for years was the key to survival where life was hard and infant mortality was high. Those babies who were fed longer were more likely to survive. When artificial feeding became "easier" in affluent societies, and fat babies desirable, breastfeeding started to fall out of favour.

Indeed, pediatrics became a medical specialty at the beginning of the 20th century as the "science of infant feeding" and pediatricians began suggesting supplements as "nutritional insurance." In order to make infant feeding "scientific," pediatricians started to establish "scientific" standards for infant feeding, inventing rules such as "Feed the baby X number of minutes on each side" and "Feed the baby every Y hours." These rules were based on how bottle-fed babies often fed and, forgetting that breastfeeding might be different than bottle-feeding, pediatricians imposed these rules on breastfeeding mothers and babies. Because of these unnatural rules, more and more mothers "failed," and thus more and more were giving supplements or stopping breastfeeding altogether. Because babies often did okay on formulas (formulas that are considered completely inappropriate nutritionally today, incidentally), the idea started to spread that breastfeeding was not necessary or, at most, necessary for no more than a few months.

In fact, formula started to be seen as better than breastfeeding. When I first started the breastfeeding clinic in 1984, many of the mothers bringing babies to the clinic had been born in the 1950s. When grandmothers accompanied their daughters to the clinic, they often answered for their daughters when I asked whether the mother herself had been breastfed. They frequently said, "I wanted to breastfeed, but the doctor told me formula was better." Is it necessary to reaffirm that those formulas the doctors insisted were better than breastfeeding would, today, be considered completely inadequate because formula has had "so many improvements" since then?

The overall effect of more than 100 years of "scientific" infant feeding was a degrading of the importance of breastfeeding in the minds of both physicians and other health professionals and in the minds of the lay public as well. The bottle became the symbol for babies. Bottle feeding and formula became the "normal" way of feeding babies. The attitude became "Why breastfeed at all"? And if breastfeeding wasn't important, then why would you ever breastfeed a baby for more than a few weeks, if at all? Breastfeeding became something similar to Aldous Huxley's "pregnancy substitute" in his futuristic novel *Brave New World*, where babies were made and grown in test tubes, while women were injected with drugs to relieve their biological and psychological need to feel pregnant. Breastfeeding for a few weeks was fine if you felt you needed to, but let's not get carried away.

A very good friend of mine was told by her pediatrician that her six-month-old baby no longer needed breastfeeding and that she should wean him and put him on formula, even though she had no problems with breastfeeding at all. She did. She didn't question the advice of the pediatrician, who obviously "knew." And she didn't need to be told this for her second child, whom she also weaned at six months. This same paediatrician told a friend of mine who was pregnant with twins not to bother breastfeeding because it was "impossible" to breastfeed twins. This pediatrician, incidentally, would consider himself "breastfeeding friendly" and knowledgeable about breastfeeding. This was 30 years ago. Have things changed? No, mothers are still getting this sort of advice.

The tide turns

But many women didn't follow the crowd and somehow, despite all of society's messages that breastfeeding wasn't important, they didn't agree. They knew their babies needed to breastfeed and they knew they needed to also. The low point in breastfeeding initiation rates was 1972 in most affluent countries and then the rates increased until, in a survey of Toronto mothers in 2009, 96% of women initiated breastfeeding. However, things are still far from perfect.

One-third of the babies in 2009 received formula in the hospital, which illustrates how far we still are from having good hospital practices that don't undermine breastfeeding. Many mothers had stopped breastfeeding by a week after birth and many more by a month.

Nevertheless, many mothers found they loved breastfeeding, especially if they didn't follow the rules and just fed the babies when the babies needed it. And they didn't agree that it was a good thing to stop after only a few weeks or after six months or after a couple of years, despite pressure from all sides to stop because it wasn't normal to breastfeed so long.

There were reasons the mothers continued breastfeeding into toddlerhood.

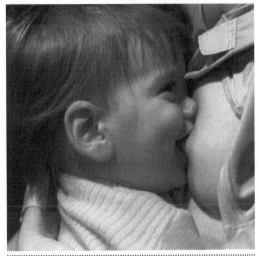
A happy 20-month old enjoying breastfeeding.
CREDIT: JACK NEWMAN

1. It was easier to continue breastfeeding than to stop.
2. The baby didn't want to stop.
3. The baby was waking up at night, and it was much easier to put him back to sleep by breastfeeding.
4. The baby wouldn't accept a bottle as he was "supposed to."
5. The family was going through a stressful time (illness, separation of the parents, financial problems) and breastfeeding helped the toddler through it.

But more and more mothers just listened to their hearts and breastfed as long as the baby or toddler wanted to, and they realized that this was all right. Better than all right; it was wonderful. Sometimes they needed to know that they weren't alone in this, and mother-to-mother support groups like La Leche League were invaluable in helping them realize it was okay to listen to your heart and your child and not the artificial norms of a society that had forgotten what breastfeeding was all about.

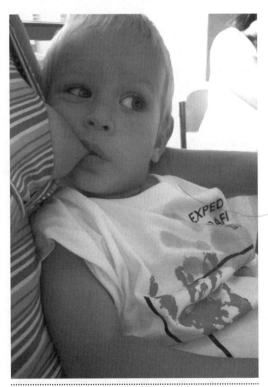
A mother and toddler at an early childhood education school.
CREDIT: ANDREA POLOKOVA

The positions of government and pediatric societies

Most pediatric societies in the world, including the Canadian Paediatric Society, as well as governments, now recognize the importance of breastfeeding. Most, including Health Canada (2004, updated in 2012) and the Canadian Paediatric Society (2005), as well as the World Health Organization (WHO), use more or less the same wording with regard to breastfeeding. They recommend exclusive breastfeeding to six months of age and continued breastfeeding, *with addition of appropriate solids*, to two years *and beyond*. The American Academy of Pediatrics (2012) states it somewhat differently, recommending exclusive breastfeeding to six months of age and then continued breastfeeding (with addition of appropriate solids) to at least one year and *then for as long as the mother and child desire without an upper limit*. The American press, in general, completely misinterpreted this statement to mean that mothers should breastfeed for a year, completely ignoring the part about no upper limit to the length the Academy recommended.

Interestingly, many Canadian women who contact me assume breastfeeding to a year is what they feel is recommended. Obviously, this is better than a few weeks or six months, but why one year? I think this is partly due to the large amount of publicity the American statement (breastfeeding for one year) got, compared to the Canadian statement, which seems to have gotten no publicity at all. Also, with new mothers getting one-year maternity leave, too many assume that breastfeeding and working outside the home are not compatible, so they believe they should stop at a year. But for many mothers the best part of breastfeeding is breastfeeding a toddler. Even if they are working outside the home, putting the baby to the breast can help make the fatigue and worries of the day melt away as mother and child reconnect

after an absence of many hours. See the chapter "Breastfeeding and Mother–Baby Separation."

Incidentally, WHO makes a point of stating that under normal circumstances there is no need for solids or formula before six months of age. And the statement make it clear that there is no need for "follow up" formulas under any circumstances.

Religious teachings?

The Talmud (the Jewish commentaries on the Torah) states that a mother should breastfeed for two years, four years if the mother and child desire and five years if the child is sickly. The Quran (Koran) teaches that mothers should breastfeed two years.

A contemporary anthropologist's view

In 1995 Kathy Dettwyler, in a book written with Patricia Stuart-Macadam called *Breastfeeding: Biocultural Perspectives*, tried to figure out how long it was "normal" to breastfeed by looking at what was "normal" for our closest relatives, the large primates (gorillas, chimpanzees, orangutans, etc.). She felt this might be helpful since presumably the length of time a gorilla or other ape might breastfeed would not be influenced by "cultural pressures."

It is important to be careful about interpreting any information about animals, especially apes. If the information is based on studies in zoos, it is likely their behaviour *is* influenced by an unnatural environment and by the "cultural pressure" of the zoo. For example, a gorilla mother born in a zoo might not ever have seen another gorilla mother breastfeed. We know that even for great apes, breastfeeding is a learned behaviour. There is a story about a gorilla that gave birth in the Milwaukee zoo. The staff were very concerned that the baby wouldn't survive because the mother wouldn't feed him. In desperation they contacted the local La Leche group and several mothers went to the zoo and breastfed in front of the gorilla mother. The gorilla mother got it, put the baby to the breast and the baby survived and thrived.

In any case, here is what we learn from Dettwyler's book:

1. Gorillas breastfeed for four to four-and-a-half years
2. Orangutans breastfeed for three years
3. Chimpanzees breastfeed for four years
4. Humans: ?

Animal biologists have tried to show a relationship between age of weaning and:

1. the baby's quadrupling of his birth weight
2. the baby's attainment of one-third adult weight
3. the adult female body weight
4. the length of gestation
5. the age of eruption of the first permanent molars

The relationship between these various biological "determinants" is only rough. In conclusion, though, Dr. Dettwyler states that based on these characteristics, the "normal" age of weaning for humans would be between two-and-a-half and seven years of age. Indeed, this tends to correspond to the age of weaning in various tribal societies around the world.

Some bizarre notions have been suggested with regard to "prolonged" breastfeeding:

"There is no nutritional value in breastfeeding after six months!"

I have discussed in the chapter "Late-Onset Decreased Milk Supply" why some physicians or other health professionals might believe this. They have seen babies who, despite spending very long periods of time on the breast, simply do not gain weight and may even lose it. The problem, once again, comes down to their not knowing how to

tell if a baby is actually drinking from the breast or not (see the video clips at www.breastfeedinginc.ca).

When one sees a baby of eight months, for example, spending much of every day sucking on the breast and yet not growing, the problem is not that there is no nutritional value in breastmilk after a certain date, but rather that the baby is not getting much milk. For some reason, the mother's milk supply has decreased (see the chapter "Late-Onset Decreased Milk Supply"). One outcome might be that the baby spends little time on the breast, often sucking his hand much of the day. Another is that the baby sucks on the breast much of the day but in fact is not getting much milk. It is possible, of course, to have babies who sometimes spend long periods on the breast, but other times only short periods. If one took the trouble to observe the baby at the breast, one would see the baby is nibbling most of the time and drinking very little. These babies, especially the ones who spend very long periods of time on the breast, get pleasure from sucking and this sucking may substitute for eating solids. By taking in so few calories and nutrients, they may become ketotic (some popular diets for weight loss use the development of ketosis to decrease appetite) and not want to eat solids.

Basically, if one does not know how to recognize that the baby is drinking rather than sucking without drinking, then the following conclusion makes sense: The baby is on the breast 24 hours a day and yet does not gain weight. It is obvious that there is no nutritional value in breastmilk. But this is an *incorrect* conclusion that derives from the fact that medical students, interns and residents learn virtually nothing about breastfeeding and learn absolutely nothing *practical* about breastfeeding in their training. And it does not get better once they are working with mothers and babies. In fact, most of the information they get about infant feeding comes from formula companies. This message is basically: "Breast is best, of course, but our formulas are almost as good. Actually using them may sometimes be better, for the following reasons . . ."

Sometimes mothers have healthy, happy toddlers who sleep, eat and drink well but breastfeed once or twice a day, perhaps before naps and bedtimes, and yet they are advised to wean. One woman was told by her doctor that her milk had no nutritional value now her baby was 18 months, so she should stop. We still tend to forget, as does this pediatrician, that even if there were not a single calorie or nutrient in the milk this toddler was getting, even if there were not a single gram of protein or fat or carbohydrate, not a single mineral or vitamin in the milk, there is much more to breastfeeding than milk. And why would this pediatrician care if this 18-month-old still breastfeeds? Where is the harm?

Another mother told me that her child's pediatrician scolded her because she was breastfeeding her two-year-old. The doctor told her that breastmilk was no longer beneficial for the little girl, and the mother felt guilty and upset that she might somehow be harming her child. She added sadly that her child still loved nursing. There are a number of interesting points here. This pediatrician is actually scolding the mother for still breastfeeding. What exactly is *his* problem? What baggage is he carrying with regard to breastfeeding? And what business is it of his if the mother is still breastfeeding her two-year-old? After all, the mother is merely following the recommendations of the Canadian Paediatric Society and of the World Health Organization, though probably without knowing it. Likely she is still breastfeeding because her daughter still loves breastfeeding; and she still loves breastfeeding, but maybe she is afraid to mention it because she will be accused of "doing it only for herself." Incidentally, why is the pediatrician not aware of the WHO and Health Canada recommendations?

Also, this pediatrician is probably among the many who say things such as, "Don't make mothers feel guilty for not breastfeeding" and yet does not hesitate to make a mother feel guilty *for* breastfeeding. He harasses her to the point where she does not admit to breastfeeding her toddler anymore, thus interrupting what should be an important doctor–patient relationship.

Finally, he speaks about breastmilk not being beneficial, which shows his lack of knowledge about breastmilk, but even worse, he does not seem to understand the importance of the breastfeeding relationship.

The toddler still loves breastfeeding, the mother says. She knows breastfeeding is still very important, but finds it difficult to resist the "all-knowing" pediatrician as "god."

In fact, there is still much nutritional value to breastfeeding after six months or a year of age. Breastmilk still contains appropriate fats, including the long-chained polyunsaturated ones (PUFAs) that the formula companies tout as being so important, but I guess they do not seem important when they are in breastmilk. It still contains protein and carbohydrates. It still contains minerals and vitamins. It still contains growth factors and colony-stimulating factors that help the toddler's various organ systems and immune system and brain to develop and mature and which, incidentally, are missing from formulas. Breastmilk still contains hormones and prostaglandins, which have benefits for the baby and toddler and, incidentally, are not present in formulas. And there is much more, including various proteins, white blood cells, and a host of immune factors that are not present in formulas.

A study we mentioned earlier that was published in *Pediatrics* in August 2005 showed that the milk of women breastfed for over a year had a high percentage of fat, sometimes 10% or more.

(Homogenized milk we buy has 4% fat, as does infant formula.) So there is still some nutritional value to breastmilk, is there not? The authors, however, came to a bizarre conclusion, that perhaps this elevated (normal!) amount of fat might predispose babies to develop atherosclerosis later on in spite of accumulating evidence that breastfed babies are *less* likely than artificially fed babies to develop atherosclerosis as adults.

What is so fascinating is that many health professionals believe the nonsense that there is nothing in breastmilk after six months or a year, but push the "need" for formula to a year or even longer. Formulas are supposed to imitate breastmilk yet they are being marketed so that parents believe they are necessary for longer and longer periods of time. Soon we will be on formula from birth to death.

Don't think that formula manufacturers have forgotten about pregnant women and breastfeeding mothers. There are not only formulas for pregnant women, but also for pregnant women who have high-risk pregnancies and even for pregnant women who are Muslims. And yes, formulas for mothers who are breastfeeding. I am surprised there are no formulas for the husbands of pregnant women and breastfeeding mothers. As of this book's publication, at least, there is no formula for men between 13 and 51 years of age. This is discrimination. I demand my formula too! Oh, I keep trying to forget—I'm over 51 so I'm not being discriminated against.

"Breastfeeding exposes the toddler to toxins for too long a period of time."

Ah, there is nothing in breastmilk of nutritional value, but there are toxins. At least there is *something* in breastmilk. Well, yes, there are toxins in breastmilk, as there are in *all our food*, and that includes formula. Formula is not as pure as the driven snow. Actually the driven snow is no longer as pure as the

driven snow, now that we have managed to pollute our environment to the point that no food is free of contaminants. The reason that we hear so much about pollutants in breastmilk is that breastmilk is an easy sample to obtain. No need to puncture a vein and take blood. Every time a study is published on the contaminants found in breastmilk, the media go crazy with reports on how dangerous it is. And many women decide not to breastfeed and many who are breastfeeding stop.

Formulas also contain toxins and it's important to bring this out, though the press reports on contaminants in breastmilk rarely mention this, probably not wanting mothers who "choose" not to breastfeed to feel guilty. Formulas contain heavy metals in quantities much higher than those in breastmilk. Lead, manganese, cadmium—all metals that can damage the central nervous system—are found in much greater quantities in formulas than in breastmilk. In a recent study, researchers Shelle-Ann M. Burrell and Christopher Exley seemed shocked that the formula companies had not taken seriously previous warnings about the high concentrations of aluminum in formulas. Note the first sentence, which shows that these researchers are not crazed breastfeeding radicals. Their August 2010 study, published in the medical journal *BMC Pediatrics,* put it this way:

"Infant formulas are integral to the nutritional requirements of preterm and term infants. While it has been known for decades that infant formulas are contaminated with significant amounts of aluminum there is little evidence that manufacturers consider this to be a health issue. Aluminum is non-essential and is linked to human disease. There is evidence of both immediate and delayed toxicity in infants, and especially preterm infants, exposed to aluminum and it is our contention that there is still too much aluminum in infant formulas."

Infant formulas are *integral* to the nutritional requirements of preterm and term infants? Integral is a very strong word and especially with regard to term babies and *most* preterm babies is simply not true. Incidentally, aluminum is particularly harmful to premature babies. Did you read anything about this problem in the newspapers, or hear about it on the radio or television? Of course not. Formula, unlike breastfeeding, is not a favourite target of the media. See the chapter "Breastfeeding While on Medication."

"If a child is breastfed 'too long,' he won't develop his own immunity."

This is a bizarre notion. It seems that the person saying this (often a pediatrician, I'm afraid), believes that if breastfeeding protects the baby against infection, the baby's immune function will not have a chance to react and therefore will not form antibodies.

This is complete nonsense, of course. First of all, breastfeeding stimulates the development and maturation of the baby's immune system; it does not inhibit it. Second, the immune system does not work in isolation. If a virus, say, is being blocked by breastmilk immune factors from entering the baby's body and thus preventing infection in the first place, it does not mean that other parts of the immune system are somehow shut off. A baby exposed to a virus or bacterium will mount an immune response anyway. An example of this is the case of a breastfeeding mother who got the West Nile Virus and the virus was found in her milk. The baby did not get sick, but he did develop antibodies to the virus. So in spite of the breastmilk "blocking" the entrance of the virus into the baby's body from the gut, he nevertheless developed antibodies against the virus. Perfect, exactly what we want to happen: the first known baby immunized against West Nile virus, but not with an injection.

"If a baby breastfeeds 'too long' he will not become independent."

And why would this baby not become "independent," whatever is meant by that? Why should breastfeeding inhibit the development of the baby's independence? On the contrary, breastfeeding helps the toddler develop independence. Independence does not come from forcing it. You can't make a child "independent" by making him sleep alone in a separate room. He may get used to sleeping alone in a separate room, but that does not mean he feels secure in this so-called independence. Independence can be achieved only by a child who feels secure. And that's what breastfeeding provides, security when the child feels ill, when he has hurt himself, when he's unhappy. The security of knowing his mother loves him. Nothing provides security like knowing you are loved and that's what breastfeeding, as opposed to "breastmilk," truly is: a reaffirmation of the love between the mother and the child, which occurs several times a day, every day.

There will come a time, without any doubt, when the child will decide it's time to leave breastfeeding behind. That may be when the child is two or three or four years old. Maybe even five or six years old. But when he makes that move, he will make it with the knowledge and the security that his needs have been filled: "I was a baby and now I'm not; I have moved on to other things, but I know I'm still loved." The child may not think of it in those terms, but gradually breastfeeding becomes less and less important to him until eventually other things take precedence and suckling at the breast is just a pleasant memory.

In any case, is a three-year-old independent? Should he get a job? Maybe he should move into his own apartment. What do we really mean by this "independence"? Do we mean that the child will not be "clingy" all the time? I think that's it. But when are children clingy? When they are feeling insecure, unhappy or hurt. Is the answer to tell the three-year-old, "Be a man. I'm not picking you up"? We do have strange ideas in "advanced" societies.

It fascinates me. We have no trouble accepting that it is "normal":

1. for a 20-month-old to suck a bottle.
2. for a 20-month-old to suck on a pacifier.
3. for a 20-month-old to have a security blanket.
4. for a toddler, or even an infant, to "self-soothe."

Self-soothing, what a bizarre notion! A baby lies in the dark and is frightened and wants the comfort of the breast or the parents' presence, but it's not allowed. The baby must self-soothe, which presumably means sucking his thumb or rocking in bed. That will make him independent. This is a throwback to the 1930s when babies were put in Skinner boxes and not allowed any human touch.

But to breastfeed, that's a problem? Why are the things above better for a child's sense of security than his mother's warm breast, the human-to-human contact of breastfeeding? What is so terrible about that 20-month-old boy breastfeeding? It truly is disgusting for some people that a toddler is breastfeeding. Why?

I believe the reason is that in our society, breasts are sexual and for many people *only* sexual. To be breastfeeding a baby a few weeks old, that is okay. But when some people see a mother breastfeeding a two-year-old, especially a two-year-old boy, they may confuse the nurturing aspect of breastfeeding with the sexual aspect of breasts. If that seems an unbelievable statement, I should point out that in some jurisdictions in North America, toddlers—as young as one year old—have been taken away from their parents because the mother was breastfeeding them. Luckily, the vast majority of case workers in most child protection agencies are not that ignorant.

We accept that the mouth can have more than one function. We eat with our mouths, we form sounds with our mouth, and the mouth is also sexual. Yet in most societies we don't refuse to eat in the presence of strangers. But in many "advanced" societies, the breast has only one function, a sexual function, and many people cannot comprehend that there is another function and that is to nourish and nurture babies and toddlers. Breasts are not sexual in this context. In one extremely popular situation comedy, which ran for several years, one of the "heroes" of the show is breastfeeding her newborn baby in the hospital. One of her friends, a man, walks in while she is breastfeeding and his jaw literally drops. It is obvious he is turned on; he can't take his eyes off her breast and the canned laughter is at 10 out of 10. This represents for many people what breasts are all about.

In the November 29, 2003, edition of *Le Soir*, they quoted a French child psychiatrist saying: "One does not share the breast; to extend breastfeeding past seven months is without doubt sexual abuse." This absurd statement is an example of where this idea that breasts are exclusively sexual leads us.

In fact, most people are not offended by breasts being exposed in public, as long as they are used to sell something, such as beer, clothing, cars or a certain lifestyle.

Breastfeeding is good; close contact is good

It is time we got away from the notion that breastfeeding a toddler is bad. It's not. It's good. What is bad is treating children mechanically, feeding them as if they were robots, not allowing them the pleasure of their mother's touch, her reassurance, her breast because "it is not time to feed yet" or they are "too old."

Loving human contact does not do harm,

We live in the logical denouement of the
Machine Age, when not only are things
increasingly produced by machines,
but also human beings . . . are turned
out to be as machine-like as we can
make them, and therefore. . . see little
wrong in dealing with others in a
similarly mechanical manner.

—Ashley Montague, *Touching*

especially not the loving human contact provided
by breastfeeding. And the feelings are often mutual:

When she first felt her son's groping mouth
attach itself to her breast, a wave of sweet
vibration thrilled deep inside and radiated
to all parts of her body; it was similar to
love but it went beyond a lover's caress,
it brought a great calm happiness,
a great happy calm.

—Milan Kundera, *Life Is Elsewhere*

Pregnancy and breastfeeding

As time passes, the mother's fertility will return.
There is a myth that you cannot get pregnant when
breastfeeding, but this is certainly not true. Once a
mother has regular menstrual periods and is ovulat-
ing she can easily get pregnant. In fact, it sometimes
happens that a mother gets pregnant before she gets
her first postpartum menstrual period because she
ovulated first.

As an aside, mothers are sometimes told they
need tests to find out what's wrong if they haven't
had a menstrual period by a year after the birth.
This, I think, is an indication of how little physicians
learn about breastfeeding.

A woman who breastfeeds into the second year
of her child's life may not get her menstrual period
back until, *on average*, 14 months after the baby's
birth. I have heard from one mother who said it
was 35 months before she got back her menstrual
period. Since a woman who does not initiate breastfeeding at all will get her menstruation back by
three months after birth, this is another "benefit"
of breastfeeding, is it not? Not only does the mother
who breastfeeds usually get her periods much later
but she also replenishes her iron stores. Iron deficiency is almost epidemic among women of childbearing age in affluent countries. Fewer menstrual
cycles over a woman's lifetime also reduce her risk of
various cancers of the reproductive system.

Speaking of pregnancy, it is interesting how
mothers are often urged by their doctors to use some
method of birth control at the six-week check-up
after the baby is born. The doctor tells them very
directly that breastfeeding does not prevent pregnancy. Actually, if the baby is breastfeeding *exclusively*
and without restriction and the mother has not had
a menstrual period yet, the chances of getting pregnant are only slightly greater than if she goes on the
birth control pill. On the other hand, if a mother is
breastfeeding a toddler, the same physician may tell
her (and yes, it has happened) that she cannot get
pregnant until she stops breastfeeding.

Does breastfeeding during pregnancy increase the risk of miscarriage?

Mothers are frequently told that they have to stop
breastfeeding during pregnancy because the risk of
miscarriage is increased. There is actually no proof
of this. It would be difficult to prove in any case.
Since at least 15% and in some reports up to 25% of
all women miscarry during the first 12 weeks, you
would need a very large group of pregnant women in
the study to see if there is, in fact, a difference in the

rate of miscarriage between those who breastfeed during the pregnancy and those who don't. A small study published in 2009 showed no increased risk of miscarriage.

The attitude toward breastfeeding may be summed up by the attitude toward miscarriage. If the mother is breastfeeding and miscarries, she is told it's because she is breastfeeding. If the mother is not breastfeeding and miscarries, one tries to soothe her; she is told, "It's just one of those things; most of the time we don't know why this happens."

In fact, a common reason for miscarriage is that the fetus is abnormal and the pregnancy cannot be maintained.

What else about breastfeeding during pregnancy?

There are issues with breastfeeding during pregnancy. Nipple and breast soreness are often the first sign of pregnancy. Thus, many women start to wonder if they should continue breastfeeding because it hurts to feed the toddler. Furthermore, as discussed in the chapter "Sore Nipples," a decrease in milk supply can also cause sore nipples and pregnancy does decrease the milk supply significantly. In other words, there are two reasons for mothers to get sore nipples during breastfeeding and pregnancy.

However, the soreness normally decreases as the pregnancy progresses while, at the same time, the production of milk increases as well. If the mother can tolerate this soreness for a few weeks, chances are things will improve.

Many mothers feel tired much of the time when they are pregnant. Breastfeeding, of course, is often blamed for this fatigue, but breastfeeding, in itself, is not a tiring process, although the relaxing hormones of breastfeeding may make a mother feel drowsy.

For some breastfeeding mothers, the decrease in milk supply can be the first sign of pregnancy.

When I get inquiries about decreases in milk supply I recommend the mothers get a pregnancy test, which sometimes turns out to be positive. When milk supply decreases, there is concern about the baby getting enough calories and other nutrients. Many young babies will stop breastfeeding with low milk. Many will continue but may be frustrated by the slow flow of milk from the breast. I don't know if there is anything that can be done to increase the milk supply in this situation.

However, it is possible to maintain the breastfeeding. If the mother is pregnant again when the baby is fairly young, say four months of age, instead of giving the baby bottles of formula to supplement the breastfeeding, it would be better to start the baby on solids. With a decrease in milk supply and poor flow from the breast, starting bottles will usually result in the baby stopping breastfeeding. Babies can be given as much as they will take of high-quality, high-density foods such as avocado, and even meat, at four months of age. Liquids can be added to the solids and, if necessary, other milk. Some babies, even by four months of age, can take liquids from an open cup (not a sippy cup, which is essentially a bottle). Often, if the baby gets some solids, not enough to fill him up but enough to take the edge off his hunger, *before* he goes to the breast, he may not pull and cry and be frustrated at the breast. Then, after feeding both sides, if he is still hungry, more solids can be given. As long as the baby is content and gaining weight well, there is no issue. Of course, this approach can be used for an older baby or toddler as well.

Many mothers have breastfed through pregnancy and ended up, in fact, breastfeeding both the toddler and the new baby. This is called tandem breastfeeding and there is no reason that it should cause problems either. The new baby, of course, gets first crack at the breast because that is his only source of food; the toddler can eat food and breastfeed more for the pleasure of it, though undoubtedly he will get some breastmilk even if the baby has breastfed just before. If the mother's milk supply is quite abundant, it is possible to feed the toddler on one side and the new baby on the other. Some mothers can certainly manage this, but need to make sure the baby gets enough. I believe tandem breastfeeding is a good idea if the mother and toddler want to continue. The toddler knows he has not been completely dethroned. He still has the breast to reassure him and comfort him. He is still welcome in the "bosom of the family."

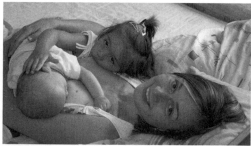

This mother is able to breastfeed two children of different ages—we call this tandem nursing.

CREDIT: **ANDREA POLOKOVA**

Breastfeeding toddlers and parental separation and divorce

When parents separate, the issue of access and custody of the child inevitably comes up. Breastfeeding complicates the issue, especially when the child is no longer a baby but a toddler. The general idea that breastfeeding does not matter if the child is 18 months of age (or *horrors*, three years old) and still breastfeeding results in many mothers being forced by the courts to stop breastfeeding, though I don't know what right they have to do this, or to allow the father (or other partner) breastfeeding-unfriendly access, which essentially results in weaning. Not infrequently, fathers are given access

for several days at a time, including overnights for 18-month-old toddlers, which makes the mother's situation very difficult, not to mention the toddler's. Sometimes the courts, in their wisdom, mandate two weeks at a time with the mother and two weeks with the father, which almost surely will result in the toddler no longer accepting the breast.

Exceptions do occur and some toddlers will return, but certainly not all. Perhaps fathers should take into consideration what it may mean to the father and child's relationship when the baby returns to the breast he longed for so much and didn't get with the father. I feel strongly that arrangements that result in long separations from the breastfeeding mother are unfair to her and, yes, to the father as well, but, even more important, unfair to the interests of the child.

Many fathers, in the contentious atmosphere of the fight for access and custody, will claim that the mother is continuing breastfeeding only in order to make it difficult for the father to have access. Although nothing is impossible, it has not been my experience that the mothers are continuing breastfeeding in order to deny the fathers access. Indeed, many mothers are willing to comply with decreasing the breastfeeding or even stopping it altogether, but they realize that the child is not ready, that it will cause him much distress and much pain to be forced to stop breastfeeding or to be denied the breast when previously they had open access to it. Whether others would agree that this is a good thing or not, the fact remains that the child suffers. In the case below, typical of many emails I receive, where the mother wishes to decrease breastfeeding, the toddler reacts in a typical fashion:

"She is still very attached to nursing, still nurses at least three times a day and during the night, since we are co-sleeping (so basically, on demand). I had tried to explain to her that we are not nursing anymore at night to start weaning her, but she will not take anything but the breast. Last night she cried until she got the breast finally, and then she would not let me go."

Forced weaning of an 18-month-old or two-year-old child from the breast can be extremely traumatic. The fact that occasionally mothers will say that they stopped breastfeeding easily, even "cold turkey," for a child this age does not mean that it would be easy for the child to be also separated from the mother at the same time. The email above is far more typical than "easy weaning."

Many breastfed toddlers wake up in the night to breastfeed. Contrary to what many think, most breastfeeding babies this age do not wake up for food, but rather for the security and closeness that breastfeeding provides. Spending time away from their mother can be very unsettling, even traumatic. Why a father would want overnight access for a child who wakes in the night, unless the parents live quite a distance apart, is difficult to understand, though I would guess the father is either not aware of the night waking or believes that the behaviour will stop if the child is weaned or adapts to the separation. I know of several fathers who, granted overnight access in just such a situation, brought the child back to the mother in the middle of the night, precisely because he would not settle and go back to sleep and cried ceaselessly. Such a change in situation for a child who receives so much comfort and security from the breast can be extremely difficult. Even if the child does not routinely wake at night at 18 or 24 months, the trauma of not breastfeeding will often result in his starting to wake again or more frequently during the night.

There are those who argue that there is no value in breastmilk after the first six months or a year, and this is said even by many who should know better—that is, physicians, and worse still, pediatricians. I feel I must repeat this here even though I have discussed this question earlier in this chapter:

breastmilk is still the best milk for children not only three months or five months or 18 months old, but also three years old, or older for that matter. It still contains the *appropriate* protein, fat and carbohydrate for the baby's developing needs. The long-chained polyunsaturated fatty acids in breastmilk (not available in cow's milk or formula until recently) have been shown to aid in the development of the child's brain, and possibly to protect against later heart disease, among many other health benefits. The antibodies and multiple other immune factors that help resist infection are still there, some in greater quantities than just after the birth of the baby. The various trophic factors are still present in the milk. Trophic factors aid in the maturation of the brain, the gut and the immune system, as well as other systems. Studies show that children who are breastfed a year or so do better in school and on cognitive tests, are less likely to get infections and are more stable psychologically (this latter point needs emphasis). Most studies have not followed children much longer than a year, but there is no reason to believe that the huge benefits of breastfeeding stop at one year just because the studies stopped following the children at this age. For these reasons, continued breastfeeding is important and the needs of the child should be considered in any decision about access.

A mother who breastfeeds a toddler is often accused of "doing this only for herself." I suppose there is some sinister suggestion contained therein that mothers are breastfeeding for some sexual satisfaction. Such is our society's lack of understanding of breastfeeding that a statement like that can be made seriously! Such is our society's messed-up notion of sexuality that a statement like that does not provoke outright laughter! But it is frequently made seriously, often in the context of parental separation and custody battles, and too often believed. Mothers breastfeed older children because they know it's best for their child, and that's the reason. They may also do so because they understand the trauma that forced weaning of a toddler causes. In our society, where breastfeeding a child even older than three or four months is not always encouraged, and is indeed often looked upon with disdain or even disgust, the mother's dedication and love is what keeps the breastfeeding relationship going. And it's not always easy to breastfeed a toddler, as much as it can be satisfying for both mother and child. This is partly because of society's disdain, but also because breastfeeding children of that age often wake several times in the night.

Often, a father will state that the child sleeps well when not with the mother, even though the mother will state that the child usually wakes during the night to breastfeed. This change in sleep is not surprising, but it does not necessarily represent a step forward for the child in the sense that many people believe—that he is becoming more independent. On the contrary, the child is often frightened, and obviously will not ask for the breast because he knows he won't get it (babies know a lot more than we give them credit for). Indeed, such non-waking nights are usually followed by a compensatory *increased* waking when the child is back with the mother and he is even more clingy than before. Independence does not come from decreasing security, but by increasing it. It was recognized many years ago that children kept alone in hospital and not allowed visits from their parents quickly learned not to protest and became "very good" patients, lying in bed quietly, sucking their thumbs and allowing procedures to be done to them. But it is still harmful to the child. I am not suggesting that being alone in hospital is comparable to the situation in the father's house, but rather that "good behaviour" is not necessarily good.

Breastfeeding is a rock of security for a child, especially when there is tension in the family. It gives the child a sense of stability when his world has been turned upside down.

A child needs his father, even at 6 months, 19 months or three years of age and I am not in any way suggesting that the father not have *appropriate* access, but forcing the child to stop breastfeeding (even if the demand is not explicitly stated) is not appropriate. However, surely some sort of arrangement can be made to allow the father reasonable access without interfering with the breastfeeding relationship. Even occasional overnight separation for a child who wakes during the night to breastfeed is not appropriate, in my opinion. It is, in my view, in the best interest of the child that both parents support or facilitate the continued breastfeeding relationship.

To be honest, I don't think overnight access for a toddler is appropriate even if the child is not breastfeeding. I don't believe an 18-month-old or a two-year-old is ready for this yet. Stability in a child's life is important and having two houses is not stable. I have heard children eight or nine or even older state, more or less, that they sometimes sleep at their mother's house and sometimes at their father's, but they don't have their own house. I don't know what to suggest about such a situation, but for the two-year-old child, I think it's not time yet.

So, after all is said and done, too often inappropriate access is given to the non-breastfeeding partner in a case of separation. Most jurisdictions in North America do not recognize breastfeeding as important nor do they understand child development. Breastfeeding is seen as expendable. The fact that a judge may decide that an 18-month-old who has never had a bottle can simply be fed with a bottle instead of the breast, and thus there is no issue about overnight access, boggles the mind.

In the first few years of a child's life, the mother is more important than the father. That is simply a fact of life, even more so if the child is breastfeeding.

One can agree with this as a good thing or disagree, one can state that it's not fair, but that doesn't change that fact. If the mother and child relationship is respected with regard to access, the father's relationship with his child will be better in the long run, not worse. Most people can be quite inventive about a solution without interrupting the breastfeeding relationship, if they want to be. Unfortunately, in the toxic atmosphere of separation and divorce, the issue is to "win." But if such is the approach, everyone loses, especially the child.

Mothers' Stories

The following are word for word what mothers have written to me about breastfeeding their older children. Possible identifying comments have been changed or removed.

Louise

I nursed my three children for a total of nine years and yours is the best article I have seen about the warmth and magic ability to comfort a toddler by breastfeeding *(referring to some information sheets on the Internet)*. This is especially true when they are sick. My pediatrician told me to stop nursing on several occasions when my toddlers had the stomach flu (not terrible cases—only mild), recommending Pedialyte instead *(an electrolyte solution made by a formula company)*. Now obviously it probably would have been better to keep their stomachs empty, but the stress they would have gone through was not acceptable to me because they obviously wanted to cuddle and nurse. So I let them nurse, figuring if nature intended anything for a sick baby, it would be breastmilk. It allowed them to sleep and rest between the times when they were sick. It gave them liquid so they didn't dehydrate. I don't believe it made things worse. It's funny, but some of my best memories of nursing are those where I was able to take my sick child and hold him and nurse him for hours, giving him the comfort he so desperately needed. To be able to truly help your small, sick child is a feeling I cannot describe and I am certain that I would not have been able to give the same level of comfort if I had only been holding him.

Louise was right about breastfeeding through stomach flu, and the pediatrician was wrong. The pediatrician learned his care of "stomach flu" in his training and/or from the formula company advertising. You may not be surprised that the formula companies also make special electrolyte solutions for rehydration of children with diarrhea. They have convinced organizations such as the Canadian Paediatric Society that these solutions are necessary for maintaining hydration when children have gastroenteritis, but in fact they rarely are. It is certainly unnecessary to stop breastfeeding because the baby has diarrhea. Occasionally adding electrolyte solutions might be useful, but not usually.

Louise understood something that the pediatrician did not—that there is more to taking care of the child than just treating a potential problem. Comforting the child is far more important, especially when comfort is all that is necessary for the majority of illnesses young children have in our society. The mother's relationship with her child takes on a whole new aspect when the child is sick and the mother "nurses" him through the illness. Some of my fondest memories as a child are of the times when I was sick and being coddled—lying on the couch, tucked in under a duvet, being brought drinks, and having cold compresses lovingly applied to my forehead.

Wendy

I think that with Jennifer, as with Jane, nursing beyond age two provided a special, intimate emotional bond that I think is at least as, if not more, important as the nutritional value of nursing at this age. Once she became verbal we could talk about nursing, which provided many precious moments. She had a nickname for nursing—"at" or "two at" when she wanted to switch. I think we got the idea of using a code word from a La Leche League mother who cited the advantage of privacy. Well, at one point we were at a restaurant with a large group of people I didn't know very well, and Jennifer piped up, "Wanna drink at from Mama's titty!" So much for privacy . . . We also had many private conversations and joked about nursing. Jennifer had quite the little sense of humour from the start. She'd tell me she wanted to "drink at" from the "squishy one," though it wasn't ever clear which one that was. Or she would say, "Mmm . . . it tastes like candy."

The emotional security provided by nursing became especially valuable and important when I separated from my husband when Jennifer was three. I think it helped her maintain a sense of security during that very difficult time. She also resumed sleeping in bed with me throughout the transition. I was a little uneasy at times about her increased dependency, but kept reminding myself to trust that nurturing her in this way would pay off, which I truly believe it has in terms of her self-esteem and independence (she is now six, in kindergarten). Also in terms of the closeness and trust between us.

Weaning was a very interesting, mutually negotiated process. We discussed it for about a year before it happened. (For about the last year or so, she nursed pretty regularly in the morning and at bedtime, occasionally skipping here and there.) Luckily, Jennifer had a friend in preschool who nursed for as long as she did. She knew when Carmela weaned, and I pointed this out to Jennifer. It gave her an incentive to wean too. She pretty much decided which day she would stop, and then never nursed again after that . . .

She still talks about nursing from time to time, and says she misses it, and sometimes cuddles my breasts as a reminder, but we both feel very good about the way she outgrew it naturally.

Ilana

I have four children. The first three nursed to about 18 months, and weaned themselves (or so it seemed).

My fourth daughter just went on nursing—every day followed the previous one, and there were days when I thought she would nurse forever. She went to daycare from the age of three months, from 7 a.m. to 4 p.m. At first I would come several times a day to nurse, later once a day, and toward her second birthday I stopped visiting her during her stay at the daycare. She would nurse when she came home in the afternoon, sometimes every hour till bedtime. She stopped nursing at night around two years, even though she slept with us most of the time. She continued nursing to the age of four-and-a-half.

As she got older, somehow she nursed less and less—in the morning we were in a hurry, and sometimes she skipped the morning nursing. In the afternoon, she started to be busy—friends, games, etc. We had interesting conversations about nursing. "Mommy, your milk tastes much better than anything else," "When I go to school, I'll stop nursing," and many other things which make nursing an older child a unique experience. Once, when she was around four years old, I asked her if there was still milk coming out when she nursed and she replied, "What do you think? Coca Cola?"

As she grew older she learned that you can't nurse anywhere, anytime, that when there are visitors it's not always okay to nurse. There started to be days when she wouldn't nurse all day, and other days when she nursed several times. Then there were several days without nursing, and I thought she wouldn't nurse anymore, but she would nurse again. In the end she nursed once every few days, and once, after two or three weeks, when she tried nursing she told me, "There is no more milk! Where did it go?" I explained that because she had been nursing less and less, there was less and less milk. She decided to nurse more, and asked me to remind her to nurse every day when she came home in the afternoon, every evening and morning, but she didn't manage to stick to this plan . . . she was weaned. Nature had taken its course. Babies don't nurse forever.

Nursing an older baby, toddler or child is a very special experience, and I would recommend it to everyone. Lately more mothers around me have gone on to nurse older babies. I think that seeing me has a lot to do with this.

Ilana is undoubtedly right. Many women do want to breastfeed, and many will breastfeed for years if only people do not tell them it is strange, bizarre, perverted. They only need a role model.

Some mothers are told they are breastfeeding "just for your own gratification." I must say this argument makes me very angry. There are few, if any, women who breastfeed just for their own gratification. This is once again taking breastfeeding as some sort of sexual activity, in a society that does not understand that the primary purpose of breasts is to nurture children. It is difficult in our society to nurse a six-month-old, never mind a toddler. A mother who does so is fighting the tide of general opinion, something that is not easy to do. And it is not possible to force a child who does not want to nurse to continue nursing. They just won't do it.

Mothers nurse past a year or two for several reasons, one of the major ones being that it is easier just to keep going than to try to force a child to stop who does not feel ready to stop breastfeeding. Some continue because the baby is not sleeping through the night, and it is just easier to nurse a child to sleep than to use any other method. But very few who continue into the second and third years later regret that they did it—especially afterward, when they see their happy, confident, independent youngsters. Independent? Really? Yes, really.

Independence and extended breastfeeding

One frequent argument against "extended" nursing (which really should be called "normal duration breastfeeding") is that the child will be over-dependent and "sucky" if nursed past a few months. This is yet another example of turning logic upside down.

Are children less independent if they are given security, comfort and love freely during their first few years? On the contrary; if they are helped to feel secure and loved, they will be independent, not dependent, because they will be secure in

that independence and know that they are loved unconditionally. I will admit that you don't need breastfeeding to two years or beyond to give them this, but the argument that continuing breastfeeding to this age causes overdependence is nonsense. It comes from a mistaken notion that nursing past six months or a year is not developmentally appropriate. In fact, it is not "developmentally appropriate" to stop breastfeeding at six months or a year. Of course, it is possible to use breastfeeding to maintain an unnatural dependence, but it is possible to use anything to maintain an unnatural

> Rejoice ye with Jerusalem, and be
> delighted over her, all ye that mourn
> for her. In order that ye may suck, and
> be satisfied with the breast of her
> consolations; in order that ye may sip
> and find pleasure from the abundance
> of her glory. For thus hath said the Lord,
> Behold, I will extend to her peace like
> a river, and like a rapid stream the
> glory of nations, that ye may suck;
> upon the arm shall ye be borne,
> and upon knees shall ye be dandled.
>
> Isaiah 66: 10–13

dependence. A mother who uses breastfeeding to control her child might use toilet training, or food, if she weren't breastfeeding.

It is possible to force "independence," to make a child sleep alone in a dark room at the developmentally inappropriate age of four months. It is possible to make a child accept being left alone with strangers for days at a time. Does this make the child more independent? Not at all. The outward appearance is one of independence, but deep down, the child is not independent—quite the contrary.

You want an independent child? Give him love and security freely. If part of the way you do this is breastfeeding until he is ready to stop, then feel secure yourself that you are doing the right thing. This does not mean letting the child do anything he wants. Children also get security from knowing what their limits are. They need to know that they can go so far but not farther.

But forcing independence does not work. How independent do you want your child to be, anyway? Do you want him to leave home at 14? Let him take his steps when he is ready. You will have your independent child.

Breastfeeding and teeth

Dentists these days make some quite negative comments about breastfeeding longer than a year, especially night nursing. The American Dental Association and the Canadian Dental Association both have policies discouraging breastfeeding after a year. The reason: children who are put to sleep with a bottle at night often have damaged teeth because of the sugar in the milk or juice.

It is quite right for us to be concerned about babies being put to sleep with a bottle, not only because of their teeth, but also because of increased risk of ear infections and aspiration of fluid into their lungs. We should also ask ourselves this: If a child needs something to help him sleep at night, is the bottle the appropriate "something"? To me, the obvious answer is that the child needs the comforting presence of a parent to help him feel relaxed and safe so he can sleep.

Unfortunately, using the bottle to keep the child happy in his crib does result in tooth decay in many cases. Nursing during the night rarely results in decay, and if any damage occurs, it tends to be mild. What dentists don't see is that the vast majority of children who are nursed during the night do not get cavities. Since those who do end up at the dentist's office, the doctor often concludes that this is a common problem for children nursing past the first year of life. It isn't. Even if the child is brought to the dentist for a routine check, the dentist will not usually ask about night nursing unless the child has cavities. Most dentists probably have no idea that some or even many of their cavity-free 18-month-old patients are still breastfeeding at night.

There is evidence, on the other hand, that nursing past a year helps prevent crooked teeth, and possibly sleep apnea, later in life. Sleep apnea (in which children or adults stop breathing at night for longer-than-normal periods of time) can cause snoring, tiredness during the day and even heart problems. Why aren't dentists concerned about these problems?

> And hence at our maturer years, when any object of vision is presented to us, which by its waving or spiral lines bears any similitude to the form of the female bosom, whether it is found in a landscape with soft gradations of rising and descending surface, or in the forms of some antique vases, or in other works of the pencil or chisel, we feel a general glow of delight, which seems to influence all our senses.
>
> —Erasmus Darwin, *Zoonomia,*
> *or The Laws of Organic Life*, 1794

But even if night nursing does cause cavities, is this a reason to force an 18-month-old or two-year-old to stop breastfeeding? By the way, this is one issue on which health professionals have no problem making mothers feel guilty: "By nursing your child at night, you have caused him to have cavities." Okay, teeth are important, but they are not all-important.

The child's psychological state matters as well. To force an 18-month-old to wean when he is not ready is likely to cause a lot more damage than continued nursing at night.

If the child does have cavities, it might be reasonable to attempt to stop the night feedings, but if this is obviously causing distress, the mother should not persist with something that is just not worth it. To stop breastfeeding altogether because of the teeth? What are the dentists thinking? Like the once-a-week hospital visits we described earlier, this is another example of causing problems while blithely thinking we are doing the best thing.

Interesting, Darwin's observation (Erasmus was Charles Darwin's grandfather). We used to build important buildings with domes that resembled breasts. Now we build phallic skyscrapers. Another sign of how breastfeeding has lost importance?

So, breastfeed a toddler? Of course, and delight in it. Don't worry; he'll stop nursing before his wedding day. You and your child will benefit from it. Go ahead. Let yourself enjoy breastfeeding until you are both ready to wean.

25 Quick Questions and Answers

My mother tried to breastfeed but couldn't. Does this mean I won't be able to?

Of course not. Many women of your mother's generation were getting even worse advice about how to go about breastfeeding than women of this generation. What is amazing is that some women who tried to feed by the clock and used other "helpful" hints of the day managed it quite well. There is no evidence that "insufficient milk supply" is hereditary, even on the off chance that your mother was indeed one of the few women who did not produce enough. See the chapter "Increasing Breastmilk Intake by the Baby."

I've heard that there are lots of environmental contaminants in breastmilk, and that if I breastfeed my baby I'll be giving him dangerous chemicals. Is this true, and if so, wouldn't formula be better?

No. It is a measure of how indulgent we are toward formula that we imagine that despite everything on our planet being contaminated, somehow formula has escaped contamination. In fact, formula has lots of pollutants—perhaps different ones from those in breastmilk and in different proportions, but lots nevertheless. The concern with contaminants such as PCBs and dioxins in breastmilk is that they diminish the baby's immunity. But babies who are breastfed have fewer infections than artificially fed babies. Another concern is that these pollutants will increase the chances of the baby getting cancer later on. But the evidence is that breastfed babies have less chance of getting certain cancers. See the chapters "Why Breastfeeding Is Important" and "Breastfeeding While on Medication."

I was told that you can't eat chocolate or "gassy" foods such as broccoli or spicy foods such as curry when you are breastfeeding because it will upset the baby. Is this true? What foods should I avoid?

Don't avoid any foods. If you find that certain foods seem to bother the baby, then try avoiding them and see what happens. But don't anticipate that the baby will react to these foods. They don't most of the time. See the chapter "Colic (The 'C ' Word)."

I'm overweight and have very large breasts. I was told that I probably won't be able to breastfeed because large breasts don't produce enough milk, and also that it's too hard to get the baby positioned on the breast. Is this true?

It is harder to latch a baby on well with large breasts, but it can still be done with good help. Most women with large breasts produce plenty of milk, as do most women with average or very small breasts. See the chapter "The First Few Days."

I'm expecting triplets. Can I breastfeed them?

Of course you can. And with good help and support you may well be able to breastfeed them exclusively.

Even if you cannot breastfeed them exclusively, you can still breastfeed. But it is best to supplement at the breast, not use bottles, because breastfeeding continues this way. See the chapter "Increasing Breastmilk Intake by the Baby."

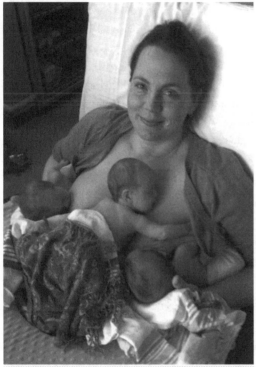

This mother exclusively breastfed her triplets. They even managed to leave the special care unit (NICU) without getting any formula.

CREDIT: DANIEL DOWER

I've heard that you shouldn't breastfeed right after you exercise, but instead should pump your milk and throw it away. Will it harm my baby if I nurse him after working out?

Not at all. Even an Olympic atwhlete can do it (there are enough of them who have proved this). Please don't listen to this sort of nonsense. Lactic acid will not harm the baby. Milk has all kinds of tastes that keep changing. At most, the baby might not like the taste. You don't have to pump the milk even then, since when the lactic acid decreases in your blood it will decrease automatically in the milk.

Won't breastfeeding for a long time—say, more than a year—make your baby too attached and dependent on you?

Attached, yes. Dependent? Well, what do you mean by that? Yes, dependent in that he needs you—but isn't that good? That's what love is all about: needing someone. Do you mean that you don't want your baby to need you? Of course not. Overly dependent? On the contrary. Babies who get the security they need are more independent. See the chapter "The Normal Duration of Breastfeeding."

I'm just 17 and my baby is due next month. I was told that I'm probably too young to breastfeed because my breasts might not be fully developed. Is this true?

What nonsense. You will probably produce lots and lots of milk. Your breasts have been fully developed for a few years. If you have what it takes to make a baby, why would your breasts not be up to the task? Nature doesn't goof to that extent.

Breastfeeding was going fine until my baby turned nine months old. Now he bites me at least once a day while he's nursing—and it hurts! Do I have to wean him? What can I do?

There are a few reasons why babies bite. Most commonly it's because the flow of milk has decreased. See the chapter "Late-Onset Decreased Milk Supply." If you can fix the problem, the baby will stop biting.

Other possible reasons: Sometimes babies bite when they have almost finished nursing, are falling asleep at the breast, and suddenly become startled. The answer is to ease the baby off the breast when he is falling asleep. Another possibility is that he is playing—trying out his new gums and teeth. This usually occurs after an initial short period of nursing, so the baby isn't terribly hungry or thirsty. Bring the baby close to you like when you were feeding him as a newborn. This often works. If not, try not to startle him too much, but just tell him no, gently but firmly. If he keeps it up, then ease him off the breast gently and let him understand that the feeding is over. (Slip your finger into the corner of his mouth so that he doesn't bite down on the nipple to prevent you from removing it!) Just as he can understand that he can't pull hair, he can understand at this age that biting is not acceptable. Usually your baby will stop this behaviour after a couple of times of being gently and firmly told it's not okay.

My baby weighed 8 lb at birth and now at four months old he's over 21 lb. Everyone tells me he's too fat, and I should put him on a diet. Am I overfeeding him? He's had nothing but breastmilk.

Some breastfed babies grow much faster than formula-fed babies. There is no concern—breastfed babies, unlike formula-fed ones, tend to slim down later. How do you put four-month-old babies on a diet? Don't worry, and don't let people worry you. See the chapter "Increasing Breastmilk Intake by the Baby."

I want to breastfeed but I don't see how I can manage it when I go out. Won't people be offended if they see me nursing?

If they are, that is their problem, isn't it? It's funny that people do not remark on billboards showing 14-year-old girls almost naked selling underwear, but are uncomfortable about breastfeeding in public. The good news is that breastfeeding in public is becoming more accepted. If you are really shy, bring a blanket to cover you and your baby. You will get used to nursing in public and you will soon stop using the blanket. Why should your baby be hidden if he's nursing? Shouldn't he be able to see you? Make a statement—breastfeed in public. Strike a blow for breastfeeding mothers and babies. Other women will follow your lead. Many jurisdictions now have legislation protecting mothers from harassment if they nurse in public. And all provincial human rights commissions have backed up a mother's right to nurse in public.

I've tried to quit smoking but I just can't. Would it be better for my baby to get formula than the milk of a mother who is smoking?

No. There is good evidence now that babies whose mothers smoke are healthier if they breastfeed than if they formula-feed. See the chapter "Breastfeeding While on Medication."

My two-month-old is gaining and content, but all his poops are green. Everyone is telling me this is abnormal and the doctor is making me very worried.

If the baby is content and gaining well, ignore the comments from well-meaning friends. Buy yourself a pair of sunglasses so you don't see the colour.

Resources for Good Breastfeeding Help

Dr. Jack Newman's Resources

My website, **www.breastfeedinginc.ca**, contains videos, articles, information sheets and other resources in many different languages including English, French, Spanish, Chinese, Russian, Portuguese, Italian, Indonesian, Arabic, Romanian, Slovenian, Slovak, Dutch, Czech, Polish, Vietnamese, Serbian, Hungarian, Croatian and German. My Facebook page has regular updates: **www.facebook.com/DrJackNewman**. If you are interested in studying with me, my institute's website is: **www.nbci.ca**.

La Leche League International

This is a volunteer organization. Leaders are all mothers who have breastfed at least one baby for at least a year and then had additional training. They have access to information about many aspects of breastfeeding. Monthly meetings are held in most communities. I am on the Professional Advisory Board of La Leche League International. Teresa has been a La Leche League Leader for 35 years (as of October 2014).

Go to www.llli.org to find a leader and/or group near you, or check the following websites:
Great Britain: laleche.org.uk
Ireland: lalecheleagueireland.com
New Zealand: lalecheleague.org.nz

The International Baby Food Action Network

This important organization works to increase awareness of the importance of breastfeeding and the ethical marketing of formula. Their website can be found at: www.ibfan.org.

Other Resources

Association of Breastfeeding Mothers (UK)
www.abm.me.uk

The Breastfeeding Network (UK)
www.breastfeedingnetwork.org.uk

The National Childbirth Trust (UK)
www.nct.org.uk

The Australian Breastfeeding Association (Australia)
www.breastfeeding.asn.au

Baby Milk Action (UK)
www.babymilkaction.org

United Kingdom Association for Milk Banking
www.ukamb.org

Lactation Consultants of Great Britain
www.lcgb.org

The UNICEF Babyfriendly Initiative
www.unicef.org.uk/babyfriendly

Ten Steps to Successful Breastfeeding
www.tensteps.org

Breast Crawl
www.breastcrawl.org

Kangaroo Mother Care (Nils Bergman)
www.kangaroomothercare.com

Co-Sleeping With Infants (James McKenna)
www.cosleeping.nd.edu

Useful link on drugs and breastfeeding:
Breastfeeding Online
www.breastfeedingonline.com/meds.shtml#sthash.Vu96ctem.dpbs

Acknowledgements

I would like to express my appreciation to La Leche League, to all the women who came to the clinics and helped me learn, and to all those who are dedicated to helping mothers breastfeed. They are the people who taught me what I know about breastfeeding today. Also, special thanks to Ruth Bacon, who kept pushing me to write a book. Thank you, too, to our editor, Kate Cassaday, and to copyeditor Nicole Langlois, whose enthusiasm and organizational skills have been much appreciated once again.

I would like to express my special appreciation to Andrea Polokova, who has added so much to this book and has made it so much more than it would have been without her input.

Dr. Jack Newman

Index

also from Pinter & Martin

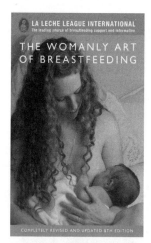

The Womanly Art of Breastfeeding
La Leche League International
The leading source of breastfeeding support and information
COMPLETELY REVISED AND UPDATED 8TH EDITION

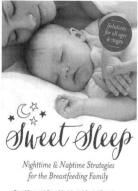

Sweet Sleep
Nighttime & Naptime Strategies for the Breastfeeding Family
Diane Wiessinger | Diana West | Linda J. Smith | Teresa Pitman
La Leche League International
Solutions for all ages & stages

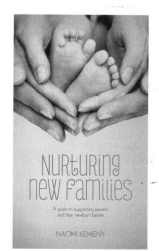

Nurturing New Families
A guide to supporting parents and their newborn babies
NAOMI KEMENY

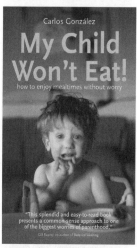

Carlos González
My Child Won't Eat!
how to enjoy mealtimes without worry
"This splendid and easy-to-read book presents a common-sense approach to one of the biggest worries of parenthood."
Gill Rapley, co-author of Baby-led Weaning

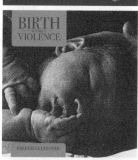

Birth Without Violence
FRÉDÉRICK LEBOYER

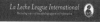
Evelin Kirkilionis

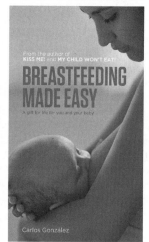

From the author of KISS ME! and MY CHILD WON'T EAT!
Breastfeeding Made Easy
A gift for life for you and your baby
Carlos González

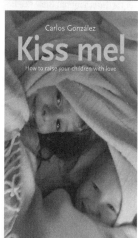

Carlos González
Kiss me!
How to raise your children with love

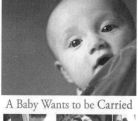

A Baby Wants to be Carried
Everything you need to know about baby carriers and the benefits of babywearing

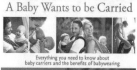

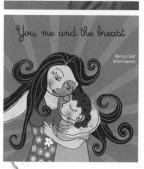

You, me and the breast
Mónica Calaf
Mikel Fuentes

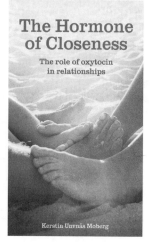

The Hormone of Closeness
The role of oxytocin in relationships
Kerstin Unvnäs Moberg

pinterandmartin.com